Politics of Pain Management:
Staff-Patient Interaction

Shizuko Y. Fagerhaugh

Anselm Strauss

University of California, San Francisco

Addison-Wesley Publishing Company
Health Sciences Division

Menlo Park, California • Reading, Massachusetts
London • Amsterdam • Don Mills, Ontario • Sydney

Addison-Wesley Publishing Company
Health Sciences Division
2725 Sand Hill Road
Menlo Park, California 94025

1/31/79 $9.95

Preface

This book is written primarily for all those who work with patients in pain. The list of them is seemingly endless. It includes physicians, nurses, technicians of all varieties, public health workers, psychologists, social scientists—even the patients themselves and their families. Social scientists and especially sociologists may be interested specifically in the concepts and theory presented here. Special features of the book include the use of case studies, case histories, and quotations from patients and staff to make the depicted situations vivid.

Those who study pain management do not often take into consideration the effect that the organization of health care itself has on the management of pain. This book shares with its readers the results of two years of field research done in several hospitals, which evolved from previous research on terminal care in hospitals. The primary task was to verify or qualify hypotheses, and new ones were developed where necessary. As a result of this work, three main themes were developed.

ORGANIZATIONAL SETTINGS AFFECT BEHAVIOR

The first theme states that pain management takes place within *organizational settings* that profoundly affect the character of the interactions between patients who are in pain and the staff members who attend them. In textbooks and journals, and at symposiums devoted to the study of pain, only the physiological, pharmacological, surgical, clinical, and perhaps psychological or psychiatric aspects of pain are studied. What is totally absent, or virtually so, is any focus on the *settings* (hospitals and clinics) where application of all that specialized knowledge is put into practice. It is as if the road from pure science to its technical application takes place in an organizational vacuum.

We maintain in this book that interactions between staff and patient, and among staff members themselves, are immensely important to the management of pain. Furthermore, these interactions are not merely interpersonal happenings, events with sociological overtones that occur between two or more persons; they take place within specifiable organizational settings, and these settings themselves profoundly affect their nature.

An organizational perspective on pain certainly does not supersede nor take precedence over the more traditional approaches. These in situ applications of pharmacological and other pain-management knowledge may ignore organizational contexts, but they can lead to at least two important consequences. The first is theoretical. One never knows for certain why a given approach or procedure does or does not work, except on faith, believing it's for purely pharmacological, physiological, or clinical reasons. The second consequence is practical. Without the study and comprehension of organizational contexts, things just "go wrong" repeatedly. From the laboratory or classroom to the hospital floor may be only a few steps; in pragmatic and programmatic reality it is miles away.

POLITICAL PROCESSES INFLUENCE PAIN MANAGEMENT

The second major theme developed in this book is: *Political* processes are involved in the interaction surrounding patients in pain. By political processes we do not mean the activities that spring most readily to mind, namely party politics or the vying for votes by aspirants to public office. Rather, we have in mind such political actions as persuading, appealing to authority, negotiating, threatening, and even employing force in order to get things done. Such political processes are clearly discernable on hospital wards when pain tasks are initiated, carried out, or fail to be completed. Even force may occasionally be deemed necessary by staff members, as when a protesting child is finally pinned down so that a painful procedure can be carried out. Far too simple is the conception that patients are relatively passive recipients of procedures done on or for them by rational, technical experts.

We need not argue that the division of labor among the staff itself will often involve political maneuvering as the staff members work on difficult or unusual tasks, including those pertaining to pain management. If this is so among staff members, it applies equally to the division of labor that includes the patients themselves; unless they are unconscious, they too, as we show, are very much part of the act. Although they have less power to get what they wish in an institution that is essentially unfamiliar to laypersons, they are neither completely powerless nor always outsiders.

ACUTE-CARE MODEL INADEQUATE FOR CHRONIC PAIN

These political and organizational issues are part of a large *ideological* issue, our third major theme. Hospitals and the activities of people who work in them are organized in terms of a pervasive ideology, variously termed the "disease-oriented" or "acute-care" model. This model is dominant in the world of Western medicine, and it is not appropriate for the majority of patients in pain, who are often suffering from chronic problems. The organization of the hospital ward is astonishingly inadequate to deal with the nonacute (medical or nonmedical) aspects of chronicity.

When patients tell us—as they did in a recent article* devoted to patients' suggestions for improving pain management in hospitals— that staff action is responsible for the failure of pain management, they may oversimplify the situation and often misunderstand the staff's perspectives. But they are not all wrong. They, too, are saying that "interaction counts." We are adding that interaction takes place inside institutions organized around some very particular assumptions and ideologies, whose relevance for pain management cannot be denied. Unless those institutions can be altered and their underlying assumptions and ideologies challenged, the new technological advances in pain management are going to be partly vitiated in practice.

The dominant practices of medical care and organization are under attack from the outside by women's movements, natural childbirth movements, bioethics movements, counter culture movements, and other health movements, as well as from inside the world of medicine itself by movements concerned with such issues as death and dying, community medicine, and primary medicine. In addition there are varied medical specialty and occupational specialty bases for further ideological differences which add to the politization, both subtle and obvious, of the work within hospitals.

All of these larger political issues show up even when researchers are focused, as we were, upon what happens in patients'

*Copp, L. A. The spectrum of suffering. *American Journal of Nursing* 74:491-495, March 1974.

rooms and in the ward's workrooms. What sociologists term the "microscopic" and the "macroscopic" are not separate realms, but merely two complementary ways of viewing the same phenomenon. The patients and their treatments become more comprehensible when seen within the totality of the hospital, while its very particular organization is illuminated by an understanding of the politics of individual treatment.

SOCIAL WORLDS AND IDEOLOGIES

In short, one of our messages is that organizations and their work cannot be understood without relating them to the larger context of the social worlds in which they are embedded. The "politics of pain" refers generally, then, to two interrelated phenomena: the detailed political processes which take place within hospitals and the influences of a pervasive medical ideology which profoundly shapes the organization of care, along with lay ideologies which secondarily affect that organization of care.

Perhaps we should add that while health practitioners commonly recognize that there are nonmedical problems of pain management, they do not understand that there is a *theoretical* problem of pain management. This pertains to the interactions of all the participants (the staff as well as the patients and their families) and the setting in which pain is suffered and handled. Of course, one could argue that the practitioners do not see a theoretical problem because they are neither trained in social science nor acquainted with its literature on organizations and ideologies. We think otherwise. In all probability, their practice (and often their research) is based on assumptions, embracing the acute-care or disease-oriented model, that prevent them from converting their common-sense problems of pain management into a theoretical issue. That issue happens to be of considerable pragmatic importance, as well as having implications for the social scientists' understanding of organizations and of the work carried out within them.

ACKNOWLEDGMENTS

The authors wish to thank colleagues and friends who helped us in a number of different ways. Above all, we are much indebted and grateful to the two members of the research team whose analyses and writings appear in this book: Barney Glaser and Carolyn Weiner, Department of Social and Behavioral Science, University of California, San Francisco. Marcia Davis, now at the VA Hospital, San Diego, also did months of fieldwork and analysis for this research project.

Earlier data were gathered by Shirley Albright Teale, then a student, School of Nursing, University of California, San Francisco. Several people listened patiently to our fieldwork anecdotes and helped to further the analyses or read parts of the manuscript; among them especially were: Melvin Sabshin, Medical Director of the American Psychiatric Association; Evelyn Peterson, School of Nursing, University of Minnesota; Berenice Fisher, School of Education, New York University; Leonard Schatzman, Department of Social and Behavioral Science, University of California, San Francisco; Rue Bucher, Department of Sociology, University of Illinois, Chicago; Elihu Gerson, Pragmatic Systems, Inc., San Francisco; Fred Davis, University of California, San Diego.

We are grateful also to the students in two classes on Social and Psychological Aspects of Pain, taught by Anselm Strauss in the School of Nursing, University of California, San Francisco, and to a sizable ten-session class on the same subject, offered in that school's Program of Continuing Education. The liveliness and interest of the students in those classes convinced us that our findings and theoretical formulations could speak quite directly to the pressing concerns of health practitioners. Like all field researchers, we are especially indebted to a great many persons who worked at the fieldwork locales. They are far too many to cite by name, but we wish at least to express our great gratitude to them and their institutions (all but one are in San Francisco) for their generosity and their acceptance of our presence. The hospitals are: Eskaton Hospital, Laguna Honda Hospital, Moffitt Hospital (University of California), Presbyterian Hospital, St. Francis' Memorial Hospital, St. Mary's Hospital and Medical Center, San Francisco General Hospital, University Hospital (University of California), and Mount Zion Hospital and Medical Center.

We wish also to express appreciation to Edith Lewis, editor of *Nursing Outlook* for generously accepting three papers from the research project and for her critical reading of them; also to *Social Science and Medicine* for publishing still a fourth paper; and to both journals for permission to republish the slightly altered materials. Appreciation also is expressed to John Johnson for his invaluable clerical assistance. As usual, we could scarcely have managed without the many-sided abilities of Elaine McLarin.

Finally, we acknowledge and thank the Nursing Research Branch, National Institutes of Health (grant number NU00457) for funding our research.

S.Y.F.
A.S.

Contents

PART 1 INTRODUCTION   1

CHAPTER 1 Politics, Organizations, and Pain   3

Medical History and Its Contemporary Legacy   3
The Politics of Treating Pain   7
The Hospital As an Organizational Setting   9
The Research and Its Presentation   12
A Final Note   15
References   15

**CHAPTER 2 Pain: An Organizational-Work-Interactional
  Perspective**   18

Organization and Work Patterns   19
Pain Work   20
Pain Trajectories   22
Assessing and Legitimating Pain   24
The Balancing Process   24
The Range of Consequences   25
Accountability and Pain Work   26
References   27

CHAPTER 3 Case History: Cancer Patient   28

PART 2 SIMPLE AND COMPLEX TRAJECTORIES   57

CHAPTER 4 Routine, Nonproblematic Pain   59

Properties of Routine Surgical Trajectories   60
The Staff's Pain Work   61

Patient Pain Tasks   63
Ward Work and Pain Accountability   63
Relief Versus Minimization: Reliance on Drugs   65
Variable Pain Philosophies: Problematic Aspects   66
The Accountability Issue   69
References   70

CHAPTER 5   Complex Surgery, Chronic Illness, and Pain   71

Multiple Linked Trajectories   72
Keeping the Patient on Course   73
The Balancing of Priorities   74
Disrupted Surgical Trajectories   76
Consequences of Extended Hospitalization   78
Staff Composure and Pain Management   79
Situations of Maximized Problematic Pain   80
Accountability and Technology   81
References   81

PART 3   INFLICTED PAIN: NECESSARY AND UNNECESSARY   83

CHAPTER 6   Inflicted Pain: Cooperation, Contest, Control   85

Work and Legitimation   86
Contract and Cooperation   86
Some Relevant Variables   87
Tactics and Countertactics   89
Two Aspects of Pain Expression   92
Variable Conditions and Tactics   93
Accusations of Incompetence or Negligence   94
Chronic Disease and Pain Infliction   97
Accountability and Control   98
References   99

CHAPTER 7   Pain Expression and Control: Burn Care Unit   101

Burn Unit Characteristics   102
Burn Pain   102
Burn Pain Expression and Control   103
Management of Burn Pain Expression   104
Learning and Enduring   106
Patient Group Support   106
Gradients of Burn Pain and Its Expression   108

A Case in Point   109
Other Variables   110
Implications for Patient Care   111
References   112

PART 4   ASSESSMENT, LEGITIMATION, AND RELIEF   113

CHAPTER 8   Assessment and Legitimation on an
   Orthopedic Ward   115

Introduction   116
Discrepant Perspectives and Their Sources   117
Assessment: Minimal Information Base   119
Interactional Assessment   120
Status-Forcing and Limits   120
The Whens and Hows of Pain Expression   121
Experiential Assessment   122
Addiction and Clock Watching   124
Psychogenic Stereotyping and "Crocks"   125
Variations and Implications   129
References   130

CHAPTER 9   The Relieving of Pain   132

Main-Job Balancing   132
Reciprocal Expectations Concerning Relief Work   135
Assessing the Pain   138
Credibility: Conditions and Calculus   140
Credibility: Tactics and Countertactics   142
Relief Work: Dimensions and Complexities   144
References   155

CHAPTER 10   Dying and Painless Comfort   156

Painless Comfort   156
"Let the Patient Die"   161
References   166

CHAPTER 11   Tractable and Intractable Pain   167

Ideological and Organizational Considerations   167
Ideology and Institutionalized Dying   168
Intractable Pain: The Interaction of New and Old Modes   171
References   177

PART 5   LIVING WITH INCURABLE PAIN   179

CHAPTER 12   Inattentiveness to Chronic Pain: Geriatric Wards   181

Illness, Pain, and Social Trajectories: Geriatric Wards   182
Social Contact: A First Priority   184
Ward Organization and Pain Work   184
Mutual Biographies   188
Social Isolation and Mutual Priority   189
The Burden of Case   190
References   191

CHAPTER 13   Living with Rheumatoid Arthritis   193

Resource Reduction and Uncertainty   193
The Hope and the Dread   195
Normalizing in the Face of Uncertainty   197
Renormalizing: The Adjustment to Reduced Activity   200
Balancing the Options   202
References   204

PART 6   TRAJECTORY AND TECHNOLOGY: COMPLEX AND SIMPLE   205

CHAPTER 14   Case History: Technology and Pain   207

The Dorsal-Column Stimulator Implant   208
Technology and Mrs. Noble   209
References   221

CHAPTER 15   Birth Process and Pain   222

General Properties of Birth Pain   223
The Potential Complexities of Pain Work   225
Medically Difficult Births and High-Risk Births   225
Ideological Versus Professional Considerations   228
Organizational Considerations   233
References   237

PART 7   JUGGLING THE OPTIONS   239

CHAPTER 16   The Balancing Process   241

Balancing and Controlling   241

Dimensions, Matrix, and Contexts   243
Balancing, Misbalancing, and Awareness   245
Crises and Fateful Balancing   246
Rebalancing: Balancing as a Process   248
References   250

CHAPTER 17   Case History: Cumulative Illness and Rebalancing   251

Rebalancing and the Cumulative Illness Trajectory   251
The Case of Mrs. Price   252
Technology, Organization, and "The Cumulative Mess"   268

PART 8   POLITICS, PATIENT CARE, AND IDEOLOGY   271

CHAPTER 18   The Necessity for Organizational Reform   273

The Paradox of Pain Management and the Acute-Care Model   273
Conditions for Reorganizing Care   275
Pain Management and Clinical Practice: Faith or Science?   285
Two Important Issues: Costs and Dehumanization of Care   286
References   292

CHAPTER 19   Social Worlds, Ideologies, Organizations, and Work   293
References   301

Appendix The Method   304

The Fieldwork   305
Theoretical Sampling   306
Theory Development as a Process   309
Theory, Case Studies, and Case Histories   313
Credibility Issues   315
References   318

Index   319

Part 1

Introduction

Politics,
Organizations, and Pain

1

MEDICAL HISTORY AND ITS CONTEMPORARY LEGACY

Behind the organizational features of the modern hospital rests a professional history pertinent to the understanding of pain management. We will present the relevant details of this history for American medicine, but they are generally applicable to medicine in most other countries.

The organizational shape of the modern hospital derives largely from medical reform movements and the evolution of "organized medicine" which emerged late in the nineteenth century.[1-7] The decades before were characterized by the prevalence of competing medical sects, many varieties of "regular medicine," and easy access to the right to practice. German and French biological and medical scientists, located mainly in the universities and research institutes, prepared the way for medical reformers who deplored the lack of scientific foundation in much of even the best-informed clinical practice. The reform drive was directed toward instituting medical practice based on research and on scientific training, hence on the building of research laboratories and the founding of research professorships in medical

schools, with an emphasis on upgrading "better" schools while dis-
solving the "poorer" ones. Spearheading these reforms in America
were physicians who taught and did research at universities such as
Johns Hopkins and Harvard, and at research sites such as the Rockefeller Institute. Later, both private philanthropists and key
foundations such as Carnegie and Rockefeller would support medical
research and lend their money and prestige to the improvement of
medical faculties.

Many elite physicians—like Osler and Welch—stood staunchly
behind reforms in the public health sector as well, and some entered
that arena full tilt. But in general the medical profession moved in
the direction of better clinical practice through sound scientific un-
derpinnings. (Later schools of public health went their own way, so
that both medical education and medical associations virtually
ignored health education and the wider community issues which
pertained to health and illness.) The development of scientific
knowledge and an improved technology, including surgical skills and
instrumentation, increasingly pushed medical practice in the direction of specialization and toward the evolution of modern
workplaces called hospitals.

The scientific research that undergirds medicine, from the
earliest decades of reform until now, is based primarily in the biological, chemical, and physical sciences. Significantly, when Flexner
(whose earlier report on medical schools had been so influential in
helping to close substandard schools) traveled Europe in the 1920s to
visit the great universities there and returned home with his influential suggestions about strengthening American medical
education, he paid little attention to the work of the famous Eu-
ropean sociologists, psychologists, and anthropologists of the era. To
this day, medical education is relatively devoid of insights from the
behavioral and social sciences. What material those sciences do contribute to curricula is typically the result of sponsorship by a
department of psychiatry, which itself finds the going rough in the
highly competitive struggle among the specialties for time in the
medical curriculum. Social work, public health, and even psychiatry
in many medical schools appear to be of marginal importance to
medical education, and understandably so, since they are peripheral
in a perspective focused so intently on biological and biochemical
disease processes. Of course that marginality is clearly reflected in
the organization of hospitals, where even the nurses usually have
little or no contact with their counterparts in the public health
departments.

The philosophy of a scientifically based medicine has meant an endemic tension within the medical profession between the "good clinician," for whom medicine is an art, and the researcher, for whom medicine must become more and more scientific. But more important for our considerations here is that, during any given era, what is judged good clinical art seems linked with the perceived state of medical science. Therefore, it is believed in all good faith that to practice competent medicine, and to judge that practice, one must be properly educated in the science of medicine and properly experienced in the art of medicine. Trained technicians and even professionals other than physicians do not have these competencies. So physicians, naturally, take precedence over paramedical personnel, allowing them little autonomy in hospitals and refusing to share the title of physician. Understandably there is not much place in this scheme of things for nonmedical personnel, except perhaps as board members to raise or contribute money, and as patients, to act cooperatively.

In all countries, physicians resent efforts by nonmedical personnel to influence what transpires on the hospital floors, even when they themselves cannot control the larger administrative and financial details of the hospital. The hospital is a medical workplace, and the physicians there have the most powerful positions. Clients tend to be regarded as having malfunctioning biological systems—otherwise they would not be clients—and they are regarded as "cases" to be diagnosed and treated as skillfully as possible. The good clinician may, of course, also be an empathetic person with insight into the psychological and familial aspects of the case at hand, but those aspects are mainly subsidiary to the primary medical ones. Understandably, the management of pain, whether diagnostic or symptomatic, is no less subject to this medical ideology and its powerful organizational expressions.

One further point to consider is the basic medical philosophy that has evolved in conjunction with the battle against disease in its acute forms. Suffering principally from infectious and parasitic disease or from the medical accidents of life, the bodies of sick individuals could well be thought of metaphorically as battlegrounds. Medicine inherited the post-Cartesian dualism of mind–body, which is perhaps why the metaphor was and is so widespread. Now the metaphor has become substantive; basic medical philosophy views the hospital as a workplace where disease is battled.

The irony is that the patients in our hospitals are there mainly because of chronic illnesses, in acute phases of chronicity, but chronic nevertheless. The major factor in this "growing prevalence of long-term illness is the impressive elimination or control of infectious and parasitic diseases."[8, 9] Probably the disease-oriented training and interests of the health professionals has led them to refer to hospitalized patients as acutely ill, although they know that many, if not most, have diseases for which a genuine cure does not exist. "What can only be accomplished is, in common parlance, mainly 'checking the progress of the disease,' 'getting them back on their feet,' 'slowing up the inevitable,' and so on. If pressed, most personnel would agree that they were not engaged in 'cure' in the old-fashioned sense of curing pneumonia or measles."[10] Yet hospital organization generally fails to accommodate this clinical fact.

Possibly because hospital staff members see patients during their worst, or acute, periods, they can continue to be disease-oriented almost to the total exclusion of any attention to the social or psychological aspects of disease, and to give scarcely any recognition of the important consequences of patient–staff interactions. Most patients will have had considerable experience with their diseases; hence they will have formed opinions on treatment in addition to having worked out modes of handling symptoms and regimens (including pain and painkillers). These opinions and modes may be quite at variance with those of the staff. Patients, many of whom have had repeated hospitalizations, compare skills and philosophies of staff members. Furthermore, if they are very ill and not responding well to treatment, patients are likely to experience problems of identity with which the personnel are ill-equipped to cope or help—ill-equipped because of their lack of specialized training. Indeed, many are even trained to be incapable of dealing with such problems by the prevalent styles of nursing and medical training.

Among the chronically ill there are, of course, those who suffer from various kinds of symptomatic pain: occasional, permanent, mild, intense, manageable, virtually unendurable. In the hospital, the staff will inevitably inflict still more pain on some of these patients while carrying out necessary tests and treatments. As with other patients, the staff seeks to control the amount and kind of its work with these patients, and it manages to do that more often than not, since like winning ball teams they have the advantage of playing on home ground. Yet winning that game with the chronically ill is not so easy, nor is it necessarily in the best interests of the patients. With perhaps increasing frequency, but certainly with much frequency, nobody wins the game. The severely ill patient with a chronic disease presents grave and intertwined medical, pain, psychological, social, and organizational problems. We shall see those problems clearly enough in the chapters that follow. Neither a focus on one-to-one nursing care, no matter how efficient or compassionate, nor on skilled medical intervention, can begin to cope with those intertwined multiple problems.

Hospital staffs are quite literally "organized" to deal with the pain of their clients. Yet we are forced to conclude that insofar as physicians and nurses are trained in an acute-care, disease-oriented model that cannot comprehend the implications of the chronicity of most hospitalized patients, their organization for pain management is often bound to be inefficient. Even when it is efficient, such organization often fails where humanistic aspects are concerned.

To assert this is not to say that pain management is always deficient—indeed it very often works well, especially in "simpler cases." What we will assert throughout this book, both explicitly and implicitly, is that major improvements in pain management must rest upon organizational innovations as well as on biological, chemical, psychological, and clinical ones. Indeed, as will be seen, medical innovation may simply exacerbate or cause new problems of pain management.

One further point will receive major emphasis: The medical ideology (philosophy) just discussed is crosscut by others. Some of these are peculiar to the world of the health practitioners, flowing from medical specialties and occupational specializations (nursing, social work, etc.). Others stem from social worlds and social movements external to health practice, but affect both the practitioners themselves (who may be black nurses or physicians who are considered "alternative-style" people) and the clients who come to the hospital and interact there with the personnel. So the ideological interplay can be complex, and often it is distinctly political in tone. It is certainly relevant to the issues of pain management.

THE POLITICS OF TREATING PAIN

The management of pain is usually attempted through appropriate drugs, medical and nursing procedures, or perhaps through the devising of sensible psychological strategies. Physicians and nurses presume that these strategies will work more or less successfully, depending on various factors, and that the degree and kind of pain are correctly assessed and countered by the correct drugs in proper amounts, in the context of a person's medical state and degree of pain tolerance, etc. Some pain, of course, is difficult to manage, so its management may be medically complex, but essentially the

management remains medical in character, with perhaps some
psychology involved.

We propose to illuminate the *political* aspects of all institutional
pain management, beginning with the assertion that behind the
standard procedures and the reasoning by health professionals about
them, there lies a basic set of assumptions. First, a person's pain is a
physiological phenomenon which can be affected by appropriate
procedures; and second, if the sufferer wishes pain to be relieved or
removed—and most people do—then he or she accepts the necessary
procedures, with perhaps a bit of persuasion to fortify courage.
These important assumptions, however, are not sufficient to account
for what happens when pain is being managed in hospitals.

Among the matters which we hope to demonstrate vividly
throughout this book is the world of difference between management
of one's own pain at home and what happens when pain is managed
in a hospital. Indeed, even when two people at home are involved in
handling a pain (let alone a patient and one or more staff members in
a hospital), political processes are likely to occur. As we shall repeatedly see, patients and staff members wheedle, argue, persuade,
bargain, negotiate, holler at, shriek at, command, manipulate
relevant contingencies, and attempt to deceive. Additionally, to get
jobs done despite the patient's pain, the staff may plainly use force
when all other tactics have failed, just as the patient, angry over the
staff's failure to relieve the pain, may sign out of the hospital.

If these matters do not seem truly political then consider also
that to get what they wish, both staff and patient will, on occasion,
plot and plan, seek out allies, and make or break promises under
duress or pressure from other interested parties. Staff members will
sometimes even be brought to informal public trial for having broken
the implicit or explicit rules governing pain management. Patients
are punished also, having knowingly or unknowingly broken the
rules laid down by the staff or the hospital administration. As in any
political arena, there are divergent philosophies for reaching common
goals, as well as different strategies for reaching divergent goals, and
there is much argument about how to attain either consensus or at
least some measure of equity for all parties. Also, in regard to pain
and illness there are personally and culturally derived differences
among patients and between patients and staff, as well as quite
divergent ideologies about illness, pain, and health which affect how
people interact in hospitals.

So it can be said that when patients enter hospitals they enter
highly politicized arenas.[11-13] The hospital is the home terrain of the
staff, especially of the physicians and nurses, and they make and

enforce the basic rules which prevail on their wards and around the bedside. The patient either abides by those rules or in some degree suffers for transgressions, unless the rules can be broken without discovery, negotiated out of existence, or at least relaxed.

The staff is, however, neither all-powerful nor completely in control of all the issues which affect patients. Otherwise there would be no politics but only total subordination of patients to staff. The staff does possess many advantages flowing from a familiarity with the terrain, greater knowledge and information, delegated authority, and legal or institutional responsibilities. Nevertheless, few patients are completely passive and none are passive about everything, all the time. Only nonsentient patients are completely passive, and their kin may not be so. Thus, medical and nursing care inevitably involves politicized action, and sometimes the politics, as we shall see, are very much out in the open.

In short, in this book we will be arguing and hopefully demonstrating that the management of pain is not merely a physiological issue, nor a simple procedural matter, nor even merely a psychological or psychiatric issue. It is all of those, but none is a central topic of this book. What is the central issue is suggested by the statement that "pain management also has *profoundly* political aspects."

THE HOSPITAL AS AN ORGANIZATIONAL SETTING

Pain management takes place within an *organizational* and *interactional* context. At home, there may also be interactional and organizational features affecting pain management, as when a mother commands her child to hold still while she applies iodine to a scratch; but clearly familial organization and interaction are not identical to the way hospitals are set up. On the face of it, a hospital setting ought to make some difference in how and with what success pain management is accomplished. But the fullest implications of what hospital management means cannot be grasped usless we understand something of the hospital as an organization.[14-18] Having explored that subject, we will be ready to examine, in the various chapters of this book, what is implied by the phrase, "pain management carried out in hospitals."

Hospitals certainly share some of their features with other organizations, but withal (to borrow a famous phrase from history) they are a most peculiar institution. Hospitals look different, feel different, even sound and smell different from most other settings. Laypeople see or sense this difference; probably most health professionals do

not. A hospital's arrangement of space is special; people are stashed
away in beds, one or two or more to a room, the rooms arranged
along corridors through which people in uniforms move with
purpose. For the visitors, there is the waiting room. There are those
special places where patients are sent for diagnosis (x-ray), for
treatment (physical rehabilitation), or for special care when exceedingly sick (intensive care units). Hospitals also tend to be
divided up into special spaces in terms of the work done "on" patients (surgery, medicine), the diseases treated (neurology), or the
ages of patients (pediatrics, geriatrics).

The hospital began primarily as a charitable institution, but
since the 1930s it has increasingly become a workshop for medical
treatment. It is where physicians do their most complicated work: diagnosis, laboratory testing, surgery, elaborate medical treatments,
emergency and other life-saving measures. Medical technology (machinery, drugs, laboratory tests, procedures) abounds and changes
continually, beginning perhaps at the most advanced urban medical
centers but diffusing rapidly even to the farthest hospitals.

Another feature of the hospital is the multiplicity of types of
workers there, ranging from those with the most expensive and extensive educations to those who deliver the food. Up front are the
administrative offices, whose occupants administer the business and
community-relations affairs, but who are not necessarily—and indeed
rarely—intimately concerned with patient care.

As everyone knows (and this is true in all countries where
Western medicine is practiced, with perhaps only China excepted),
among the personnel engaged in health care, the physicians have the
most prestige and power. This holds for private as well as state-run
hospitals. As specialization among physicians increases, there are
related hospital reorganizations and spatial rearrangements. Although
the titles vary in different nations, universally there are assisting personnel, and each major medical specialty tends to develop its own
paramedical technicians or professionals and its own types of ward
organization. Everywhere nurses tend to administer the daily
business of the wards and to give the hour-to-hour care to patients,
as well as to run a kind of day and night hotel.

Success in treatment is still frequently problematic; hence specialists often consult with each other. The patient's treatments are
then either divided up among the specialists or medically coordinated by one of them. Consequently there is not necessarily just one
physician "to" a patient, but several physicians, plus all the assisting
personnel who are resident both on the ward itself and in other specialized feed-in departments.

Hospitals have important rhythmic features. Chief among them is that the place must be manned 24 hours a day, even if with a much reduced staff. Physicians are usually absent during the night shift although perhaps on direct call. Other workers tend also to be absent at night. It is easy to see why the predominant rhythms of work vary in accordance with each of the three shifts (day, evening, night).

Related to, as well as superimposed on, each shift are various work rhythms. Patients are fed twice during the day shift and not at all at night. Surgery begins early in the day and patients are prepared during the preceding evening and night shifts. Most tests are run during the day shift. Normal, nighttime sleeping prevails, yet the staff must be alert at night to the patients' requirements and emergencies. In the United States, the evening shift often has to contend with visiting, both by physicians and by families who are otherwise busy during the day.

Longer rhythms are also evident. Residents and interns rotate through wards on monthly or other periods, as well as enter and leave the hospital annually. Where nursing shortages exist, nursing administrators spend considerable time programming the movement of nurses around the wards in an attempt to cover the site shortages. Of course, there is also, except for hospitals for chronically disabled (e.g., stroke and paraplegic), a fairly rapid turnover of the patients.

A striking feature of the hospital which derives from the way patients are "processed" is the tremendous amount of record keeping. People are admitted and discharged, and there must be records of those movements. Disease conditions are diagnosed, treated, and noted. Tests flow in from all the relevant services; specialists are consulted and write down their observations and their orders; patients are monitored and their physiological reactions entered into the appropriate records. For virtually every act (diagnosing, dosing, monitoring) there are comparable written notations. In short, to get the work done, not only verbal but written communication abounds. Some personnel share the responsibility for writing, others for reading; some must do both. Responsibility, then, is fairly specific, but it is of different types depending on one's position in the total division of labor. Clearly, however, the most responsible kinds of communication and work (from the staff's perspective) pertain to patient care.

Having now briefly noted many features of the hospital organization, it is necessary to reiterate that even in relatively small, noncomplex hospitals, the setting belongs to the staff, not to the patients. There are a host of rules which the latter must obey. Some are

laid down by the hospital administration, especially those pertaining
to finances. Some are issued as commands by the relevant physicians
in regard to treatment. Nursing and house staffs enforce (and sometimes originate) a host of explicit and implicit rules concerning space
(no loitering near the nursing station), time (pain pills every four
hours, not every three; don't take up the nurse's time unnecessarily
during the busiest hours), and comportment (no nudity, not too
much noise, no complaining about nursing care to the physicians),
and cooperation with various regimens and procedures.

Patients of course contest those rules, but it is safe to say that
the patients generally operate from positions of weakness. The hospital's personnel assume that the patient is there to be worked upon
for his or her own good and sent home as fast as possible, hopefully
in an improved state. If the patient cooperates, well and good. If not,
the work must be done anyhow, though that may involve rudeness
or "snowing" with drugs. If families help, or at least do not hinder
the work, they are relatively welcome, but if they are also uncooperative, the staff will try to control or even banish them.

We can see that the hospital is a kind of *workshop*,[19] where patients are regarded as something to be worked on, or at the least they
share the work by being sensibly cooperative. Chapter 2 examines
this workshop model in detail. The balance of this chapter describes
the research behind and organization of this book.

THE RESEARCH AND ITS PRESENTATION

Some years ago, while studying terminal care in hospitals, one of the
authors observed the interaction among staff members and dying patients who were in pain.[19, 20] As the research was written up,
analyses of the problems confronted by both the patients and the
staff in coming to terms with that pain were included. Later, when
we decided upon a focused study of hospitalized patients in pain
(whether dying or not), we began with a systematic, conscious bias
toward looking at pain interactions within the context of the staff's
work within organizational settings.

Our research design and fieldwork methods are described in the
appendix. Interested readers may wish to consult those pages before
continuing their readings. For others, it is probably sufficient to state
briefly that this publication is based on two years of systematic observations in the field, on about 20 selected wards and in 8 hospitals
located in San Francisco and 1 in a small town in Northern California. As in most field research, systematic observations were
supplemented with innumerable informal but often directed in-

terviews and occasional lengthy interviews with hospital personnel, patients, and family. In addition, considerable relevant data were available from previous research on terminal care.

We had two general purposes in doing this research. First, we wished to develop an approach to pain management that would be radically different from, but could also supplement, more established approaches—namely, those based on physiological or pharmacological research, clinical practice, and psychological or psychiatric studies of pain.[21-27] The intent was to ground a new perspective on pain in a consideration of the organizational settings in which pain management and patient care take place, rather than in consideration of the pain itself or the one-to-one interaction of patient and nurse or physician. Our perspective would supplement, rather than conflict with, other approaches, for the improved care of patients in pain should draw upon all the approaches and knowledge available. At the same time, we reasoned from our previous observations that substantial improvement in the care of patients in pain would prove very difficult unless organizational relevancies were taken into account.

Besides our pragmatic aims, we wished to develop a substantive theory about what happens in hospitals when people are confronted with pain and attempt to deal with it. From our previous experience in developing similar theories about terminal care, we believed it possible to formulate one about pain management. The latter theory pertains centrally to complex issues of balancing and controlling of pain tasks (relieving, minimizing, enduring) and medical tasks (diagnosing, treating, saving life), and other stakes (personal identity, ward morale) as they are affected by various organizational and interactional conditions.

Having accomplished our second aim, we chose to present our theory in a form partly different from those in the books on terminal care. There, the theories are presented in a discursive, though systematic, mode. Because we wish to maximize the pragmatic use of our theory by health practitioners and laypeople too, we have employed a presentation at three levels of abstraction. (It is discussed at greater length in the appendix.) Some chapters (2, 6, 9, and 16) are written at a relatively high level of abstraction. Other chapters consist of case studies—descriptions with analysis—of pain interactions on particular types of wards (burn units, geriatric wards, etc.). The third mode of presentation consists of case histories—the evolving stories of interaction around specific patients in pain (Mrs. Abel, Mrs. Noble, Mrs. Price)—where the drama of actual events is emphasized but accompanied by analytic comments.

Our beliefs about the theory can, we think, be best expressed by quoting from the preface of the research reported in *Time for Dying* (pp. iii–xiii).[28]

> *We have great faith in our theory, which is carefully grounded on comparative data. But we also strongly feel that readers must bear a responsibility for a critical review. We expect that they will variously agree with some, disagree with other specific points. Yet the theory is not to be refuted, wholly or in part, simply because it does not always fit some readers' experiences. The applicability of a general theory like ours requires that readers make the necessary corrections, adjustments, and other qualifications specific to each hospital (or ward) under consideration. An effective theory is capable of such qualifying elaboration, and indeed should lend itself readily to the alert reader's critical qualification. If some readers are motivated by our theory to engage in research on [pain management], we should both anticipate and be delighted at their transcending incorporation of our own work.*

This quotation and the later inclusion of a number of pages from *Anguish*,[19] dealing with comfort care of dying patients in pain, reflect the continuities and linkages between the respective researches on terminal care and on pain management.

The general plan of this book is as follows. Chapter 2 introduces our theoretical perspective and some of its major concepts. Chapter 3 consists of a lengthy case history of a cancer patient and is presented in a straightforward manner, without theoretical commentary; we consider it a dramatic, possibly unforgettable, way to introduce some of the main themes of this book. Part 2 deals with simple and complex trajectories: Chapter 4 on routine surgical trajectories and Chapter 5 on complex ones. Part 3 discusses inflicted pain, both necessary and unnecessary. Chapter 6 is theoretical, and Chapter 7 provides a case study of interaction on an intensive burn unit. Part 4 pertains to the important tasks of assessing, legitimating, and relieving pain. Chapter 8 is a case study of chronic back pain, highlighting problems of assessment and legitimation. Chapter 9 is about the relieving of pain in general. Chapter 10 analyzes interaction during the comfort care phase of dying, and Chapter 11 addresses certain ideological and organizational issues in management of very severe pain. Part 5 addresses a situation where a person must live with incurable pain. Chapter 12 discusses pain on geriatric wards, and Chapter 13 addresses living with chronic arthritis. Part 6 is titled "Trajectory and Technology: Simple and Complex." The former is illustrated by Chapter 14, a case history of a patient with

terminal cancer whose terrible pain was treated by implanting a dorsal stimulator; the latter by Chapter 15 which discusses childbirth.
Part 7 is called "Juggling the Options." It consists of Chapter 16,
which deals with the processes of balancing and controlling, and
Chapter 17, which is the case history of Mrs. Price, who had incurable lupus and whose prolonged stay at the hospital, on several
wards, made her the hospital's "Patient of the Year." Pain was only
one of her problems, but a central one. In Part 8, Chapter 18, the authors offer opinions and suggestions about needed reforms for
hospitals and other medical institutions, as they pertain to the care of
patients in pain. In Chapter 19, there is a discussion of larger theoretical issues raised by the book as a whole, relating to such matters
as social worlds, ideologies, work, clients, and organizations. The
volume closes with an appendix dealing with methods used in the
research.

A FINAL NOTE

It is obvious that health practitioners recognize the fact that there are
nonmedical problems of pain management (psychological and
cultural). Nevertheless, they do not see that there is a *theoretical*
problem of pain management which involves the interaction of all
the participants (the staff, the patients, and their families), as well as
the setting in which pain is suffered and handled. Of course, one
could argue that the practitioners do not see a theoretical problem
because they are neither trained in sociology nor acquainted with organizational literature. We think otherwise. In all probability, their
practice (and often their research) is based on assumptions embracing an acute-care or disease-oriented model which prevents them
from converting common-sense problems of pain management into a
theoretical issue. But the issue happens to be of considerable
pragmatic importance, both for medical practitioners and social scientists who study organizations and the work carried out within
them.

REFERENCES

1. Ben-David, J. 1960. Scientific productivity and academic organi-
    zation in nineteenth century medicine. *American Sociological
    Review* 25:828–848.
2. Brieger, G. 1976. The "new" medicine: the Johns Hopkins' in-
    fluence on education and practice. Delivered at the William
    Henry Welch-Isabel Hampton Robb Centennial Symposium,

January 15, 1976, at Johns Hopkins University, Baltimore, Maryland.

3. Lippard, V. 1974. *A half-century of American medical education: 1920–1970*. New York: Josiah Macy Jr. Foundation.

4. Markowitz, G., and Rosner, D. 1973. Doctors in crisis: a study of the use of elitism in medicine. *American Quarterly* 84:107.

5. Strauss, A. 1966. The structure and ideology of the nursing profession. In *The nursing profession*, ed. F. Davis, pp. 60–104. New York: Wiley.

6. Wiebe, R. 1967. *The search for order: 1877–1920*. New York: Hill and Wang, pp. 111–132.

7. Wordsworth, J. R. 1973. Some influence in the reform of schools of law and medicine, 1899–1930. *Sociological Quarterly* 14:496–516.

8. Gerson, E., and Strauss, A. 1975. Time for living: problems in chronic illness care. *Social Policy* 6:12–48.

9. Strauss, A., and Glaser, B. 1974. *Chronic illness and the quality of life*. St. Louis: C. V. Mosby, p. 4.

10. Bucher, R., and Strauss, A. 1961. Professions in process. *American Journal of Sociology* 66:325–334.

11. Bucher, R. 1970. Social process and power in a medical school. In *Power in organization*, ed. M. Zald. Nashville, Tenn.: Vanderbilt University Press.

12. Gerson, E. The social character of illness: deviance or politics? *Social Science and Medicine*, forthcoming.

13. Strauss, A. et al. 1964. *Psychiatric ideologies and institutions*. New York: Free Press of Glencoe.

14. Burling, T.; Lentz, E. M.; and Wilson, R. N. 1956. *The give and take in hospitals*. New York: Putnam.

15. Freidson, E., ed. 1963. *The hospital in modern society*. New York: Free Press of Glencoe.

16. Freidson, E., and Lorber, J., eds. 1972. *Medical men and their work*. Chicago: Aldine-Atherton.

17. Mauksch, H. 1966. The organizational context of nursing practice. In *The nursing profession*, ed. F. Davis, pp. 109–137. New York: Wiley.

18. Smith, H. 1955. Two lines of authority are one too many. *Modern Hospital* 84:59–64.

19. Glaser, B., and Strauss, A. 1965. *Awareness of dying*. Chicago: Aldine.

20. Glaser, B., and Strauss, A. 1970. *Anguish: case history of a dying woman*. San Francisco: Sociology Press.

21. Blaylock, J. 1968. The psychological and cultural influences on the reaction of pain: a review of the literature. *Nursing Forum* 7:262–273.

22. Crowley, D. M. 1962. *Pain and its alleviation*. Los Angeles: University of California Press.

23. McCafferty, M. 1972. *Nursing management of the patient in pain*. Philadelphia: J. B. Lippincott, Co.

24. Merskey, H., and Spear, R. 1967. *Pain: psychological and psychiatric aspects*. London: Bailliere, Tindal and Cassell.

25. Way, E. L., ed. 1968. *New concepts in pain and its clinical management*. Philadelphia: F. A. Davis.

26. Weisenberg, M., ed. 1975. *Pain: clinical and experimental perspectives*. St. Louis: C. V. Mosby.

27. Zborowski, M. 1969. *People in pain*. San Francisco: Jossey-Bass.

28. Glaser, B., and Strauss, A. 1968. *Time for dying*. Chicago: Aldine.

Pain:
An Organizational-Work-
Interactional Perspective*

2

We think of our approach as both radically different from but supplementary to the more established ones, such as those based on
physiological or pharmacological research, clinical practice, and
psychological and psychiatric studies of pain.[1-6] In contrast to
these approaches, our perspective is a three-way one: organizational-work-interactional. It is grounded in a consideration of the
organizational settings within which pain management and patient care occur, rather than in consideration of the pain itself or
the one-to-one interaction between patient and nurse or physician.

Our general position begins with an emphasis on the staff
member's work, which *includes* their care of patients in pain. To
understand the actual patterning of occurrences during that work,
we need to look closely at (1) the general *organizational setting* in
which the staff's predominant work occurs, (2) the *work itself*, including that entailed in the staff's management of pain, and (3) the

*This chapter was published in slightly altered form from *Pain:
An Organizational-Work-Interactional Perspective* by Anselm
Strauss, Shizuko Fagerhaugh, and Barney Glaser. Copyright ©
September 1974, The American Journal of Nursing Company. Re-
produced, with permission, from *Nursing Outlook*.

18

consequent *interaction* between staff and patient and among staff members themselves.

We turn now to a brief exposition of some major concepts in our perspective, all of which will be developed and perhaps all too vividly exemplified in the chapters to follow.

ORGANIZATION AND WORK PATTERNS

Hospitals consist of highly differentiated spaces; that is, the work and organization of the various wards vary considerably. For instance, the chief *organizational* features of most ICUs tend to be: relatively ample staff, machinery and drugs; critically ill patients, including those close to death; organization of staff for potential medical crises and minute-to-minute monitoring of vital signs; careful utilization of expensive space.

Correspondingly, the predominant *work* of the ICU nursing staff is: one-to-one care of patients; close monitoring of machines and biological systems (rather than "working with the patient"); intense concern with therapeutic and recovery care, in contrast to comfort care; rather close working relations between nurses and physicians; and very low priority for any work with the patient's kinsmen.[7]

Neither the work nor organization of any type of ward can be as neatly outlined as that of the typical ICU, but one has only to visualize the usual run (OB, ER, surgery, pediatrics) to understand that distinguishing patterns of ward work and organization do exist. Even when a ward has a heterogeneous patient population, this in itself sets characteristic work patterns and affects the ward setting, including the kinds and amounts of human and material resources available.

Now the staff's work on a given type of ward need not involve the handling of pain. Indeed, many, if not most, medical and nursing tasks have nothing to do with pain. So it is useful to ask: Under what conditions is pain encountered by staff? And, in a general sense: How will it be handled? Roughly speaking, the answers are as follows.

First, the patient may either arrive with pain or it may develop, because of an illness, during the course of hospitalization. But this does not at all mean that relief of this pain is of primary concern to the staff. In an emergency room, the main job may be diagnosis or immediate treatment, despite the patient's pain. Moreover, ongoing pain may be immensely useful in providing clues to the correct diagnosis, so its relief may be temporarily withheld, wholly or in part.

Second, pain may be produced by the staff's actions. Most induced pain is necessary, for it accompanies various diagnostic, surgical, or therapeutic procedures. Understandably, then, inflicted pain is very much part of the staff work and interaction. However, except when the pain is deliberately induced for diagnostic purposes, it is secondary to the staff's assigned tasks, not a main focus.

Whether inflicted or ongoing, the patterns of pain and of work with pain will vary on different wards, linking up with the predominant work of the staff on those wards. In the recovery room, for example, postoperative pain may be minimized by drugs, but pain control is usually seen as subordinate to close monitoring for potential complications. On the other hand, on wards where cancer patients are clearly dying, comfort care is the staff's primary concern, including the relief of pain to the degree deemed advisable.

Pain minimization in recovery rooms generally represents no great problem, given the available technology. However, on cancer wards (or medical wards with cancer patients), many potential problems are associated with providing appropriate relief to patients in pain while at the same time giving comfort care to those who are dying and recovery care to those in less serious condition. In other words, the work focus in such settings is diverse.

PAIN WORK

The Dimensions of Pain Work

Working with patients in pain—or "managing pain" in common parlance—tends too easily to be equated with the *relief* of pain, perhaps because of our advanced drug technology. However, even brief observation makes quickly evident that care of patients in pain, and interaction with them, involve additional dimensions of pain work: for instance, the handling of pain *expression*. Staff members can be much concerned with or disturbed by the overly expressive patient, for they are up against not only how to manage the patient's expression of pain but also, perhaps, how to manage their own reactions to that expression.

There are still other dimensions to pain work. *Diagnosing* the meaning of pain can be a task, either simple (a sprained thumb) or complex. Some procedures (setting a broken arm) may involve *inflicting* pain. Then there is the work of *minimizing* or *preventing* pain. If the pain is of the inflicted type, the work consists of exerting care to keep it to a minimum. If the patient already has pain, attempts are made to avoid increasing it. If a patient has no pain but has the potential for developing it in the course of his illness, then staff members need to try to prevent or lessen the probability of its occurrence.

Finally, there is the work centered around the patient's *endurance of* pain. The staff's task here is to get the patient to come to terms with pain, whether this involves living with it through only a short procedure, for several days, or even forever. The staff members may have work to do, also, in controlling their own reactions to a patient who may be either excessively expressive or fantastically stoic.

Quite clearly, the salience of these different dimensions of pain work will vary in accordance with the kinds of illnesses experienced by the patients and the organizational features of the particular ward. In the total work of one ward, the relieving of pain may loom large while the problems of managing inflicted pain are negligible. On another ward, persuading the patients to undergo painful procedures may by salient tasks, while problems associated with pain relief may be peripheral. Pain management, then, is not all of a piece: it is highly but determinably variable. Any ward can be analyzed in terms of its *salient dimensions* of pain work.

Cooperation in Pain Work

Patients, of course, are rarely passive objects to be worked upon as the staff is carrying out its pain-related tasks. The patient's cooperation is nearly always called for, if only implicitly. If the patient does not cooperate, does not assent, or actually resists, the task won't get done or will be badly done. At the most extreme, coercion may have to be used, as when screaming children are held forcibly while a necessary procedure is carried out. Or cooperation may be "automatic," if the patient's view of the task is identical with the staff's; that is, it's necessary despite the pain. But cooperation may have to be elicited through persuasion, appeal to good sense or to authority, and perhaps most of all by negotiation.

The negotiation can be explicit:

> *"This won't take long,"* I said to her. . . . *"It's not going to hurt. . . . I think I can inject it right into the IV tubing and not have to stick you."*
>
> *She looked unconvinced.*
>
> *"Honestly I won't stick you unless I have to."*[8]

Or the negotiation can be implicit, bordering on subtle appeal.

The staff's frequently used adjectives, "cooperative" and "uncooperative," represent its views of properly acting patients—where "properly" may signify maximally obedient patients—but we mean something quite different by cooperation. In our concept of pain work, the patient has a part in the total division of labor and is a necessary participant. Of course, participation may consist only of lying still and not interfering with or protesting against a painful procedure, or it may involve more active cooperation, like breathing deeply after a cardiac operation.

PAIN TRAJECTORIES

On almost all wards, there are what we may term *expected* pain trajectories; that is, the staff has repeatedly experienced, and so anticipates, "more of the same" courses of illness and pain and is prepared to work with those standard trajectories. On surgical wards, to give an example, patients commonly arrive with some pain or no pain; after surgery they will be sedated through a few hours or days of considerable pain; and then, providing no complications arise, the pain will drop off at a rate appropriate to the type of surgery.

When an *unexpected* pain trajectory appears, the ward may not be organized nor the staff psychologically set to handle it. For instance, a cancer patient who keeps insisting that relief measures are not controlling pain; an expectant mother wanting natural childbirth in the years before staff members knew about or would accept the philosophy; or a postoperative patient who complains about genuinely *intractable* back pain, on a surgical ward organized to care for *manageable* pain.

An unexpected trajectory—unexpected for a given ward, that is— carries a potential for staff and patient disturbance and ward upset. Both the sentimental order and the work order of the ward are threatened. (As described elsewhere,[9] the term "work order" pertains to the overall organization of the staff's work, and the term "sentimental order" to "the intangible but very real patterning of mood and sentiment that characteristically exists on each ward.") Patients with an unexpected or atypical trajectory tend to be labeled as "uncooperative" or "difficult," and relations between them and the staff are likely to grow progressively worse. Psychiatrists are frequently called in, but often fail to help, either because it is too late to break the vicious cycle of worsening relationships, or because they do not understand the complexities of the work situation.

As a consequence, the nursing and sometimes the medical care of these patients may suffer. In such instances, it is evident to researchers like ourselves that nobody is at fault. Rather, everyone has been trapped into a "no exit" situation, understandable only or primarily in terms of organizational inadequacies.

Trajectories: Illness, Pain, Medical Care, Social

As we remarked earlier, many persons who come to hospitals and other health facilities arrive not as emergency cases nor as cases of an acute illness that requires only a single visit. Chronic disease is what brings most of them there. This means that, unless it is the very first visit, the patient has had previous experiences with health professionals, facilities, and medical care. It also means that the patient has had an illness career or trajectory, with its characteristic symptoms and associated experiences.

If the symptoms include pain, then there has been plenty of pain work associated with the particular trajectory; the patient may, for instance, be very knowledgeable about how to use pain killers. Thus, what the staff encounters most frequently is a patient with a biography that includes considerable experience with (1) *illness,* (2) *pain,* and (3) *medical care.* However, the staff may either be ignorant of or have only limited knowledge of one or more facets of the patient's biography. Also, what is frequently termed the patient's "social background" does not figure very prominently in the staff's work concerns.

Each facet of the patient's biography can present interactional problems, some of major magnitude. As a minor but frequent instance, consider the psychological and physiological difficulties of someone who has been accustomed to taking pain medications of a certain kind and certain strength at certain intervals of time. This person then comes to the hospital where the staff takes over the relief work and, without being consulted finds one or more of those variables are changed. Several patients have told us that they warned nurses and physicians about specific drugs which they knew to be ineffective or to trigger allergic reactions, only to have their warnings ignored, at cost to themselves.

In general, the nursing and medical staff know little or nothing about a patient's pain trajectory, other than the currently evolving portion of it. Patients with severe, chronic back pain, for instance, often come into hospitals for operations, hoping that "this one" may accomplish what one or more others did not, but highly mistrustful of health professionals who previously have misdiagnosed, misoperated, or just plain scoffed at their complaints. So they often prove to be difficult patients, as we shall see.

As for those with considerable experience in hospitals, they can cause plenty of bad feeling when they compare different hospitals' handling of medications or comment pointedly about what they think is incompetency producing unnecessary pain. And concerning patients' social trajectories, about which more will be said later on, note here that a poignant and constant feature of burn wards is patients who lie gloomy and silent, contemplating their dubious futures, or more immediately being frightened of returning home to have their wounds entrusted to the unskilled hands of well-meaning relatives. Ward workers who comprehend this and the other chronic types above will be better equipped to successfully manage the pain.

ASSESSING AND LEGITIMATING PAIN

Only the person who is experiencing (feeling) pain can directly perceive it. Others must either rely on verbal report, or judge gestures as indicators of pain. When the onlookers expect pain, then crying, groaning, grimacing, wincing, perspiring, or the clenching of teeth may easily convince them that pain exists. If they do not expect pain, then the patient must make the pain plausible, or in effect, legitimate it. Under ordinary household circumstances, a person can remark on a headache and others will believe it exists. But if "wolf" has been cried too often, there may be trouble. In the hospital, patients are sometimes suspected of claiming more pain than they have, or of claiming pain when they have none.

Thus, assessing and legitimating are associated processes. Assessment has several dimensions, one or more of which may be salient in any given case. We can express these dimensions as queries: Does she really have any pain at all? How much pain does she have? It's pain, but is it "real" or "psychological"? What does the pain indicate diagnostically? People use different kinds of tactics for different types of assessing. Sometimes the tactics work well, sometimes they do not. As for legitimation—depending on specifiable conditions, sometimes pain or degree of pain are relatively easy to prove but sometimes not. The legitimating tactics are varied. We shall see a fair number of them in operation.

THE BALANCING PROCESS

Among the most important features of pain work is the balancing of priorities. The staff, as well as the patient, must frequently make a choice between or among alternative options, basing the decision on what is believed to be most important. Some decisions are made easily: for instance, to produce (or endure) minor pain during a procedure that will increase the chances of an accurate diagnosis. But some choices are excruciatingly difficult: whether or not to banish daily migraines with an operation that will leave the patient blind.

The staff members may not always agree among themselves, and the balancing done by the patient may not agree with the staff's. Patient and staff may even opt for opposite choices, disagreeing over the value of living a bit longer versus enduring terrible pain. They may be balancing quite different considerations. The staff may be balancing more work versus quicker pain relief, while the patient may be balancing pride in not complaining about pain versus difficulty of enduring it without more medication.

Staff members may not know or care that those balancing options are discrepant, so we can see that the balancing situations can lead to great misunderstanding and controversy. They can also lead to unforeseen consequences, including heightened mutual antagonism, staff withdrawal, a patient's rejection of the staff, even leaving the hospital or attempting suicide.

Consider also that balancing is a process not necessarily confined to a single instance of decision-making. If a person is in pain for very long or an illness trajectory changes very much or other contingencies occur, then the patient and individual staff members may all balance again, that is, they rebalance their respective priorities.

THE RANGE OF CONSEQUENCES

Clearly, the organizational, work, and interactional features of wards have consequences for the nursing and medical care of patients in pain. "Care," when used by staff, usually means something that pertains to recovery from illness, or at least to the blocking of further deterioration. However, if one thinks not only of the patient's illness but of pain, medical care, and social trajectories, then it becomes apparent that there can be consequences for all those trajectories, too.

Indeed, a positive impact on illness may have negative impacts on one or more of the *other* trajectories. For instance, the patient may end up by disliking hospitals and nurses, or may be markedly improved in actual health but facing what seems to be an even more hopeless future because of the severe disabilities accompanying an illness. In a genuine sense, all four trajectories (illness, pain, medical care, and social) pertain to patient care, whether or not the staff is cognizant of this more extended meaning of the term.

There are also consequences for staff members, and these can be conceived in terms of at least a few distinctions. Depending on how the pain has been managed, for instance, a nurse's work may be disrupted or, if unnecessary pain has been inflicted, there may be some loss of professional stature. Of course, personal identity may be affected deeply, not merely by displayed incompetence but by having gone through intense involvement with a patient in pain. Those are negative consequences, but positive ones can also accrue, as when challenges in pain work are successfully met.

We have previously suggested that the ward itself, either in its sentimental order or in its work order, can be affected by various episodes of pain work. Most of the examples given here were of disruption of those two types of order. But there can be positive consequences, too. The successful management of a potentially painful death through skillful comfort care and appropriate medication can bring gratification to the staff, as well as to the patient and the family.

There may also be consequences for the hospital at large, such as law suits by outraged patients. And of course there can be consequences for members of the patient's family, such as anger toward the staff or a patient's blaming the family for not pressuring the staff for effective pain medication.

ACCOUNTABILITY AND PAIN WORK

Chief among the difficulties facing anyone who would reform current practices of pain management in our hospitals is the far from obvious fact that most aspects of pain work are peripheral to the attention and the responsibilities of the staff. By responsibilities we mean not merely the staff's perceived responsibilities, but also its actual legal and organizational ones. We are asserting, in other words, that *the staff is not genuinely accountable for much of its interaction with or behavior toward patients in pain.*

It is evident from even cursory inspection of medical-nursing records, or from listening to reports made by personnel to their superiors, that staff members are responsible only for communicating about certain actions—say, the giving and carrying out of orders about medications—and not for many others. There are also communications (not necessarily required) concerning the assessment of pain, about certain problems with the patient, about complaints of pain, and so on.

The larger array of detail in relation to pain and its management (regardless of whether the information reflects well on the staff or not) is reported only fortuitously. Staff is not really accountable, in the explicit, organizational sense of the term, for the information it provides and the actions it takes in regard to the patient in pain.[10]

Everyone has done more, observed more, knows more, than he or she reports or talks about to colleagues, and certainly much more than goes into the official records.

Genuine accountability concerning pain work could only be instituted if the major authorities on given wards or clinics understood the importance of that accountability and its implications for patient care. They would then need to convert that understanding into a commitment that would bring about necessary changes in written and verbal communication systems. This kind of understanding and commitment can probably come about only after considerable nationwide discussion, such as now is taking place about terminal care, but that kind of discussion seems to lie far in the future. The imagery of "acute illness" is deep-seated and built irrevocably, and directly, into the fabric of medical institutions. We shall see the consequences of that nonaccountability in every chapter of this book, and we shall address the issue explicitly in our closing pages.

REFERENCES

1.   Blaylock, J. 1968. The psychological and cultural influences on the reaction to pain: a review of the literature. *Nursing Forum* 2:262–273.

2.   Crowley, D. M. 1962. *Pain and its alleviation.* Los Angeles: University of California Press.

3.   Knighton, R. 1966. *Pain.* Boston: Little, Brown.

4.   Merskey, H., and Spear, F. 1968. *Pain: psychological and psychiatric aspects.* London: Bailliere, Tindall and Cassell.

5.   Way, E. L., ed. 1968. *New concepts in pain and its clinical management.* Philadelphia: F. A. Davis.

6.   Zborowski, M. 1969. *People in pain.* San Francisco: Jossey-Bass.

7.   McIntyre, H. M. 1968. Intensive care nursing. *Nursing Clinics of North America* 3:1–93.

8.   Glaser, R. 1973. *Ward four hundred two.* New York: George Braziller, p. 130.

9.   Glaser, B., and Strauss, A. 1965. *Awareness of dying.* Chicago: Aldine.

10. Strauss, A.; Glaser, B.; and Quint, J. 1964. Non-accountability of terminal care. *Hospitals* 38:73–87.

Case History: Cancer Patient*

3

The substantive part of this book will begin with a case history. It is by no means typical of hospitalized patients in pain, but it does bring out clearly—and we hope unforgettably—many features of our perspective on pain management. Interaction with and around the patient takes place in a specifiable organizational setting, a cancer ward. Certain dimensions of pain work are salient—notably relieving by the staff and endurance and expression control by the patient. Problems of assessment and legitimation abound. Lack of accountability is a highly pertinent issue. Consequences for ward work, staff relationships, staff mood and morale, and consequences for personal identities, let alone for patient care, are dramatically evident.

This case history is meant to serve as a curtain raiser to the chapters which follow. For that reason, it is presented with only the briefest analytic commentary. The remainder of the book will be enough of a commentary, we believe. Thus one can have the enlightening double experience, first of reading the book and ana-

---

*This chapter is excerpted from Strauss, A. and Glaser B. 1970.
Anguish: case study of a dying trajectory. San Francisco: Sociology Press. pp. 33–105. Reprinted by permission.

lyzing it on one's own, and second, after finishing the book, re-reading the case history, reacting, and analyzing again. It will not be the same case history!

A word about the history and its style of presentation: Mrs. Abel proved to be what we researchers dubbed "the patient of the year" for the staff of a cancer ward at a large metropolitan hospital. The narrative covers her brief initial stay and the first two months of her second and final hospitalization. During all these weeks, Mrs. Abel is enormously preoccupied with her pain, reacting to it in such ways that cause the staff first to react strongly against her, finding her bothersome, then troublesome, then impossible. From those reactions follow a host of consequences: for the nurses, for their relationships with the physician involved, and of course for the evolving relations of all staff and the patient. This phase of Mrs. Abel's illness ends when the nurses finally realize that she is dying—and will die on their ward. The months covered here include a few days in September, then the weeks from early November until the end of December.

Three persons tell this story: S. A. (Shirley Albright), a nurse, trained in field research, who followed the developments occurring around Mrs. Abel; S. Y. (Shizuko Yoshimura Fagerhaugh), a graduate student in nursing, who had chosen to give special care to Mrs. Abel as part of her class assignment, and so was drawn irrevocably and deeply into the case; A. S. (Anselm Strauss), who appears occasionally as listener and questioner.

S. A. When I started in September I asked the nurses to describe patients on the floor who had pain. They mentioned several. Mrs. Abel was about 54 years of age and had had radiation for metastasis of the breast. She had an enlarged endematous right arm and bandaged chest. She cried frequently. When I went to see her, she explained about being in the hospital and gave some of her personal history, even about her girlhood. She brought out a picture of herself as a young woman—in her early twenties. She was then very beautiful. Her second husband is a salesman. Sometimes business is good, sometimes poor. At the moment they are having financial problems. There are no children.

Mrs. Abel spent quite a bit of time weeping off and on, telling about these things. The nurses didn't come in to see her very often—she frequently put on her buzzer, but no one would come. The nurses told me she kept a notebook; everytime she had medication, she would jot down what she had had—the kind of medication, the timing, and whether an

patient breaks
staff rules

injection or pill. She was getting both. She was on methadone, Percodan, and Darvon. She had a schedule she reg-
ulated so as to get something every hour for pain.

There were frequent notes in the cardex in these first two or
three weeks about Mrs. Abel wanting pain medications
around the clock. Finally Dr. Colp wrote orders that she
could have the medications, but the nurses didn't want to
wake her up at night. Then Mrs. Abel started setting an
alarm clock so she could wake up to receive pain medication. This did not go over very well with nurses who felt it
was wrong to wake up patients to give pain medication; if
they're sleeping through all this, then they don't have pain!

**patient has had
previous pain
experience**

Mrs. Abel's explanation was that if she waited until morning
to get the medication, the pain got such a start the medication then didn't take care of the pain. She wanted a consistent dosage of medication; she was very frightened of
pain. The nurses said the first thing in the morning—6:30—

**patient's
reputation
begins**

Mrs. Abel was on the buzzer for her medication. They were
annoyed, they were irritated, and they complained among
themselves.

This had been Mrs. Abel's first admission prior to her final
admission. She'd been here about three weeks. During this

**patient–staff
disagreement
over
timing of drugs**

early period, "she was on the buzzer all the time." There was
a note about this in the cardex. Mrs. Abel was trying to get
them to come right on the dot when the medication was due.
She was handling her medications—ordered every three
hours—and arranged her schedule to get it once every hour.

Mrs. Abel also complained of previous experience with a
private doctor. She had gone for a lump in the breast; he
had told her to go home and exercise her arm and it would
go away. She waited about four months and went back. He
sent her immediately to a surgeon, because the lump had
continued to grow. She complained bitterly that he had not
done a biopsy, that maybe if he had done something she
would have been spared all this. If only it had been caught
in time. "I have an adenocarcinoma, which is one of the fast-
est growing tumors. But they think they can stop it with medications." She also showed me her radiation wound lesion
which had not healed: open, raw, irritated, ulcerated—a very
ugly thing. Later her shoulder became very painful looking,
very black.

Soon after, she went home for a week. I talked to Dr. Colp
about pain thresholds. I asked, "How did you determine

assessing the
pain

this?" He answered, "I used a No. 25 needle and she
jumped. This patient has a very low threshold, and so she
will need medication. I also told her she was on narcotics,
hoping she wouldn't take very much. This isn't, usually, anything that is painful." Dr. Colp hoped Mrs. Abel would stop
taking medication but she didn't.

differential
assessment

is the pain
legitimate?

There was a note on the cardex to use a No. 25 needle. Mrs.
Abel was getting IM injections and should have had a larger
needle than a 25, but they were using the smaller. She was
still jumping and complaining about how much the injections hurt. The nurses were beginning to have some questions about how much she actually hurt because normally a
patient does not jump with a No. 25 needle.

During this early phase of her hospitalization, I have very
few notes about her. She was not mentioned much.

On October 20, I discovered Mrs. Abel had been readmitted
on the preceding day. The head nurse said that Mrs. Abel
was still constantly complaining and had returned because
her husband could not take care of her. The doctor admitted
her in spite of turning away of others because of his di-
minishing budget. There seemed to be a great deal of feeling by the RNs that the doctor was in a bind. The head
nurse told me the patient was admitted specifically for reasons of pain.

beginning of
doctor–nurse
conflict

Mrs. Abel was still complaining, and asking for medication
throughout the night. She was still waking up at 6:30 AM and
asking for her shot. Dr. Colp said to keep her comfortable
but not to wake her up, and this was the bind—how to keep
her comfortable when she was constantly complaining. She
slept all night and set the alarm to wake herself up, and yet
she wanted medication during the night. The doctor said to
give the medication but not to wake her up. He told the patient one thing and the nurses another: "They'll keep you
comfortable" and "Don't wake her up."

patient's
"demand"
schedule

The patient began to complain of drowsiness from the medication and to sleep most of the time. One way nurses determine the amount of pain patients have is by how much they
sleep. Are they sleeping through the pain? If they are sleeping, they are fairly comfortable at the moment. Mrs. Abel was
still insisting on medication every three hours. The head
nurse said, "The doctor has now ordered the medication for
every two hours, but we haven't told Mrs. Abel that so she's

still running on the three-hour schedule." She was on Sparine and Morphine. Some of the nurses found that simply talking to Mrs. Abel for a while made her forget to ask for her
medication.

patient
complains
about
competency

On October 20 I talked with Mrs. Abel. She again complained about the RNs forcing her to space the timing of her
medication. "They all give injections differently." She had
begun to play one nurse against the other, and one shift
against the other by complaining about one to another while
both were there. "You do a better job of this," she would remark to one or the other. She would try to manipulate or co-
erce them into giving the medication and try to make friends
by siding with people. She had great faith in her doctor, in
his being able to handle the pain, but she questioned
whether the nurses could. She felt that they weren't giving
medication properly.

playing staff
against staff

staff feels
rejected

The same afternoon, when the evening shift arrived, a discussion developed about Mrs. Abel. The evening nurse,
Fran, said, "I just can't get along with her. I've never had a
patient who rejected me so."

nurses' bind

legitimation
of patient's
claims

She mentioned the bind they all felt the doctor was putting
them in; he was telling the patient one thing (he could manage the pain, he could control it) and telling the nurses another thing (to keep the patient comfortable but don't wake
her up, and so forth). Fran said, "Certainly she is in pain."
There was not really much question that she was, although
the staff had begun to question whether there was as *much*
pain as Mrs. Abel said there was. But they all had the feeling the woman was certainly in pain.

staff tension
rises

During our discussion Elaine, the second night nurse, said
Dr. Colp had gotten to where he was saying: "You girls can't
do anything right." He complained the nurses couldn't even
collect 24-hour urine correctly. Communication began to
break down at that point. Until then there had been fairly
good communication. They had worked together for at least
a half year.

medication
routines

Around that time, Dr. Colp complained about being called at
night. "Why don't you call me earlier in the evening if you
know a patient is going to need something or other?" Dr.
Colp wrote a list of medications that would cover everything
Mrs. Abel might possibly need so he would not be disturbed

at night or called on a weekend. This was his normal way of doing things and becomes significant later.

On October 21, the day after Mrs. Abel's return, the head nurse told me Mrs. Abel had set her alarm for 4:00 AM. Although the nurses were frustrated, they felt in control of the situation.

staff still
in control

"We were running at an even keel. Now she is getting morphine every three hours, and her last dose was at 5:45 this morning." The night nurse told me Mrs. Abel said she didn't mind dying because she was afraid of too much pain. She had talked about suicide to me before, but this is the first time that I began to pick up that the patient didn't mind dying so much but couldn't tolerate the pain.

first mention
of dying

That afternoon another nurse said Mrs. Abel was euphoric, and that this was due to the amount of morphine she was getting. We tried to evaluate this euphoria. How much was due to organic reasons and how much to psychiatric reasons and tensions that might be within Mrs. Abel, leading to the amount of pain that she had and her reaction to pain? Mrs. Abel was put on Ritalin, a mood elevator.

psychological
or real pain?

preparation for
going home

On October 28 Elaine and I talked to Dr. Colp about teaching Mrs. Abel to give herself injections so she could go home. She was requiring so much medication that a nurse would have to be there 24 hours a day. Mrs. Abel's finances wouldn't allow this. But how were they going to get her home? They hadn't yet tried teaching Mrs. Abel to give her own medication, since her right arm was so edematous that she could not manage a syringe. This put them in a final bind. She simply couldn't give herself medication and she was not getting relief from anything oral. I had begun to realize, as had the nurses, that the physician didn't want to send Mrs. Abel home.

more
doctor–nurse
disagreement

sedation
routines

By this time, Mrs. Abel was on increased amounts of morphine and also on Leritine, a synthetic narcotic. She could alternate the drugs so as to have one of them every hour.

does patient
know she's
dying?

At this point it seemed that Mrs. Abel was more afraid of pain than of dying. For the nurses, the psychological aspects of death were becoming a part of the picture. They felt that Dr. Colp, in his usual manner, was sidestepping the issue and not really being honest with the patient about her real prognosis and outcome. The nurses knew he only gave Mrs. Abel a 10% to 20% chance.

Mrs. Abel's "pain" began to affect every aspect of her care in the hospital. One nurse explained, "I tried to cut her fingernails and ran into such a problem that I couldn't do *anything* right for her. It had to be done *her* way, and just *exactly* that way." She added, "I just don't know what to do with her." It was very frustrating.

orders contrary
to normal
procedures

Mrs. Abel was on Leritine and Sparine around the clock, every two hours. The nurses didn't have the alternative of choosing at night whether or not to give medication to Mrs. Abel—they had to give it by order. The dosage was contrary to the feeling on this floor that there is very little pain connected with cancer. Patients were started out on gradual dosage of aspirin and so forth. Yet this specific patient was getting massive doses of narcotics and also sedatives. She was getting these medications on or around November 4.

relief routines

The nurses were extremely busy during November. There were quite a few critically ill, terminal patients. A note on her chart said Mrs. Abel could have whatever kind of schedule she wanted for pain medication at bedtime, and by the doctor's orders she was allowed the privilege of scheduling things to some extent. A note in the nurses' planning care sheet on the cardex noted: "Patient is very frightened about pain and keeps her own schedule. To be given medication every three hours. Awake and use No. 25 needle."

new symptoms
of new phase
of illness
trajectory?

I visited Mrs. Abel the night of November 4. A nurse came in with pills. Mrs. Abel asked if her pain medications were among the pills she was about to receive. The nurse said no, and that she would be back in about a half hour with the pain medication. I stayed about an hour and a half, but Mrs. Abel did not mention the medication again. About half an hour or forty-five minutes after that she finally said, "Where's the nurse?" She hadn't realized that forty-five minutes had elapsed since the time she was scheduled to get the medication. I had been standing there talking about many things. As previously, she had been crying off and on. Also she began to tell about the increasing appearance of new nodules, particularly around her neck, and she began to point them out. Her shoulder had begun to look very black and necrotic.

doctor's
dilemma

On November 6 I saw Dr. Colp and asked what he was going to do with Mrs. Abel. Was he going to send her home or keep her in the hospital? What were his plans? We were in the hallway. He spent a half hour explaining. He seemed to find a need to talk to somebody about this problem. He didn't know what he was going to do. He was going to see his supervisors and the social worker and find out what could be done, because there wasn't anyone at home to give medication; the husband was a salesman and away from home most of the time. He knew she was having pain, and he felt something had to be done. She just couldn't go home with no one to take care of her, and he didn't want to just send her to the county hospital or any place like that because nobody would take care of her there. He didn't know *what* he was going to do, but he was at least going to talk to his supervisor to find out what could be arranged.

legitimate
pain

animosity
toward
physician
grows

The nurses still felt Dr. Colp was not aware of the basic problem. The problem was that Mrs. Abel was asking for medication and he was telling her that they were going to keep her comfortable, ignoring the fact that she was sleeping through the schedule yet still demanding medication and still complaining. As we spoke, I realized that Dr. Colp *was* aware and actually attempting to say something to the patient. The nurses were not seeing clearly what he was doing. He was thinking, "That's right, what am I going to do with her, as she only has 10% to 20% chance of cure?" He was estimating roughly six months to live. Yet almost a month would pass before the nurses would realize Mrs. Abel was a terminal patient.

dying
trajectory,
but "closed
awareness"

"patient of the
day"

She was beginning to become the "patient of the day" for the staff (i.e., the patient who gets the lion's share of the staff's attention). I realized that this was the beginning of an expanding mushroom of staff focus upon the pain of one patient.

On November 8 I talked again to Dr. Colp to find out what had transpired in the interview with his supervisor. The only way to keep Mrs. Abel in the hospital was as a research patient, because the budget was getting so low they couldn't keep her in simply because she had pain. There was no bed space, and no budget for her. This is the first time Dr. Colp mentioned the possibility of having Dr. Tree—who was doing research on new drugs for control of pain—do research on

Mrs. Abel. This would legitimate her stay in the hospital. So within two days' time, he had this arrangement made. Dr. Tree was going to compare new drugs against morphine. He would substitute his new drugs in place of morphine. Dr. Colp had tried to convince Mrs. Abel that she would stay just as comfortable with the new research drug and that this was the only way she could stay in the hospital. She had become very worried about the possibility of pain but took his word for it. She still had a great deal of faith in him. In fact, I think she never did lose that.

It was the first I had ever seen such tactics used to keep a patient in the hospital, and I began to wonder what Dr. Colp's motivations were for keeping this patient in. Did she really need to be in the hospital? I had begun to recognize, first, it was pain that had first brought this woman *to* the hospital; second, pain was keeping her *in* the hospital; and third, one man now had control of *keeping* her there.

physician's comfort care measures

Mrs. Abel had begun to be very sleepy and to complain that she was never really pain-free in spite of the medication. Dr. Colp said, "I keep her on high levels of sedation and high levels of morphine, and I'll keep increasing." He didn't know what else he was going to do, because I asked him: "What are you going to do when you reach the limits of morphine? What's happening? What can you do for this woman?" I was envisioning that he was saying to Mrs. Abel, "I'm going to keep you comfortable," while she was saying, "But he isn't keeping me comfortable now." And I thought, "How much morphine can you give a patient?" He began to indicate to me—this was the second time—feelings of guilt about the massive dosage of narcotics and medications that she was getting. This amount was very unusual. By this time he knew she was terminal, but he was still looking at her in terms of his six-month prognosis rather than as immediately terminal. He never was concerned with her becoming an addict.

physician not concerned with addiction: balancing

tactics for reducing contact with patient

I began also to watch the nurses. They'd walk into Mrs. Abel's room and do something or other to get the other nurse out—get her off the hook. They were getting caught in there and couldn't easily get out, so one nurse would call the other out. Mrs. Abel was making more and more demands, utilizing everything she could think of to keep nurses *in* the room. She began to take a long time swallowing her medication. A couple of times when I was there, it took a half hour.

The nurses really began to be unable to tolerate Mrs. Abel. They were saying they couldn't stand to take care of her because her need for patterned activity was bordering on ritual. "We can't tolerate working with her for more than a day at a time." They worked out a pattern so no one would be stuck with the patient for too long. They assured me that they all spent an equal amount of time with her.

When I talked with Mrs. Abel on November 10 she was crying a lot. "I've been out of bed since 9:30 this morning." The nurses had gotten her out of bed and taken her down to the window. This was when they started the tactic of getting her down to the view window; she'd sit there all day long. They were hoping she would focus less on her pain if there were more things for her to watch.

patient
balances life
against death

About now Mrs. Abel really began to say she was not being kept comfortable, was never relieved of pain. Most pain was during the day; she didn't complain much of staying awake at night. The sedatives were keeping her fairly comfortable at night. She began to describe this pain as a tight, drawing sensation, mostly in the right arm, which was very edematous. She began to say, "I don't want to live. The few moments I'm free of pain aren't worth living for."

issue of
legitimacy

patient accuses
staff of
improper
care

The nurses felt Mrs. Abel was demanding more attention and more medication than needed because she slept a great deal of the time, even through meals. She'd sleep down at the window. They had begun to feel they couldn't tolerate her, and Mrs. Abel was not legitimating her pain completely. They knew she had some pain—they all say this—but the amount was doubtful. The nurses began to spend more time with other patients to legitimate their avoidance of Mrs. Abel. Around November 14 Mrs. Abel decided she didn't want to be so sleepy and asked Dr. Colp to decrease the sedation. He decreased the phenobarbital. But Mrs. Abel still complained bitterly about the staff. One day she was crying and complaining that on the preceding night, although she was supposed to be getting medication every three or four hours, she hadn't gotten it even though she had repeatedly asked. It turned out that the night nurse had gone back to check but Mrs. Abel was asleep, so the nurse hadn't given the medication to her. The next morning Mrs. Abel was complaining they weren't giving the medication.

crying: credible
as legitimating
signal?

I don't think the aide was as much involved as the nurses, although she did say Mrs. Abel always cried to get procedures done the way she wanted; also that she had to give Mrs. Abel's bath exactly the same way every day. This bothered her. "It isn't as if I didn't know how to give a bath."

more demands:
the patient's
strategy

On about the 17th Mrs. Abel was asking for pain medication about ten or fifteen minutes ahead of the time she was actually supposed to receive medication. It took the nurses that long to get there. And she wanted to make sure the medication actually was *there* on the appointed hour. She would put the buzzer on to remind them just in case they had forgotten. "I like to give them advance warning."

patient now
in control

At this time, Mrs. Abel was on 15 mg of morphine every three hours and was on Percodan "prn." Helen said Mrs. Abel had put herself on a one and a half hour schedule, so that every hour and a half she got something or other. Helen was still complaining that Dr. Colp was telling the patient one thing and telling the nurses another about how much medication she could get and how often. "We've sort of given up, we give her anything she wants."

On the 18th Dr. Tree started doing his research. The nurses really began to question whether she was responding realistically to pain. They had been giving her IM injections with a No. 25 needle, but Dr. Tree was giving injections with a No. 22, the normal procedure. "I don't understand how he can get away with it. She wouldn't ever let us do it." They began to question Mrs. Abel's tolerance to pain. Dr. Tree was increasing the amount of research drug and comparing that to the response of morphine and the response she was getting. He was also using placebos, while she thought she was getting the research drug; however, the placebos followed the research drug by about three hours, and so there was some question about whether he could interpret whether his research drug was having a lasting effect.

I spent half an hour with him and his assistant at the bedside watching everyone's reactions. She would cry one minute, then ask to have the window either open or closed, or talk about how awful her condition was and how much pain she was in. She was using the same tactics she had used on the nurses. He listened, but with one ear open and one ear closed. He spent a half an hour, then left his assistant to spend the other half hour with her. Immediately after,

another case
of "I can't
stand her!"

he said, "I just can't stand a whole hour with her." He said, "I leave my poor assistant." So *he* also pulls out! Although he planned to do further work with her later, he never did.

In the middle of November, Elaine was complaining about the nurses' inability to tolerate Mrs. Abel, and the rotation of people answering her light. "My turn, your turn." Then they actually had a team conference, discussing their inability to tolerate Mrs. Abel and the fact that she always irritated them so much that they walked out of the room. They then took it out on the next person, whoever it might be. They were all getting mad at one another since they couldn't openly get mad at Mrs. Abel. Although there was a breakdown in com-

consequence
of interactional
downward
spiral

munication between them and Dr. Colp, there was no real breakdown among the nurses themselves. By the next week, Dr. Colp was really pulling out of the situation. The communication between him and the nurses *really* stopped.

The final break came when Dr. Colp would not dismiss Mrs. Abel from the hospital. That was in December. The nurses got to where they asked the supervisor to get rid of Mrs. Abel, but the physician said, "No." That was just prior to Christmas vacation, when I took the message back to Elaine that Dr. Colp was going to keep Mrs. Abel in. But the real break came with their getting the supervisor in on the situation.

"patient of the
month"

The patient had by now become "the patient of the month." She preoccupied the staff members, providing the major talk and gossip among them.

Elaine was talking in November of her complaints about Dr. Colp and the misery that all the nurses were going through, and the anticipated misery that was going to develop for them because of the research study. They did not know quite how Mrs. Abel was going to relate to Dr. Tree. They didn't know enough about the research project he was on, but neither did I, then, to know whether this was going to affect Mrs. Abel's routine schedule. And wouldn't the research pull her off some medications? Would she, therefore, become more complaining, more weepy, and so forth? Was this drug

anticipation of
ineffective
relief measures

going to be as effective as morphine or wasn't it? If it wasn't, Mrs. Abel was going to be in real trouble and would cause many more problems for the nurses. Elaine said, "Next week it's going to be awful for the patient *and* for *us*." The emphasis was on *us*, and "we" are going to get her constant complaints.

A. S.: Could even Dr. Tree have told the nurses what would be the effect of their own tasks of his research? Was there any way of knowing then?

S. A.: Not at that point. In fact, that drug had not been used here before. This was the first patient he had used it on.

I mentioned before that Mrs. Abel had mood swings. When I was there, she complained about the pills that now were due but that she hadn't gotten, and with the next breath she asked the nurse who had come in to water the plant. The nurse started to do it with water from the pitcher, and Mrs. Abel said, "Heavens no, not with ice water." It was as if she said: "Even *I* know that you don't water the plants with ice water." So she went from one thing to another, complaining about how much pain she had and then she worried about

*more
assessment
of degree of
pain*

her plant. I think this is where the nurses started to question how much pain Mrs. Abel really had. Of course, when the affair with the placebo began (and *they* were supposed to make descriptive notes that Dr. Tree could use as a reference for his research, which meant that the nurses had now to spend much time in Mrs. Abel's room), they really began to question the amount of pain.

*another phase
of trajectory*

As Mrs. Abel's edema became worse, the right hand got puffier and puffier, and she couldn't even straighten her hand. "Do you think I'll ever be able to straighten my fingers out again?" Her arm looked as if it was ready to split the skin, it was so edematous. She would focus on her inability to use it, along with the amount of pain, and the heaviness, the weightiness, of her arm. So I began to notice how localization of a particular body part should so engulf her attention that virtually her total life was focused around it.

*pain
expression . . .*

During Dr. Tree's research, Mrs. Abel was beginning to complain about the tension building up: "I just have to cry." She began to talk about crying as a relief from pain. I remember the nurses talking about how *they* began focusing on the pain, too. In fact, June said, "With some people, crying helps, but with Mrs. Abel it doesn't." But it was Mrs. Abel's feeling that crying actually relieved her tension, pain, and the whole frustration that she had built up. She said, "It's within my chest," where her lesion was anyway.

When June said this, she had a great deal of feeling in her voice, because she had begun to tell Mrs. Abel to stop

... nurses' response

crying. The nurses began to change. All of a sudden they were beginning to be very aggressive. "Look, crying just doesn't help you, so stop it!" It is unusual for a nurse to stop a patient from reacting in this fashion. They now felt they were more helpful if they became authoritarian, and very openly so. There was an interchange between June and Elaine and between June and me: We just *have* to make her do things and to become very authoritarian. June wasn't using the word "authoritarian" really; what term *did* she use ...? "Setting limits." They had to set limits for this patient.

"setting limits"

routines: staff and patient

Actually, they never really did set limits. They were going to set limits concerning her taking pills, but they really stuck with her pattern. They had become used to her routine and did realize they were sticking with it. But they always talked about how it would be better for Mrs. Abel to be moved off this floor so limits could be set. Yet Mrs. Abel had them wound around her finger. She continued to cry frequently.

A. S. When they are talking about moving in to set limits on her crying, what is the mood?

using the nurse as a relief messenger

S. A. Anger. They've had it up to their teeth and they're going to stop this. It's, "I did this and found it worked, and I've *had* it." In fact, June later describes herself as doing something when Mrs. Abel had finally gotten to her. She called Dr. Colp one night after Mrs. Abel had pushed and pushed her. So June thought she'd better check with him about symptoms. The next day, Mrs. Abel was not bothering any other nurses, but was calling for June and pushing her to ask Dr. Colp for more medications. June: "I laid the law down again. I'm not going to do it." June had begun to set limits because she *had* to or the patient would use her.

A. S. Did other nurses, or aides, talk at any time in terms like, "She's using me as an agent to get something?"

S. A. June is the only one. I don't think the others were that aware of what was going on. They were mad and angry, but not completely aware of the reason. They had the beginnings of awareness, but not to the extent that June did.

husband cannot help with pain tasks

This night her husband was in the room. She began to talk about not getting any relief from her medication, not getting her pain pills, and she began to cry. The husband got up and left. He just couldn't tolerate this. He came back in a few minutes. She had continued crying. He sat down. "Are you having pain now?" She answered very angrily, "Yes, I told you, I'm always in pain."

Fran felt Mrs. Abel was very angry at her. Fran was the nurse who believed Mrs. Abel considered her incompetent. Mrs. Abel was constantly complaining. This bothered Fran because she wanted to feel she was a competent nurse. She just could not work with Mrs. Abel, and Mrs. Abel constantly complained about her ability. In the next breath Fran said she felt sorry—that she wanted to help her but couldn't seem to. "Everything I do for her is wrong." This was about November 20, and Dr. Colp was saying that because of Dr. Tree's coming up, he himself could escape a little more. (He said that to Dr. Tree and me.)

accusation
of
incompetence

Mrs. Abel was not, at this point, talking about death as such. June said, "She's not focused on death." But the nurses thought her pain was heightened by her feeling that maybe the pain was related to death. But in fact Mrs. Abel concentrated more on her disfigurement. Mrs. Abel didn't then feel that she was terminal and neither did the nurses. Only the doctor knew it.

another
interpretation
of pain

A. S. Did Mrs. Abel ever show a genuine comprehension of what the nurses were going through and their difficulties with timing, and so on?

S. A. No . . . She took a good half hour to take medication one night when I went in with June. June slipped me the pills so that she could go on to her other jobs. You're not supposed to leave pills at the bedside with a patient, particularly narcotics. She could stockpile them. I don't think the nurses were too careful about that with Mrs. Abel; they would leave medication at the bedside. Mrs. Abel was annoying June because she was spending too long taking the medication. Not until the middle of November did anyone actually start expressing this. "Look at the number of times we *have* to be in there, just to give her medication!" Somebody had to be in there almost every hour because now Mrs. Abel had it scheduled so that at every hour she had her medication. It took her a half hour to take the medication, so the medication nurse was in there a half hour of *every* hour. Then the bath would take longer than that, and Mrs. Abel stretched this out. There was very little time when Mrs. Abel did not have some member of the staff in there for legitimate reasons. There was very little time when she was actually alone.

interfering
with work

stockpiling
drugs

I talked to Dr. Colp about the stockpiling of drugs; she had asked him a couple of times for an overdose. The nurses were not paying too much attention to Mrs. Abel's medication. Nor were they asking questions when they went in her room. They stayed a very short period of time. The pills might be left there. She could have stockpiled. If she had wanted to commit suicide, it would have been very easy. She knew all the drugs she was on—pill by pill, name by name. She was *asking* to die and considering suicide, although she never mentioned it to me at all. There was some concern about her committing suicide.

suicide

S. Y. Was this just before she knew she was terminal?

S. A. Yes. She knew the possibilities. She didn't know it was a 10% to 20% chance, but she knew the probabilities were poor. Dr. Colp had said he had been telling her that, and she knew it was a very fast-growing cancer, but she kept saying, "*If* they cure me, *if* they can control this. . . ."

A. S. Did she ever take any extra drugs by herself illicitly?

S. A. None that we were ever able to pick up.

S. Y. I don't think she had stockpiled.

staff rotation
as tactic for
handling
demands

S. A. The medication nurse, by the way, was a different nurse each day. The team leader is usually the medication nurse, so rotates also. Team leaders pass out medication, so the team leader was also Mrs. Abel's personal nurse. It was foolish to assign another nurse when you were in there all day giving Mrs. Abel medications anyway. When the team leader was out of the room, the aide was there with Mrs. Abel. I was never alone in the room and the chaplain was complaining someone was always in the room. Out of necessity. By and large.

S. Y. They did things she requested: taking her to the commode, moving the arms this way and that, getting her a drink of water. Once you got into the room there was a steady stream of requests. There was a new request before you finished the last.

legitimate
pain work
demands

S. A. The staff couldn't pull out altogether. There were specific doctor's orders that somebody *had* to be there. Mrs. Abel was on massive doses of medication which would disorient her. If she started to get out of bed, she could fall and hurt herself. Since Mrs. Abel was in the process of suing for a whiplash injury, there was a possibility of a suit for negligence against the hospital. This complicated the picture, and they were afraid; they had to obey doctor's orders, they had to be there, or else the bedside rails had to be up.

Mrs. Abel had begun to get so much medication that she was nauseated and unable to eat very much. There was no real encouragement by the nurses to get her to eat.

My next notes on Mrs. Abel simply say that she was the same. I remember there was nothing really new during this time. It's then that Shizu (SY) starts working with her.

challenged by
an interesting
case

S. Y. For about a week prior to taking care of Mrs. Abel, I began to hear a lot about her, in reports, in careful conversation—mostly griping about Mrs. Abel. I just introduced myself to her. Then "It" just poured out. She made a special point that she could not go home because of the pain and because of the situation at home. She talked about the new drugs the doctor was looking forward to trying. I felt, "I'll take a whack at caring for her." She would certainly be a challenging patient. I announced to the head nurse that I would be taking care of Mrs. Abel. She immediately wanted to know how many mornings I would be going up there, although she already knew. She said "good" because the patient was so impossible they had to rotate the staff around. No one could stand being with her for days on end. I became curious to find out what this patient did that made everybody react so violently.

So I read through the patient's chart, gathering as much information as I could about her history. There was a clear schedule worked out for her narcotics: every one and a half hours narcotics were given, and the schedule had been going on for some time. I decided I wasn't going to fight it. I was going to follow this routine. Another thing the staff had been telling me was that she sat with a book marking down very carefully when her narcotics were due. Mrs. Abel would turn on the light 10 to 15 minutes before the drug was due in anticipation of the drug and also of warding off the pain.

pulling out

S. A. It was on November 25, the day Shizu was coming in, that Dr. Colp pulled out—in the sense that there wasn't anything more he could do for Mrs. Abel. He did all he could. He knew there wasn't anything that was going to help her.

He was going to hold her on the medication she was now on, because when he changed drugs then her level of hope would drop noticeably. He felt he could no longer stand to be involved with Mrs. Abel . . . could no longer "take her problems home" with him. He didn't even want to talk about her case.

new pain nurse

S. Y. The following morning I was greeted very cheerfully by the assistant head nurse and the staff. Previously they had been pretty much ignoring me. I thought, "Well, I guess I'm in like Flynn now because I'm taking care of this 'ward pill'." I offered to be responsible for the narcotics. They very gladly and happily relinquished the job.

pain talk

As soon as I entered her room, she began to tell all about her aches and pains. She complained bitterly about not getting her injections at night, that she had to call for them, and by the time she called for the nurse the pain had really gotten a good hold of her and it took at least an hour to overcome. "I have pain *all* the time, my dear," she said, and went into a long description of where it was and pointed out that she was getting a few more nodules and hoped they would not continue.

The first few days I was just going to sit back and let Mrs. Abel do all the talking. Actually that wasn't very difficult because it was a monologue. I was also fascinated by the injection. I went into her room with her injection *on time*. She brought out her little book (which was carefully hand-lined). It had the time the drug was due, and on it was *right, left,* indicating in which hip each injection was to be given. Then she wrote the time down in red; after the drug was given it was carefully crossed out with blue ink. She said that previously she used to do it all with blue ink, but then she couldn't see the last time she wrote on it. I was fascinated by all of this. "What an elaborate system of controlling the environment and the means of warding off pain." I realized I was not going to argue with the book; I was going to let her write in the book, and I was going to give her the drugs exactly on time.

I was fascinated by this record keeping, and I asked if this helped in keeping account of the drugs. She said that if she didn't keep an account, the anticipation of pain became so great that she couldn't stand it any longer and it took some time for the drug actually to work. Then she mentioned things that the doctor was hoping to do to slow down the cancer process; at the same time she said being kept alive was no help because one had to consider how one lived, and being kept alive was all pain and ugliness which wasn't worth it. She vacillated back and forth about the new drug, full of hope and at the same time wanting to die.

balancing

The following day I ran into Dr. Colp. I asked what the plan of care was, and he said nothing more could be done for her. He was more concerned with trying to keep her free of pain. At the same time, he was thinking of playing around with another hormone. I thought this was very strange. He felt he had carried Mrs. Abel as long as possible beyond what was reasonable in terms of research. Mrs. Abel's stay must be terminated. But he was "up a tree" because the only recourse open to Mrs. Abel was to go home, and he was petrified of the idea. He could not accept the idea of her going to the county hospital. He described the whole situation as poor and Mr. Abel as being beat down, and that he probably would be beat down too if he had a wife like Mrs. Abel. He appreciated what was happening to the husband, and said the awful part was that there was nothing you could do except to tolerate it. "I know. I went through an experience just like this with an immediate relative of mine." He described this relative who had the whole family in an uproar.

"nothing more to do"— comfort care

mutual biographies of physician and patient

Then he complained that he got it from all sides, from the nurses and from the patient. I asked if he had contacted the social worker and he had; she was looking for some place to discharge the patient. I wondered if he was running into difficulties in getting her discharged because of his personal experience. The following day I took care of Mrs. Abel again and typically she immediately began to complain about the previous night. I was greeted with a steady stream of complaints. I thought this must be the thing that really gets the nurses down because it makes them feel inadequate. I almost wanted to say, "Please don't do it this way, you make the nurses so angry."

sentimental order deteriorates

S. A. The nurses were now very angry. Elaine kept saying to me, "I'm just living for my days off." They all got very irritable, very sharp with each other.

S. Y. This was the second morning I was taking care of her, and I was going through the supreme test of one request right after another. Even though I kept telling her I was going to be with her all morning, she needed to use these tricks. Later she didn't have to do this, but I was really put through the paces that morning.

S. A. I noticed, too, that it was then Mrs. Abel began to sleep and couldn't remember when she had medication. She started to ask the nurses to remind her to cross out the medi-

nonlegitimate
pain

cation in her notebook. The nurses felt she was no longer legitimating her pain; she was sleeping through it. The nurses couldn't tolerate the notebook in the first place and when Mrs. Abel started asking them to remind her to take care of the notebook, this was the last straw. They had really begun to question the amount of emotional pain and the amount of physical, organic pain. They believed she was emotionally overreacting. This continued until December 6, when they actually pulled out.

S. Y. I ran into the chaplain that morning, and his comment was, "Isn't she something, though?" We exchanged information, and it was pretty much the same information that the patient had rattled off to me.

At the end of the week I wrote: "Mrs. Abel is indeed a disturbed and disturbing patient. This illness with all its fearful meaning exaggerates her past neurotic behaviors. It is obvious her behavior has regressed—dependency, with whining, and wanting constant attention. The nurse must play a mother surrogate role, but it is time-consuming and sometimes very, very hard to take. The breast cancer is a further threat to her already badly damaged body image. Her elaborate record keeping is a method of controlling the environment. Pain seems to be symbolized in guilt, punishment, and aggression which intensifies pain. The rituals are very important to her, and I am up a tree, not knowing where one interferes with it and where one does not. I need help in trying to know what to do in relating to the patient and also in terms of managing the patient."

A. S. Did they ever call in a psychiatrist?

more balancing

S. A. When Dr. Colp was telling me about not knowing what to do—before he made her a research patient—he said he had decided not to have a psych consult because of the length of time that she would live. It wasn't worth it for her to undergo therapy at this point. It would take too long.

S. Y. Then I saw the social worker. She had announced to the nursing staff that Mrs. Abel's stay might be extended. The nurses moaned and groaned saying they couldn't possibly put up with Mrs. Abel any longer.

S. A. I have in my field notes, Shizu, that you had already begun to see Mrs. Abel as terminal. You felt more and more agitated as the end came closer. This was December 4.

desire to "get
rid of patient"

This was when Elaine had talked about their having to give pills, changing her dressing—the whole ritual. "I don't know how long they're going to keep her here. Breast tumor isn't the burning problem any longer, and the tumor board isn't learning anything from her." Dr. Colp was just keeping her in. This was December 4. Two weeks later, she was really pushing to get this patient out and was telling the supervisor about it.

amusement as
outlet for
aggression

S. Y. Their amusement, pretty high amusement, began to appear around the middle of December. "Did you hear about the other particular thing that she did?" This sort of thing.

During a team conference on December 5, I asked if they had any suggestions about what I or they might do to relate better to the patient. This drew no suggestions. I got the feeling that they were up a tree. And I was up a tree. I gathered they were fed up and didn't want to discuss it. They would laugh derisively about it, and so forth, but not discuss the situation in terms of what actually could be done.

repetitious
pain talk

Again I stayed with her. Mrs. Abel talked and talked and talked, pretty much about the same things. She would repeat the same things over and over. "It drives you nuts. The same old story morning after morning," said one nurse.

Periodically Mrs. Abel would complain about pain and weep about its uselessness. However, I did notice that she did not complain about it as much as the week before. Again, the medicines were given exactly on time, and I allowed her to record them. It occurred to me: What could the nurses have done earlier during the course of her care? If they had done something differently would her focus on pain be less? Yet I couldn't decide what they could have done. Such things were running through my mind.

"nothing
works"

Later I reported to the team leader who was merely interested in knowing when the next narcotic was due and not really about what went on with the patient. I asked what she had done in terms of trying to relate better to Mrs. Abel. "Nothing works. Do whatever you like. You do whatever you think is right. I don't care what you do."

This was when I wrote "I feel very frustrated. I'm getting nowhere. I feel like I need psychiatric help." Then the chaplain came to the student seminar and a good portion of the discussion was spent on Mrs. Abel again. I don't think we came to any solution though. The gist of the seminar was mostly his role in helping the dying patients, and how the chaplain and nurses could work as a team in helping patients. Mrs. Abel was brought up as an example.

sedation tactics
juggling
medication

On December 6 Mrs. Abel was quite nauseated from all the drugs, so promazine was given. Doctor Colp wrote on her chart: "Possible discharge. Discussion with patient in a few weeks. The patient might become anxious." Mrs. Abel was getting more depressed, so he gave her some mood-elevating drugs.

S. A. This was when Elaine really started wanting to get rid of Mrs. Abel. Dr. Colp had started pulling off the floor—because Elaine was asking *me* for information. Elaine was the assistant head nurse and was really running the floor. Elaine

collective
desperation

said Mrs. Abel had them like puppets on a string. "She's really gotten to us and we just act like puppets and do whatever Mrs. Abel wants us to do. Dr. Colp doesn't want to discharge her . . . I can't see throwing her out in the cold snow, but . . ." and her "but" just hung. She said Dr. Colp felt sorry for Mrs. Abel and was really vague when he talked about her. "We can't pin him down to anything." That day she wanted me to pin Dr. Colp and Dr. Tree down to find out exactly what was going on.

The nurses hadn't yet realized Mrs. Abel was terminal and thought there would be no end to her stay on the floor; the research could go on forever. And they would all be in anguish if it went on forever.

stereotyping

They were getting really desperate. One said, "Mrs. Abel is so self-centered," and they began to describe her with this type of terminology.

S. Y. I remember Elaine saying, "She's *so* selfish." With great anger I think she said to the patient, "I think you're so selfish!"

S. A. In fact, the chaplain got around to telling Mrs. Abel, "Try. Maybe you could set a better example for the other patients on how to accept suffering." This was December 1.

S. Y. On December 9 I finally located Dr. Colp. He had just told the patient about eventual discharge. He expected the patient now to become quite agitated. He was waiting for Dr. Tree's return from vacation to discuss the possibilities of new pain studies, and, therefore, Mrs. Abel's discharge would be delayed for about a month. He had questioned Mrs. Abel at great length about the pain in her arm. He felt it was not pain but actually a heaviness, like a dullness experienced after Novocain injection in dental work. There was no pain as such but one could feel the pulling and tugging. He assured the patient that no matter what drugs they gave her, they could not stop this feeling.

admission: no real relief possible

S. A. This is the first time *this* point came up. Before, he was reassuring her that they could take care of her pain. Now he said they couldn't.

reassertion of claim to pain

S. Y. The following day I questioned her at length about the pain, and she kept saying, "It's a real pain." She kept saying, "I really have pain," over and over again.

S. A. She probably did not believe the "heaviness" explanation because she used the same tactics to prove that she had pain. And Dr. Colp said, "Even if I had this tightness, I, *too,* might have expressed this as pain. She always expressed this as pain."

S. Y. Then I asked the doctor about getting psychiatric consultation. He sounded quite hostile, "Do you think it's going to help her now?" I answered that I certainly didn't think it would help her in any long-term way, but I did feel the consult might be able to help her. Also, the nursing staff needed it, and I, too, needed help in terms of relating to the patient. He didn't think it would help: "Maybe *you* take your problems home with you, but *I* don't because I forget her the minute I get off the station." I thought to myself, "The hell you do." I thought he must really find this a threat and wondered if he was running into problems with pain pills and all the related moral and ethical problems.

Then he looked down at the medication charting sheet and said, "Well, there are a few more free spaces available to order more drugs. She's getting enough pills now, but there are three more spaces." I was getting pretty irritated with him. "You keep treating her and treating her, giving her a lot of false hope, and probably are just relieving your own conscience." The doctor was getting irritated with me, too. He looked at his watch and said he had to see another patient on another ward. I wrote in my notes, "I wish I knew what to do; I'm stuck."

That same day, he indicated to me a feeling of depression about county hospitals: she just wouldn't get as good care there because those places are always so depressing. He constantly mentioned this. He said he was definitely going to wait for Dr. Tree's return. Dr. Tree was the justification for keeping Mrs. Abel in the hospital. He emphasized this again; he's keeping her despite the nurses and the fact that the budget is getting very low. He was actually turning other patients away, not admitting them, and cutting corners with other patients.

"presence" as
tactic

On that day the doctor discontinued some of the other drugs he had been treating her with for cancer—ACTH and the tyroid—and started estrogens. On December 10 I debated whether to continue taking care of Mrs. Abel as I didn't seem to be getting anywhere very fast. But I decided Mrs. Abel probably could tolerate some unirritated nursing care. I decided that I would have no plan of care but merely be with her and give her what little comfort I could. I told the team leader that I would take care of her total medications (where previously I had only been responsible for the narcotics).

When I questioned Mrs. Abel about the pain in her arm, she said again it was dull, aching, never went away, and was really very painful. The medications I administered were taken without the usual fuss and crying. I left troubled with her silence because I didn't know what it meant.

negative
reputation
spreads

On December 11 I saw Mrs. White, a faculty member of the School of Nursing. I told her about my needing psychiatric consultation. She said she had posed the subject of psychiatric consultation to the nursing staff, and the assistant head nurse (Elaine) to whom she talked rejected the suggestion completely, saying the nursing staff could adequately solve their problems through the team conference. What did this conference with Mrs. White do for me? Nothing. I ran into Shirley and we discussed Mrs. Abel at great length; Shirley reassured me that I was doing my best and not to feel bad about it. Then I ran into A. S. who said (in so many words), "You can't beat the system. The system is creating the problems and *don't feel bad* about it." At the end of the day I thought, "By God, three people in the past hour have told me not to feel bad, that I have done my best. Well, I'm frustrated in the situation, but probably I'm the only one who *shouldn't* feel too bad about it because I'm the only one that's actually going in and *doing* something with this patient."

S. A. *Later on that day I found that the nurses realized they were never going to get rid of her.*

S. Y. I wasn't ready to buy that yet. Partly because I had been talking to the social worker who had been working on plans, although Dr. Colp was saying, "We're running out of funds," and so on.

thoughts of death

Mrs. Abel was talking to me about her arm and its dull, aching pain. Then she was silent for quite a long time and kept looking at her arm. I said, "It must be very difficult for you." She cried and said, "I pray and I pray, but it doesn't seem to help." I said, "The praying doesn't help you?" and she said, "It helps sometimes but most of the time it doesn't." Then as if talking to herself, "I wonder what happens to the soul, it must look for something and not find it, just as we seek something in life and not find it." I answered "yes" and kept nodding my head and encouraging her to talk, but she would not talk any more. Then I asked if she had been able to talk over these matters with the chaplain. "He's very nice, but I think I can preach as well as he can." So I said, "Do you feel you could preach as well as he can?" She answered that she could and talked about her religious beliefs and reincarnation.

S. Y. Then the social worker decided they would not meet with the patient, only with her husband. I went down to the office where Mr. Abel was agitated and wringing his hands. He just could not have Mrs. Abel at home because he was upset and had had a nervous breakdown before. If it were not for tranquilizers he would fall apart. He kept saying over and over and over that Mrs. Abel upset him; he didn't know what he was doing.

"giving up"

A. S. By now the patient had been relatively abandoned by everybody except Shizu and the doctor. The doctor was the person who somehow kept the whole situation going, and Shizu was sticking by Mrs. Abel in her room. I assume the chaplain also was not giving up yet. The husband had given up. The nurses had pretty much given up, probably the interns also.

S. Y. The social worker was beginning to see her more frequently.

S. A. The chaplain hadn't given up. He was frustrated and not able to acknowledge that maybe he couldn't stand the situation. He said there was always someone in her room; that other terminal patients needed him also. He began to spend more time with other patients and was comparing them with Mrs. Abel. He was also complaining (December 13) about the inability of the nurses on the floor to relate to Mrs. Abel. He said they are having difficulty because they identified with her; they too could have cancer, could have this kind of pain, and so forth, and therefore they became hardened and hostile. "It's a crying shame. They just can't stand her making demands on them. I haven't had time to spend with her, there are so many terminally ill making demands on my time."

S. Y. The social worker stated there were three possible discharge avenues open. One was to discharge the patient home, which the patient rejected, even though Dr. Colp kept suggesting she be sent home with a vocational nurse.

an impossible balancing

S. A. Somebody, he said, who would be willing to work around the clock, because of medications. He didn't see this as feasible unless it were a paid nurse, but this was not financially possible. He was really on a hot spot. He never did get off it. Somebody kept the pressure on him right up to the end.

S. Y. A second possibility was the county hospital, which Dr. Colp rejected. A third was the nursing home, a pretty good possibility. The social worker instructed the husband to call the welfare department for an application. On December 12 the assistant head nurse told me Dr. Colp had definitely made arrangements to keep the patient for several weeks more, awaiting a pain study. "I could have cried when I found that out. You know Dr. Tree isn't coming back for several weeks and so the pain study will be delayed, and we will have to tolerate her that much longer."

S. A. Elaine was just beside herself. "This will ruin my Christmas vacation if she is going to stay with us. We can't get rid of her." This was about December 16.

S. Y. I asked if there was any change in Mrs. Abel, she was so quiet the last time I saw her. The answer the nurse gave was that she hadn't changed a bit and was getting more and more demanding—and more and more unreasonable.

hallway conferences

S. A. It was on December 16 that you and I and the chaplain had a three-way conference in the hallway. Remember? Dr. Colp had been to see the patient, and the three of us had gotten together. (By this time the nurses couldn't tolerate the sight of me.) All three of us stood in the hallway and everybody just passed us as though we were just so much furniture. Dr. Colp almost did also, but I snagged him as he went by. He changed the subject after two words about Mrs. Abel. In the meantime, Shizu and the chaplain stood there talking about Mrs. Abel. They were both deeply confused.

S. Y. We were talking of her becoming more and more agitated with nothing and nobody able to help her. She was avoided more and more by the staff, so getting more and more agitated. Mrs. Abel was a "bad, bad girl" but bad, bad

collective mood: helplessness

girl attention is better than no attention at all. The mood of the conversation was general helplessness. I just needed someone to talk to because nobody else would listen to me.

S. A. I knew that I couldn't press the nurses because they couldn't tolerate me any longer. But I was trying to keep some form of relationship. So I decorated a box of homemade cookies for them as a Christmas gift to show appreciation. They had just been putting up the tree on that floor. I gave the box of cookies to them, and a couple commented "thank you" and left. You know, they looked at the note on the Christmas card and put the box under the tree—and literally just left. I was fascinated. They *just could not* tolerate being around me at all. They simply left. Well, this left me with the secretary who said Mrs. Abel was "snowed" all the time. She was still crying. "She could stay here for a year, I guess." The nurses asked Dr. Colp when Mrs. Abel would go. He told them she would be there as long as she was of use (meaning research), and she could stay as long as a year. The secretary said, "I guess she will be here until she dies." This was the first one who really said what we had anticipated.

EPILOGUE

So that our readers will not be left without some closure, we will briefly discuss what finally happened to Mrs. Abel. She died on February 18 after two months of virtual isolation. The staff members could neither suffer her nor withstand the ordeal through which she was going and in which they were participating. Her death finally occurred after even the most empathetic nurse had pulled away and her physician had, because of his own feeling of helplessness, abandoned her to a last-ditch, and quite possibly fatal, surgical operation. He left her so that she had to make her own decision. Mrs. Abel understood the riskiness of this operation but was almost beyond caring. She could stand neither her almost unendurable pain nor the almost total isolation which staff had imposed on her. Surgery represented more of a potential release from her impossible situation than a chance to live—if live it really was (since she saw herself as "a vegetable")—a bit longer. She died (some of us think it was merciful) during the operation.

We should add that Mrs. Abel went off to the operation without a farewell from any of the ward personnel, and the night before, in preparation for the operation which involved her head, an appointed stranger came to shave off the one remaining feature of her body which she could still prize: her hair.

Although we have chosen to forego extended analytic comment on this case, we do wish to say to readers that if they have blamed particular actors in this sad drama, then they have missed its essence. Nobody is to blame for this downward spiral in events. The organization itself is at fault. Faced with a very difficult situation rendered more difficult yet by a ward principally organized, and a staff trained, for medical work, everyone—every single actor—is caught up in the inexorable downward spiral of events. That spiral *might* have been broken in its earlier phases by skilled psychological interventions, but certainly not later, at least not without concerted and sustained effort.

Part 2

Simple and
Complex Trajectories

Routine, Nonproblematic Surgical Pain

4

In any acute-care hospital, a large percentage of the patient population is composed of surgical patients who must suffer pains and discomforts. The types of surgeries performed there may vary from the relatively routine, where the surgical and pain courses are predictable and nonproblematic, to the very complex, where the illness and pain courses are highly unpredictable and very problematic. The management of a given surgical patient's pain may occur in the context of clinical settings organized in terms of highly specialized medical disorders (chest, cardiac) or broader categories (general, surgery).

Whether the given setting is specialized or general, it tends to be organized around the staff's expectations that, for certain types of surgeries, there are anticipated surgical and pain trajectories. Ward work, routines, and medical technology are geared to carry the patient successfully through the surgical course and manage the accompanying pains. When the patient's condition is highly unstable, there are intensive care units for managing such critical states. Hence, a typical statement made by nurses about surgical patients on their units:

We don't have many pain problems with most surgical patients.
They have severe pain for a couple of days after surgery, but we
can generally control the pain with drugs. We're generally liberal
with pain drugs the first couple of days postoperatively and gradu-
ally taper off the drugs.

Implied in this statement is, first, that the staff members perceive surgical and pain courses as nonproblematic for many of the
surgical patients. Second, with appropriate medical technology the
pains can be adequately controlled. Third, there is little tension between the patients and the staff. Because the patients usually do not
complain or challenge the staff, they are assumed to be satisfied with
the way their illnesses and pains are managed. In large part the personnel see themselves as handling surgical patients and their pains
quite well.

One might assume, then, that with the more familiar, run-of-
the-mill surgeries (appendectomies, hemorrhoidectomies, her-
miorrhaphies, cholecystectomies, uncomplicated fractures, etc.)
where the surgical and pain courses are usually predictable and entail
few medical risks, there are well-organized procedures for managing
pain. Our observations indicate quite the contrary. Indeed, neglect of
these patients often results from the competitive presence on the
same ward of patients who had more complex, unpredictable, problematic surgical conditions. This latter aspect will be discussed in the
next chapter.

This chapter will focus on routine, nonproblematic surgeries.
These highlight the lack of organizational accountability in relation to
important aspects of pain management. Let us consider the properties of routine surgical trajectories and their associated pain tasks,
before discussing the organizational shortcomings.

PROPERTIES OF ROUTINE SURGICAL TRAJECTORIES

Routine surgical trajectories can be characterized as predictable, involving few risks, unambiguous, and of short duration. Barring
complications, the recovery courses and their accompanying pains
are predictable and nonproblematic. Both the hospitalization and the
pain courses are anticipated to be short. The hospital stay is usually
from a week to ten days, and sometimes even shorter. Staff anticipates that pain will be relatively high for 24 to 72 hours postoperatively and will then quickly taper off.

There is a relatively high degree of specificity as to the causes of
physiological (as opposed to psychological) pain and discomfort. So,

patients generally need not legitimate the presence of pain, although there may be questions as to the degree of pain suffered by individual patients. Because of the physiological bases of pain, specific drugs and specific nursing and medical measures are utilized to relieve pains.[1-6] Of equal importance to relief, however, are the prevention of complications and the returning of the patient to physiological equilibrium, both of which may unavoidably require inflicted pains and discomforts.

Because of the familiar nature of the surgical trajectories, patients, too, are generally aware that they must endure some pains and discomforts from both the surgery and treatment. Usually they are aware that severe pain will last a few days, but that all pain will eventually end.

THE STAFF'S PAIN WORK

The pain tasks of the staff include assessment, prevention, minimization, and relief. The approaches to these pain tasks may be physiological, pharmacological, or psychological. The tasks are an integral part of the overall work done to accomplish a successful surgical outcome. The division of labor involved is the usual one in medical organizations. The surgeon and the anesthesiologist determine the preoperative drugs, treatments, and anesthesia for a successful and painless surgery. The surgeon prescribes the drugs and treatments appropriate for relieving postsurgical pain and discomfort. The professional nurses administer the drugs and treatments and assess, observe, record, and communicate the patient's pains and responses to the various pain-relieving approaches. When the approaches do not control the pains, or when new pains and discomforts develop, the nurses consult personnel such as head nurse, medical house staff, or surgeon, for appropriate action. Auxiliary nursing personnel are accountable to the professional nurses, to whom they report the patient's pain and responses to the pain-relieving approaches.

Preoperatively, the staff attempts to minimize the degree of anticipated postsurgical pain by relieving the patient's apprehension about the impending surgery and pain. This is accomplished by talking with the patient about pain tolerance and anxieties concerning the surgery. The necessary preoperative procedures are explained, as are the surgical course, the accompanying pains, and the measures available for relief. The staff explains painful but necessary procedures which require patient cooperation and tolerance in order to avoid complications. In nursing vernacular this stream of information is called "preoperative patient teaching." Its purposes are not only to relieve patient apprehension and thereby reduce pain perception[7-8] but also to assure a cooperative patient for a successful surgery.

For the first 24 to 72 postoperative hours, the staff is concerned with returning the patient to physiological equilibrium after the effects of anesthesia and surgical trauma. Staff members monitor vital signs, maintain fluid and electrolyte balance, prevent complications, and do other treatments specific to the surgery. Together, the treatments require a multitude of tasks, some involving no pain (taking blood pressure), others giving some discomfort (intravenous infusions, irrigations, or dressing changes). Circulatory, respiratory, and other complications associated with bodily immobilization must be minimized at the cost of "patient-induced pain" caused by deep breathing, moving around in bed, and early ambulation. Achieving patient cooperation is vital.

Incisional pain will probably be high for the first 24 to 72 hours postoperatively, but it depends upon the type of surgery and an individual's pain tolerance. This pain is minimized by narcotics given at three- to four-hour intervals, as required. The nurses' tasks include assessing the pain and giving the drugs at appropriate intervals. When the dosage or frequency of administration of drugs does not "hold" the pain, then the surgeon or house staff is notified about changing the drug order. The pacing of drugs must be sufficient to control the worst pains, but it must not cause sleepiness or drowsiness when cooperation with treatment is necessary. Antinausea drugs are administered if needed. Appropriate drugs are also available for "gas pains." Other drugs, such as antispasmodics, are used with certain types of surgical courses.

There are many additional pain-minimization tasks such as splinting the incision when the patient coughs, vomits, or changes body position. A variety of discomforts can be anticipated: dry mouth, headache, urinary and bowel retention, irritations from tubes placed in various body orifices, sore throat from an endotracheal tube used for the anesthetic. For each of these discomforts there are appropriate discomfort-minimization measures. Reassuring and encouraging the patient are, of course, related pain-minimization tasks, as is relieving of the family's apprehensions. There is much in medical and nursing literature about medical, nursing, and psychosocial approaches for the relief of surgical pain and discomfort.

Usually by the third or fourth postoperative day, the patient is expected to be "over the hump" and is encouraged to be more physically active, take foods by mouth, and be more self-sufficient. As pain decreases, less potent drugs are used.

PATIENT PAIN TASKS

When the patient accepts the decision to have surgery, an implicit contract is made with the staff. The patient must, first of all, trust the physician's judgment that surgery is necessary; the physician is responsible for as successful a surgery as possible and as comfortable a hospital stay as possible. The patient is to cooperate with the physician and other health personnel for this common goal. From the perspective of the staff, two of the patient's pain tasks are to apprise the personnel of existing pain and to give appropriate information (where, when, and the character of the pain) as requested. Using this information the staff assesses the pain and takes appropriate action. The patient also must keep pain expression within reasonable limits by avoiding prolonged loud crying and moaning which might disturb other patients. One of the patient's major tasks is to cooperate with and endure painful but necessary procedures, such as insertion of needles. Noncooperation can unnerve the staff members and affect their technical performance.

WARD WORK AND PAIN ACCOUNTABILITY

Considering, then, the properties of routine, low-risk surgical trajectories (predictable, unambiguous, short duration, and finite) and the specificity of approaches to pain prevention, minimization, and relief, we can assume that much of pain management is nonproblematic—as perceived by the staff. We can also assume that when the surgical trajectory is routine, there are well-developed, well-organized approaches for managing pain. There is a discrepancy, however, between what is possible and what is neglected in effective pain relief. This discrepancy can be understood only when viewed from the combined impact of (1) the work demands of the clinical setting, (2) the institutional accountability surrounding pain management, and (3) the complexity of patient–staff and staff–staff pain interactions.

Surgical units are usually very busy places, with innumerable and complex tasks requiring much skill, frequently involving a considerable use of machinery. Compared to medical units there is a constant flow of new patients, and the rate of patient turnover is quite rapid. There is a mixture of routine and complex problematic cases which require more or less of the staff's attention. When emergencies occur or when there is a shortage of staff or when there are several critically ill or problematic surgical cases, attention is naturally focused on the critical or problematic patients at the expense of the routine, low-risk surgical patients who are recovering on schedule.

The neglect of the latter is due in part to competing tasks and time and staff shortages, but also to the lack of institutional accountability for some important aspects of pain work. Take, for example, the patient's induction into the hospital. Considerable staff accountability is demanded on matters related to medical tasks associated with the preparation for surgery, but the same accountability is not demanded for psychosocial considerations. If a nurse were to neglect a preoperative medical procedure, there would be repercussions from superiors; there would be no repercussions if the nurse neglected to exchange information with or to prepare the patient psychologically for the operation. Related to this neglect in many hospitals is the phenomenon of elective and nonemergency surgical admissions occurring between noon and 4:00 P. M. The nursing staff is caught up in attending to preoperative tasks for large numbers of new surgical patients. These tasks involve not only carrying out procedures but also coordinating the work of such departments as laboratory, x-ray, and surgery.

When we asked nurses what kinds of preliminary information were routinely given to patients about surgery and pain, the answer invariably was, "It depends. . . ." It depended, in fact, largely upon the amount of competing ward work and the number of patients admitted to the unit. Nurses who were more psychosocially oriented complained to the researchers about having so much work they had little time to interact preoperatively with the patients.

The consequences of work pressures and the high priority accorded medical and procedural matters relegated informational exchange and the psychological preparation of patients to a catch-as-catch-can basis, determined by individual inclinations and the pain-management philosophies of the nurses or the competing work priorities on the ward. Yet the nurses all recognized that the relief of a patient's preoperative apprehension was important. Most of them also assumed that because doctors and nurses are professionally trained, each would attend to the psychological needs of the patient.[9] The nurses assumed that the surgeon would handle the matter with the patient; the evening nurses assumed that the day-shift personnel, who admitted the patient, would take care of the matter. The evening shift also assumed that the time when a patient is groggy from preoperative sleep medication is hardly the proper time for extensive patient–staff interaction.

RELIEF VERSUS MINIMIZATION: RELIANCE ON DRUGS

Not only did we find a lack of psychosocial accountability in pain relief but also a lack of pain minimization through nursing-comfort measures. Paradoxically, this dual neglect is due partly to the very properties of routine, low-risk surgery. Because the causes of pain are unambiguous and of short duration, there is high reliance on manipulating either the frequency or the dosage of drugs in order to relieve pain. After all, the pain is anticipated and specific drugs can be ordered for pain relief.

Thus, when patients complain of pain, the nurse's immediate response is to check when last a shot was given and whether the drug can be administered again within the limits of prescribed frequency. The reliance on drugs for relief is also due to the fact that patients, like nurses, tend to see drugs as the only solution to pain relief.[10, 11] Consequently, patients tend to initiate pain interactions by saying, "I need a pain shot." This reinforces the nurse's stereotypical responses: "Let me check the last time you had a shot;" "It isn't time for your shot yet;" "You just had a shot an hour ago." These responses also reinforce a patient's perception of drugs as the major means of relief. When asked their reactions to the nurses' stock answers, patients replied: "It made me angry;" "I felt devastated;" "It made me feel stupid;" "I felt the nurses weren't very sympathetic;" "I knew I had to stand some pain, but not this much."

The anticipated short duration of the surgical pain also encourages reliance on drugs. Anxiety or no anxiety, when there is no danger of complications or problems of drug dependency, such as those that might arise with an extended trajectory, the severe pain will last only two to four days at the most. Adding a tranquilizer or increasing the dosage or frequency of medication will control the pain. Even if a given patient is overly expressive about pain, it lasts for a few days and does not ordinarily upset the ward's sentimental order.

Nurses have other measures available to minimize pain and give comfort, such as splinting an incision when the patient has coughed or turned, giving a back rub, positioning, or pacing the drug to minimize the pain in ambulation. But these are volunteered rather than mandated, due to the great emphasis on drugs as the relief measure.[12] The exceptions that we observed were in situations such as involved cardiac or respiratory surgery, when coughing was

absolutely essential to avoid complications and when the surgery itself caused much coughing with pain. Here the main minimization
measures were "ordered."

Although the patients we queried were critical of both the staff's
management of pain and care in general, they were not likely to express disgruntlement or to voice criticism directly to the staff. Several
factors contributed to the lack of overt critical expression on the part
of patients. Generally knowing that severe pain would be short-lived,
the patients were concerned with getting past the acute phase of surgery and back on their feet to resume their former social roles and
were, therefore, willing to endure the pain. They were also concerned about staff reprisal should they voice their criticism. Enduring
pain and discomfort was also related to their comparisons of themselves with others who were more critically or seriously ill; they
considered themselves more fortunate. The relative absence of overt
fussing and complaining by patients tended to encourage the staff's
assumption that their management of pain was adequate.

VARIABLE PAIN PHILOSOPHIES: PROBLEMATIC ASPECTS

What may be routine and nonproblematic to the staff because a patient does not complain may be very problematic for the patient.
Patients know they must cooperate in the recovery process, but *how*
they are to behave is not made explicit by the staff. This is due, in
part, to the routine nature of certain surgeries which fosters a taken-
for-granted attitude, so that the who, what, when, and how of patient–staff informational exchange and interaction are not considered
essential. This results in each staff member interacting with the patient in terms of his or her own philosophies about pain. These
philosophies may vary widely on issues like threshold assessment,
pain legitimation, giving of information, kind of control administered to the patient, pain trajectory, and limits of endurance.

The staff usually assumes that drugs can control surgical pain,
yet the effectiveness of drug control calls for a complex set of staff–
staff and patient–staff interactions. The patient must know the appropriate times and ways to request pain relief, the amount of pain he
or she is expected to endure, the rules governing drug administration, etc. Unless the patient has had previous experience in hospitals
or has been given explicit cues by the staff, drug transactions can become quite problematic.

The varied philosophies of pain greatly influence transactions
involving drugs. Wide variations were noted in the decisional pre-
rogatives of doctors and nurses regarding drug-related tasks. Some

nurses thought that giving information to patients about pain medication was solely the responsibility of the surgeon; others thought it
was a shared responsibility. Variations were noted concerning how
much information should be shared with the patient about anticipated pain and about pain drugs, and who should give this
information. When a patient asked about pain drugs, some nurses
would respond, "You'll have to ask the doctor." Others freely gave
information about the drug, its dosage, and frequency of
prescription.

A nurse who believes that patients should be told about anticipated pain may have difficulties with a physician who believes that
informing only increases the patient's "anticipatory pain." Variations
were noted on the degree to which nurses adhered to the prescribed
frequency of dispensing drugs. Variations were also noted on how
much pain the patient had to endure before a nurse would consult a
physician for changes of a drug order. And physicians varied in the
discretionary latitude they allowed nurses in dispensing drugs. For
example, a drug order might be specific—"50 mg of Demerol every 3
hours"—or allow more latitude—"50–75 mg of Demerol every 3–4
hours." Given this latitude, however, some nurses consistently gave
the lower dosage while others gave the higher dosage. Some lowered
the dosage earlier than did others. The degree of discretion allowed
by the physicians, and the acceptance of responsibility by the nurses,
were related partly to their degree of consciousness of legal consequences and restrictions.

The consequences of varied philosophies such as these can strain
patient–staff and staff–staff interactions. For example, a nurse tells a
patient to wait for a pain shot. Immediately afterwards, the surgeon
visits the patient who complains of pain. The surgeon asks the nurse
when the patient last had a shot. The surgeon then decides the patient can have a shot and orders the nurse to give it immediately.
The physician thinks the nurse has shown poor judgment. The nurse
feels betrayed; her reasons haven't been taken into account. After all,
she sees the patient for eight hours a day while the surgeon is in
only a couple of minutes a day. The patient begins to think the nurse
is neither trustworthy nor sympathetic.

There are also staff variations on the amount of control patients
are allowed to have, the willingness to act on patients' suggestions,
and the degree of adherence to bureaucratic rules. In one instance, a
patient was confounded by a nurse who rigidly adhered to the rules
and could not tolerate any suggestions. The patient explained that
the ordered drug was too strong and was causing sleepiness which
interfered with the coughing up of mucus—something the doctor had

said was important. The patient requested the dosage be decreased. The nurse insisted the dosage could not be altered. Since the doctor was not available, the patient, knowing about possible respiratory complications accompanying surgery, balanced the options and decided not to take the dosage at all, but rather to endure the pain resulting from coughing up the mucus.

The staff may assume that a patient has been given adequate information about his or her responsibilities in the drug transaction, but in fact the information may be far from adequate. Take, for example, a surgeon's assurance to the patient that pain shots will be available for controlling postsurgical pain. The patient is then faced with the problem of whether to ask for pain relief or to wait for the nurse to exercise judgment. The surgeon may have said the drug would be available every three hours. If three hours have passed, should the patient ask for the next shot or wait for the nurse to act? One patient we observed suffered unnecessarily because he assumed the nurse would automatically deliver the drugs on schedule without his asking for pain relief. A related question is: How *much* pain is the patient expected to endure before requesting relief? Would it not be more efficient to tell the patient that pain drugs are available at intervals of three to four hours; that drugs will control the worst pain but some pains must be endured; that since patients vary in their pain tolerance he is to report his pains to the nurse and that together they will evaluate the pain and make the necessary adjustments in consultation with the physician?

Among the consequences of the many unshared, individual pain philosophies is a tendency for patients to become very confused and generally dissatisfied with their care, or to develop distrust of professionals. Here are some common statements made by patients:

I don't get it. One nurse says don't hold off asking for pain shots. Another says hold off.

Some nurses offer pain shots. Others give the shot only when I ask for it.

Some nurses are regular time nuts, giving the shots to the minute. Others are not so exacting.

When I complain of pain some nurses try to find out more about the pains. Others say, let me check the last time you had a shot.

Some nurses plan the drug so it won't be so painful to get up and walk around. Others just come in and command: "It's time for you to walk now."

In addition to variations among nurses, there are group variations among work shifts on the same ward. The latter depend upon
the pain-management philosophies and the degree of accountability
demanded by the charge nurse for the given shift, on the numbers of
staff assigned to the shift, and on the kinds of competing work demands. In one situation we found problems of pain management
stemming largely from two charge nurses who had opposing pain
philosophies. The day shift charge nurse was psychosocially
oriented, allowing the patients more control over their pain
management than the evening charge nurse. The patients were
caught in a conflict of opposing philosophies.

It is noteworthy that when patients complained to the researchers about the ways their pains were mismanaged, they
attributed many of the problems to personality defects in the ward
personnel, calling them unsympathetic, unkind, mean, and so on.
The patients were totally unaware that the personnel were acting on
the basis of their individual pain philosophies. Nurses criticized each
other on the same basis. We should add that the patients often had
their own pain philosophies, which they might or might not openly
express. Later, we will deal with this additional interactional and
consequential complexity.

THE ACCOUNTABILITY ISSUE

Although this chapter has focused primarily on surgical situations,
the same kind of nonaccountability (as defined earlier in this book) is
found in other clinical situations. Routine, everyday, taken-for-
granted situations often reflect glaring shortcomings of hospital organization. The acute-care model underlying that organization tends
to encourage little attention—even blindness—to the interactional aspects of pain management. Yet, to the patients those aspects are
among the most confusing and certainly the most important.

A major implication of our research is that a critical examination
of pain management in routine situations might provide an opportune starting point for improving psychosocial accountability. This
accountability is crucial, for without it the hospital and its personnel
are ill-equipped to cope with certain issues of reduced management,
let alone with pain in more complex surgical situations. Indeed, effective coping with routine situations may well prevent the
phenomenon of problem pain patients. (In Chapter 18 suggestions
will be made about how routine situations might become a starting
point for the improvement of accountability.) In the next chapter the

more complex trajectories will be discussed, with emphasis on the crucial need for accountability.

REFERENCES

1. Dodson, H. C., and Bennett, H. A. 1954. Relief of post-operative pain. *American Surgery* 20:405–412.

2. Gilden, J. 1968. Relief of post-operative pain. *Medical Clinics of North America* 52:81–89.

3. Keats, A. S. 1956. Post-operative pain: research and treatment. *Journal of Chronic Diseases* 4:72–83.

4. McBride, M. A. B. 1969. The additive to analgesic. *American Journal of Nursing* 69:674–676.

5. McCafferty, M., and Moss, F. 1967. Nursing intervention for bodily pain. *American Journal of Nursing* 67:1224–1227.

6. Moss, F. T. 1966. Effects of nursing interaction upon pain relief in patients. *Nursing Research* 15:303–306.

7. Bruegal, M. A. 1971. Relationship of preoperative anxiety to perception of post-operative pain. *Nursing Research* 20:26–31.

8. Healy, K. M. 1968. Does preoperative instruction make a difference? *American Journal of Nursing* 68:62–67.

9. Strauss, A. et al. 1964. The hospital and the negotiated order. In *The hospital in modern society*, ed. E. Freidson. New York: Free Glencoe Press.

10. McBride, M. A. 1967. "Pain" and effective nursing practice. In *ANA Clinical Sessions*. Paper presented in the ANA convention held in June 1966 in San Francisco. New York: Appleton-Century-Crofts, pp. 75–82.

11. Whiting, J. F. 1959. Patients' needs, nurses' needs, and healing process. *American Journal of Nursing* 59:661–665.

12. Schatzman, L. 1966. Volunteerism and professional practice in health professions. In *Sociological framework for patient care*, eds. J. Folta and E. Deck. New York: Wiley, pp. 145–155.

Complex Surgery,
Chronic Illness, and Pain

5

If organizational shortcomings result in staff inabilities to cope effectively with relatively routine surgical pain trajectories, one can
imagine what happens with more complex and problematic ones.
Increased longevity and the consequent increase in chronic illness
bring into our hospitals a growing percentage of surgical patients
who are middle-aged or elderly.[1] Their presence creates many
problems for the wards as they are currently organized, even when
nurses and physicians anticipate that a given surgical trajectory
will be problematic or difficult.

These patients and their surgeries are usually of a character
which complicates medical and nursing care. (1) The probability
is high that patients will have multiple disorders, often of a
chronic nature. (2) The surgeries frequently are done to correct
chronic conditions, or as palliative measures to control the rate
of bodily deterioration and to prolong life. Thus, as a disease
progresses, there may be a series of surgical operations and
treatments, and any given operation may be a "desperate" one.
(3) The patients may have had surgery for other conditions as
well as for the current illness, and so they may have already had
wide experience with illness, pain, and hospitalization. (4) The

71

surgeries may in fact be performed specifically in order to control pain. (5) Other disorders may complicate the surgical outcomes, or the surgeries themselves may be done to control the complications of drug technology used in treating other illnesses. (6) The operations may be very difficult and have a high probability of accompanying complications or the surgical trajectories may be unpredictable and uncharted, especially when the surgeries are of a pioneer or experimental nature. (7) Hospitalization is frequently an extended affair for these patients.

The presence of a number of middle-aged or elderly patients with multiple disorders, undergoing surgeries for chronic conditions or as palliative measures, increases the problematic aspect of pain management. Prevailing conditions in the ward situation further increase that problematic aspect. Those conditions include the following: (1) Pain management is closely intertwined with the patient's illness, pain, and social career, and these factors are often invisible or of secondary importance to the hospital staff. (2) The age of the patient, together with the multiple-illness conditions, increases the possibility of problematic and unpredictable surgical and pain courses with their attendant problems of balancing and juggling priorities—priorities which may differ not only among the personnel but between them and the patients. (3) The ward and hospital organization, and also the work focus, pose difficulties in coping with multiple-illness conditions. The interaction of these three preceding conditions greatly increases the problematic aspect of pain work and the consequent interactional problems for both the patient and the hospital staff.

MULTIPLE LINKED TRAJECTORIES

The middle-aged and older patients who come for surgery often have multiple illnesses, each with its characteristic trajectory. In chronic disorders, furthermore, the illness and its management (including pain management) are closely intertwined with the person's social trajectory. By social trajectory we mean life style, social identity, family and social relationships, and work (see Chapter 2). If pain is present in these illnesses, there has often been a long history of managing pain, and considerable experience with medical personnel and hospitals. Such pain experiences are varied and unique from patient to patient. Moreover, chronic disorders present themselves in a multitude of combinations, each with its characteristic pain pattern.

Thus, we can expect great variance in how a surgical patient will assess, minimize, prevent, express, and endure pain during a surgical course. Influential factors include: (1) the nature of the surgery as it affects life style and social identities, (2) the point at which the surgery occurs in both social and illness trajectories plus its effects on them, (3) the character of the pain which accompanies the surgical course, (4) past experiences with pain (i.e., pain biography), and (5) other existing disorders which might compromise the success of the surgery while the patient is in the hospital.

For the staff to "properly" assess, prevent, minimize, and relieve pain requires an awareness of a patient's medical and social trajectories, and their relationship to the prevailing approaches in pain management. Such information is crucial for the management of pain. Personnel recognize the importance of that information, but their recognition is often more philosophical than operational. Indeed, it is safe to say that patients' psychosocial and pain histories are usually deemed unimportant. This is not surprising considering ward organization, the staff's work focus, and the competing priorities associated with the surgery itself.

KEEPING THE PATIENT ON COURSE

Understandably, the main work focus of the staff is directed toward successfully carrying patients through the surgical trajectories. The focus tends, also, to be on the surgical conditions for which the patients are hospitalized. Certainly, the existence of the patients' *other* illnesses are known, but that does not necessarily mean that they are taken into account and acted upon. Whether they are or not is related to how these illnesses impinge on or compromise the surgical trajectories.

The staff is particularly concerned with keeping the older patient with multiple disorders on the proper surgical course, without complications. The possibility—and even probability—that such a patient may go off the scheduled course is ever present and recognized. Staff members are constantly vigilant, especially when a patient has other conditions—such as cardiovascular, pulmonary, or endocrine disorders—which may endanger the surgical outcome. This aspect of staff work becomes increasingly important with current medical technology, which makes surgeries possible on patients who a decade ago would have been considered high-risk cases. When a ward has a number of these patients, energy and time are taken up with tasks that contribute to keeping each patient on an appropriate surgical timetable. Controlling the surgical trajectory can be an extremely complex undertaking as in a case where a patient having surgery for cancer of the ovaries also has asthma, diabetes, and hypertension.

As for pain management, the staff's customary focus on routine surgery coincides with its focus on the pain course that accompanies the surgery, hence staff members rely heavily on drugs and other treatments for pain prevention and relief. This is so partly because the surgical pain is relatively unambiguous and physiologically based. So marked is this focus that even when patients with a known and long history of pain such as chronic low-back pain, are admitted for surgery specifically for pain relief, there is generally a neglect of pain histories. Staff members get bits and pieces of the patient's psychosocial history, but often they do not share or assemble them, or they simply do not consider them salient to their pain work. Only when the pain cannot be managed by the usual routines (mostly through the juggling of drugs), and the patient creates problems in pain management, are efforts made to seek psychosocial information relevant to the pain.

Even with uncomplicated surgical conditions, however, a multitude of specialized personnel and services must be coordinated to keep patients on their surgical timetables. For complicated cases, the necessary amount of coordination increases drastically because of possible complications. The temporal ordering, priorities, and main work focus of these multiple services and personnel are likely to pose great difficulties with regard to pain management, especially for nursing personnel.[2] For example, painful or uncomfortable diagnostic procedures and treatments cannot be coordinated in accordance with the pacing of drugs which are designed to minimize or prevent pain —as with physical therapy or x-ray studies—because the ward personnel have limited jurisdiction over the temporal ordering of other services and personnel. Diagnostic testing or the carrying out of painful treatments by physicians tends to occur at times inconvenient for the ward staff. Even when nurses are cognizant of the alignment of drug pacing with treatment timing needed to minimize pain, they tend to disregard this because of work pressures. Moreover, the time and energy required for negotiating with many departments and personnel can be overwhelming.

THE BALANCING OF PRIORITIES

An important aspect of pain work is the balancing of priorities (see Chapter 16). Both the patient and the staff choose between or among alternative options, and these choices are based on what is believed to be more or less important. Problems arise when the patient and the staff are balancing different considerations. Not only does the staff confront many balancing problems in keeping the patient on a scheduled course, but the multiple conditions of chronic disease increase the likelihood that the patient and the staff members will have discrepant pain priorities. They may have different disease priorities as well.

In multiple-illness conditions, the patient suffers from surgical pain as well as the various pains from other illnesses and all these pains are likely to peak at different times during the current surgical episode. Those pains may even be intensified by the surgical experience. A common example is arthritic pain, intensified both by the patient's being bedridden and because methods of controlling pain used at home are not possible in the hospital. Put another way, there is primary pain associated with the surgery itself, along with the possibility of secondary or tertiary pain from other disorders. Over a given hospital period, what might have been primary (concerning pain or illness) may shift and become secondary for the patient, but not for the staff.

Interactional difficulties between staff and patient arise if staff members are not alert to the patient's altering hierarchy of pain concerns or if they have pain hierarchies which differ from the patient's. Often, staff members will focus on the surgical pain course and be alert to those pains and discomforts which might indicate probable complications, but tend to neglect the pains from other disorders if they are not complicating the primary surgical trajectory. Not infrequently, several days of complaining by the patient are necessary before definitive action is taken by the personnel. Such pains and discomforts (for example, painful joints), while not signalling life-threatening disorders, nevertheless can result in full-blown episodes of normally more manageable chronicity. When this happens, the patient's trust in the personnel consequently decreases, and the patient may accuse the staff of negligence. One woman who had suffered through acute pain from surgery for lung cancer later complained of extreme discomfort from hemorrhoids. After five days of complaining without action from the staff, she sent her husband to buy Preparation H, a remedy she had used at home. Here was a situation, then, involving a pain-message failure because of the staff's other concerns. Such failures may involve not only patient and staff but also staff and staff, because each person can have competing hierarchies of concern. A common source for such failures of communication is the ward's constant flow of new surgical arrivals; this results in such expenditure of staff energy and time that patients who seem to be progressing on schedule are somewhat neglected.

DISRUPTED SURGICAL TRAJECTORIES

The staff is ever vigilant to keep chronically ill patients on course without complications. Compared to relatively healthy patients, the chronically ill must suffer more inflicted pains from diagnostic and treatment procedures, such as frequent blood withdrawals, intravenous infusions, and inhalation therapy. Also, larger numbers (and classes) of hospital personnel (each with his or her own time schedule) are involved so that the nurse's work is often interrupted, and her control of drug pacing can easily be lost. If the patient perceives inflicted pains as legitimate in the recovery process, then he or she will try to endure them and keep expression of pain within reasonable limits. Thus someone who may have exhibited much anxiety prior to surgery, and was anticipated by the staff as likely to create pain-assessment problems, may actually be quite manageable providing surgical recovery is on schedule.

The problematic aspect of pain management increases, however, when the patient goes off the scheduled course because of surgical complications, or because of an acute flare-up from other disorders. Efforts to control and reverse such complications vary widely in accordance with their life-threatening potentials, residual disability, reversibility, and medical complexity. There are variabilities in the character of the pains and discomforts which accompany complications and also in the character, frequency, and duration of inflicted treatments and diagnostic pains, which the patient must endure so that an illness can be controlled and reversed. Each of these variables results in altered priorities, with considerations that patient and staff must take into account in their balancing processes. As complications arise the probability increases that discrepancies will appear between the patient and the staff. Patients are more apt to weigh and balance psychosocial considerations while the staff is busily weighing medical considerations.

When a complication is accompanied by minimal pain, when reversal can be accomplished with little discomfort, or when the outcome of medical treatment is fairly predictable, the patient cooperates and creates minimal problems pertaining to pain or interaction. There may be some anxiety, but a reassuring word from the staff and the prescribing of a tranquilizer can usually control this. However, pain work becomes very complex when reversal and control of the complication involves pain accompanying frequent treatment, when the outcome is unpredictable or the reversal is not on schedule, or when the outcome involves leaving the patient with residual disability.

The complexity of such pain work arises because multiple considerations necessarily are being juggled and balanced in relation to the work. Psychosocial problems must be dealt with because they affect pain and recovery, as well as the staff's ongoing work. A patient's depression and anxiety about his or her condition and future commonly affects perception of pain, making it seem greater than it actually is. Assessment problems emerge because of the increase in "psychological overlay." Patients may begin to doubt the necessity for their surgeries and the wisdom of the staff. A previously cooperative patient may become uncooperative and demanding.

The staff is caught in a major dilemma: simultaneous and complex medical and psychosocial problems demand attention. Not infrequently a reversal of complications requires numerous treatments and monitoring that monopolize patient–staff interactions, leaving little time available for attending to the patient's psychosocial requirements. Pain interactions then typically occur only when someone is complaining about pain, which encourages the staff to develop a narrow and biased picture of both the patient and the pain.

Because of the aforementioned factors and the staff's predominantly medical perspective, the prevalent pain and anxiety-relieving approaches tend to be medical: the juggling of analgesics, tranquilizers, antidepressants, and the like. But an individual's depression and anxiety may become more and more serious when treatment fails to bring about the expected reversal and in turn creates other medical-balance problems. Antibiotics used for controlling infection can cause a sore mouth and severe diarrhea plus subsequent problems of maintaining adequate hydration and nutrition. Still more treatments are required and the patient becomes increasingly hard-pressed to maintain equanimity.

When the reversal is perceived as taking an inordinately long time and is accompanied by frequent albeit necessary therapeutic pain, then older persons with severe chronic disorders, who have suffered years of discomfort and pain, are likely to weigh enduring the pain against living only a bit longer. Depending on the person's condition and probable outcome in relation to his social trajectory, "death work" by the staff may be of equal or greater importance than their pain work or curative work. Even when staff members are troubled about the wisdom of continuing their efforts to reverse the illness, treatments are often continued because most wards are organized around a determination to save lives.

The weighing and balancing of life versus death, and the enduring of pain in a life decreasing in quality, are frequently problems with older surgical patients who have severe chronic disorders.

To further complicate matters, such "precarious" patients are often transferred to intensive care units which emphasize even more than surgical wards the saving of lives "no matter what." The "what" is very frequently further reduced attention to psychosocial considerations.

CONSEQUENCES OF EXTENDED HOSPITALIZATION

Other pain and interactional problems can arise as a result of hospitalization being extended because of complications. (This is not to say, however, that when a patient is well liked, there cannot be a good, long-range working relationship with the staff for the management of pain.) A common problem emerging from weeks of hospitalization is the staff's concern over drug addiction, especially when the pain accompanying the complications is handled through extended use of narcotics. Like Mrs. Abel, the patient often begins to demand pain drugs on schedule and becomes a clock watcher. A struggle for control of drugs ensues. The patient is faced with a pain-legitimation problem and the staff with an assessment problem. Arguments occur within the staff itself not only about assessment of pain, but also about the timing and the timeliness of weaning the patient from narcotics. Not infrequently, nurses accuse physicians of not being attentive to the problem of addiction.

Even in situations where the staff and the patient mutually agree that addiction is a problem, weaning might not be so easily accomplished because of the patient's anxiety and because of the temporal hitches deriving from the organizational structure of the hospital. The patient may be writhing in pain, but the nurses are unable to reach the doctor to obtain a change of drug order because he or she is "tied up" in the operating room. If weaning begins on weekends, immense problems can occur because nurse staffing tends to be low and physicians are not readily available. In one observed case, for instance, the nurses were upset when someone with a complex illness became dangerously addicted to narcotics while numerous doctors continued to write contradictory orders for pain drugs. Each physician was reacting in accordance with his or her own private pain philosophy and hierarchy of concerns. Only after weeks of numerous informal, *ad hoc* discussions among individual nurses and physicians, while the general "mess" continually increased, was a meeting of the total staff called to discuss the issues.

With extended stay a patient also becomes familiar with the staff, the ward routines, and the effects of the pain drugs and so attempts to prevent and minimize pains by making demands or negotiating with the personnel. These demands may disrupt the ward routines and the work schedule of the nurses, who, of course, must care for many other patients. More moderate requests may involve implicit trade-offs of cooperation with the staff in its work.

A patient's familiarity with the staff may also result in rating of the staff members in terms of their pain-inflicting potential. Interactional difficulties can arise because the patient refuses to have a specific staff member do a painful treatment or makes invidious comparisons, saying that one nurse doesn't hurt as much as another or doesn't make the wait as long for the painkiller. In an effort to minimize the treatment pain, the patient may make suggestions about how to do the procedure, which can irritate and even enrage staff members who may interpret such remarks as questioning their competence.

Concurrently, what we term a "patient reputation" emerges among the staff. Often individuals are stereotyped as "manipulative," "uncooperative," "infantile," or "paranoid." These negative definitions profoundly affect the patient–staff interaction, especially when new psychosocial information about the patient further justifies the stereotypes. And the patient faces more problems of legitimating pain and getting staff cooperation in the control of pain. Anyone who comes to the ward with or develops a negative reputation has a most difficult time in altering this image. An individual physician, nurse, or aide who disagrees with the prevailing image is unlikely to be able to change the views of the rest of the staff.

STAFF COMPOSURE AND PAIN MANAGEMENT

When a patient is not recovering on schedule, the staff members' composure can become upset.[3] The continued deterioration of a patient's condition may make it difficult for them to cope with their own feelings. Touchy and difficult interactional situations arise when a patient presses for definite answers, not knowing (as the staff does) that the outcome is highly unpredictable or that there may be severe residual disabilities. The staff's physical or interactional avoidance of such a patient results in a failure to gather psychosocial information, such as anxiety level, relevant not only to general care but to pain management. Meanwhile, pain may be used as a mechanism to gain staff attention, which is only likely to lead to further staff withdrawal.

Another common surgical situation where the personnel's composure is upset involves a surgery some perceive as unnecessary—one that leaves the patient with a disfigurement that will severely af-

fect the quality of his or her life. Concerned with their own feelings
of helplessness and discomfiture with such a patient, staff members
will often rotate their assignments, spreading the misery as evenly as
possible.[4] In such a case the staff is holding its composure and emotional equilibrium higher in priority than its care of the patient.

SITUATIONS OF MAXIMIZED PROBLEMATIC PAIN

There are at least two different surgical situations which maximize
the problematic aspects of pain management, (1) experimental or
pioneer surgeries and (2) surgeries done to alleviate chronic pain. In
experimental surgery, the problematic aspects of pain management
increase because the outcome of surgery itself, the surgical course,
and the pain course all tend to be highly unpredictable. Problems involving interaction and composure affect all personnel. The medical
staff is concerned with mapping out the surgical course and the technical details of medical management. The nursing staff is learning the
complex medical details. At the same time, the patient's anxiety is
high because of the pioneer nature of the surgery; it is often a final,
desperate option. In pioneer surgery, pain-management problems
stem primarily from the fact that medical matters are deemed of far
higher priority than pain, whether organic or psychosocial in origin.
The balancing and juggling of many medical considerations is
complex.

The second type of surgery, that which aims to alleviate chronic
or intractable pain, also almost invariably creates problems of pain
management. Many conditions which complicate the management
prevail. The patient has had a long history of pain and many disappointments with a variety of pain-relief approaches, including
other operations. Such a patient may also have had difficulty legitimating pain to medical and nursing personnel—even to family or
friends. Usually most if not all of this history is invisible to the staff.
The patient anticipates the current surgery with additional anxiety
because of previous disappointments. In many instances, this surgery is the last option available, and its outcome is not only
unpredictable but may pose still other problems. Anxiety also heightens the patient's perception of postoperative pain.

When surgery for chronic pain is also experimental, these problems are even more intensified. This kind of patient is often
dependent on pain drugs prior to surgery; hence there is a three-way
tension—the patient's anxiety, the staff members' assessment of pain,
and their juggling of medications.

Based on their respective previous experiences, both the patient and the staff usually anticipate problems with each other, starting virtually at the time of the patient's admission. Complaints from nurses in anticipation of pain-management problems is not unusual when they are told of a certain type of surgical admission. This mutual, negative, and anticipated response often results in a good deal of distrust and antagonism, and often in open warfare for the control of pain. The staff's juggling and balancing of its pain work, along with keeping the patient on a correct surgical course, can then become most difficult problems.

ACCOUNTABILITY AND TECHNOLOGY

Although this chapter has focused primarily on surgical pain management, our analysis is applicable to nonsurgical wards wherever there are patients with chronic disorders. The acute-illness orientation of the medical and nursing staffs and the multitude of tasks and procedures necessary to maintain these patients on their recovery courses prevent the personnel from taking into account the patient's multiple biographies (illness, pain and social) as each affects pain during the hospitalization. This omission results from the lack of organizational accountability in those aspects of care.

On the current hospital scene the coordination of a multitude of medical specialists with specialized hospital services and personnel is required in order to give proper care. This coordination is a major task in itself, and much has been written about the consequent fragmentation of care and its ill effects for the patients.[5-8] In addition, new technologies are rapidly being introduced without sufficient anticipation of their organizational consequences. The new technologies can be adapted to old organizational forms, but they create *new* kinds of tasks, *new* kinds of professional–professional relationships, and *new* staff–patient relationships.[9, 10] If the old forms of organization are inadequate in management of even routine, nonproblematic pain, then they are quite clearly—as we have just seen—unable to cope with more complex problematic illness situations where new technology tends to be used.

REFERENCES

1. Moien, M. 1975. *Inpatient utilization of short-stay hospitals by diagnosis, U. S. 1972.* Department of Health, Education and Welfare, Series 13, no. 20, Public Health Service. Rockville, Md.: National Center for Health Statistics, pp. 1–8.

2. Mauksch, H. O. 1957. Nursing dilemmas in the organization of patient care. *Nursing Outlook* 5:31–33.

3. Glaser, B., and Strauss, A. 1965. *Awareness of dying*. Chicago: Aldine, pp. 226–256.

4. Menzies, I. E. P. 1960. A case study in the functioning of social system as a defense against anxiety. *Human Relations* 13:95–121.

5. Shep, C. G., and Bachar, 1964. Changing pattern of practice— nursing and medical. *North Carolina Medical Journal* 25:435–438.

6. Duff, R. S., and Hollingshead, A. B. 1968. *Sickness and society*. New York: Harper and Row.

7. Mechanics, D. 1967. Human problems and organization of health care. *Annals Academy of Political and Social Science* 399:1–11.

8. Freidson, E. 1967. Review essay: health factories, the new industrial sociology. *Social Problems* 14:493–500.

9. Hays, D., and Oken, D. 1972. The psychological stress of intensive care nursing. *Psychosomatic Medicine* 34:109–118.

10. Edelstein, R. 1966. Automation: its effect on the nurse. *American Journal of Nursing* 66:2194–2198.

Part 3

Inflicted Pain:
Necessary and Unnecessary

Inflicted Pain:
Cooperation, Contest,
and Control

6

Health personnel usually understand the management of pain to mean the relief of ongoing pain and the prevention of new pain. A more implicit understanding requires patients to exert reasonable control over excessive expression of their suffering and to endure whatever pain cannot be relieved. One of the often unrecognized ironies attending the work of health personnel is that they who minister to pain also may inflict pain. Indeed, this may be a fairly inevitable part of their jobs. A considerable proportion of work with and around patients involves the inflicting of pain. It is associated, of course, with a host of essential tasks: with diagnosis, surgery, various therapies, regimens, and even with the mechanics of giving adequate nursing care. Most of such induced pain is necessary although some of it surely is not.

Part 3 will address this phenomenon. Some events discussed here will be relatively uncomplicated and easy to understand; others will not. Together, the next two chapters should present a vivid idea of the political nature of the main issues attending inflicted pain. In the present chapter, central questions pertaining to inflicted pain will be discussed. In the next, we will describe and analyze pain work on an intensive burn unit where an immense amount of inflicted but necessary pain must be endured by patients.

Among the critical issues that pertain to inflicted pain are: the grounds for its legitimation; an implicit staff–patient contract and the division of labor for carrying it out; the tactics and countertactics utilized by personnel and patients; the balancing of infliction of pain against other considerations; and the question of how much and what kinds of pain expression are expected and acceptable. Perhaps the central issue is the question of control—who, how, and why— over the entire infliction and response process.

These are critical issues because until both health personnel and patients come to understand the complexity and interrelationship of these issues, there will be a continuance of the current situation, which frequently involves both too much unnecessarily inflicted pain and, more importantly, the cycles of resentment and distrust generated by even quite necessary pain.

WORK AND LEGITIMATION

The first step in comprehending this complex issue is to realize that in hospitals and clinics (doctors' offices also), the primary work may not involve dealing with any pain whatever, but when it does, the inflicting or relieving of pain is almost invariably secondary to the primary diagnostic, therapeutic, rehabilitative, or comfort-care work of the staff. It is the *work* which is of central importance to the staff. The patient may be more interested in the relief of pain, or in the prevention or minimizing of now-to-be-inflicted pain, but he or she generally shares the staff's definition of the medical goal as primary. The patient, like the staff, wishes the disease properly diagnosed, treated, cured if possible, and the symptoms alleviated.

It is understood then by both parties that to accomplish primary tasks some infliction of pain may be necessary. Implicit in the situation is that the pain should be kept as minimal as possible. It is also implicit that, unless special circumstances intervene, the potential sufferer should be warned and told of its necessity. Said another way, the actual production of pain is viewed as legitimate because it is either a by-product of medical/nursing tasks or even, as in diagnostic work, an important means toward attaining the desired medical end.

CONTRACT AND COOPERATION

There is an *implicit contract* between the person who inflicts the pain and the person who receives it. Sometimes the contract includes explicit promises about relief of the pain "afterwards," as well as specific information about the anticipated degree and duration of the pain. Unless coercion is used, this contract implies that the patient's cooperation is needed in order to accomplish the primary activity, which only incidentally results in the infliction of pain.

Cooperation is needed in all of the various kinds of pain work. In tasks which involve production of pain, the patient may have to cooperate very actively as when, in the days immediately after a cardiac operation, he must breathe deeply despite the pain caused by such activity. Or a patient may be asked to report the degree of pain, so that personnel can take effective steps to minimize or temporarily relieve it while still accomplishing their primary work task. Or, knowing his own body better than the personnel, the patient may have to make a task easier, quicker (and not incidentally less productive of pain) by directing the actual pain-inflicting procedure. Less obviously, the patient may not be required to participate in the primary task but must at least control excessive expression of pain which could disturb the staff in its work.

The necessary level of cooperation, however, is really much more subtle. It involves a trade-off—usually, though not always, unspoken —between the staff and the patient. The personnel can promise to keep at a minimum the intensity and duration of pain and actually to prevent the production of unnecessary pain. In turn, the patient is obligated to perform competently two other separate but related types of pain work. First, the patient must endure the inflicted pain as much and as long as possible. Second, the expression of pain must remain within proper bounds; the patient must be able to groan without moving, for example. These obligations are as real as the reciprocal ones of the staff members. If the staff fails to perform competently, the patient can complain of incompetence or negligence, but if he has failed in his part of the bargain, he runs a range of risks from scolding to severe reprisal, such as the staff's thereafter pulling away because, in their common parlance, he is downright uncooperative, even an unpleasant or disturbing presence.

SOME RELEVANT VARIABLES

Faced with a multitude of events related to the infliction of pain, we will find it useful to think first about some relevant variables. These will help us to understand the relationships among those events. There are four sets of significant variables.

First are *the properties of the inflicted pain*. These include its predictability, intensity, duration, whether it is one-shot or repeated, and, if repeated, the frequency of infliction. Clearly it is easier, other things being equal, to persuade someone to undergo induced pain if it can be promised that "it won't hurt much" or "it won't last long," or "only this once." Also, there may be multiple pain inflictions (biopsy plus a painful x-raying) or multiple and simultaneous inflictions of pain (three nurses debriding a burn patient).

Second are *the properties of the work* (diagnostic, therapeutic) during which pain infliction occurs. These properties include the degree of difficulty of the work, how long it takes to complete, how many persons are involved in its accomplishment, whether it is one-shot or repeated, and how often and how urgently it needs to be done (for example, a genuine emergency which precludes minimizing the extreme infliction of pain through prior medication).

Third are *the properties of the staff and the patient*—the "workers on" and the "worked on." Among the most important staff properties are their degrees of skill with the pain-inflicting tasks and their experience with particular kinds of patients. (A physical therapist remarked that in school, students practice procedures on each other and feel fine, but they don't realize such practice is different from working with a patient who has an incision and is already in pain.) There are also more variable characteristics, such as how fresh or how tired staff members are when doing the tasks, and their degree of interest (bored, challenged) in the work itself or in the patient (concerned, indifferent, hostile). Similar variables pertain to the patient. How much previous experience has there been with undergoing the particular procedures? How many different persons have done the tasks "on" the patient? What do the tasks and the expected pain mean to the patient (frightening, shameful, absolutely necessary for saving life)? And there are more variable characteristics, such as how tired or sick the patient feels. Additionally there is the important matter of whether there is ongoing pain to which inflicted pain will be added. What are *its* properties?

Fourth, are *a number of organizational (ward, clinic) properties* which can significantly affect interactions involving pain infliction. They relate directly to whether the staff is in a rush, feels overworked, and so on. These organizational properties include the following: the size and rate of turnover of the staff and patient populations; the relative proportions of different types of personnel; whether the staff is thoroughly familiar with the tasks which incidentally induce pain or whether these are relatively new tasks (because of new technologies or new types of patients). Important organizational properties also include those which pertain to working and sentimental relationships among the staff itself, based on experiences they have had with each other, and the length of time they have worked together, plus other relevancies of professional and personal biographies.

One can imagine what different constellations of the preceding variables might mean by comparing, even sketchily, pain infliction by nurses on a typical burn unit with that inflicted by technicians whose specialty is the drawing of blood. On a burn unit (as described in the next chapter), patients undergo exceedingly painful debridement by a team of nurses, and they suffer other treatment procedures done by only a single nurse more than once daily for a number of days or even months. Usually, the same staff nurses are involved throughout. Also, all patients on the ward are going through different stages of the same procedures. Everyone knows the painful procedures are necessary to insure some degree of recovery. The patients as a group socialize new patients, helping them to endure pain and control expressions of pain.

On the other hand, technicians who draw blood tend, during their daily work, to move from service to service. They do not meet the same patients repeatedly. A patient going through the procedure more than once is likely to encounter different technicians who possess varying degrees of skill.

TACTICS AND COUNTERTACTICS

The preceding variables, then, bear quite directly on the tactics which both staff and patients use to gain some measure of control over the work activities which entail pain infliction. The number of such tactics is great, and there is not much point in simply listing them. However, it is useful to think about how such tactics relate, on the one hand, to variables just mentioned, and on the other hand to such specific considerations as: (1) how the primary task and the pain inflictions are legitimated, (2) how the patient is alerted to the anticipated pain and its properties, (3) how the pain is minimized, (4) how pain endurance and pain expression are made to relate to noninterference with the primary work task. Said another way: the implicit (and sometimes explicit) contract between staff and patient involves them in tactics and countertactics. While sometimes the participants, especially the staff, become so habituated to the work that they scarcely think of their actions as tactics, tactics they nevertheless are.

The specific task of legitimating an anticipated and potentially painful procedure generally amounts to explaining its purpose and, if need be, arguing its necessity. The physician or other personnel may have to field sharp questions from the patient or the patient's family.

When the procedure is done repeatedly, and the patient has suffered much pain, the question will probably arise: "Must we do it again?" Alternatives may be sought. Some patients will, of course, simply refuse to cooperate. The staff member might become desperate or perhaps disgusted and may resort to a tactic like the one used by a surgeon with an adolescent in pain from probable dystonia who refused a painful diagnostic procedure: "Okay, Janet, if you're so goddamn smart, go back to Idaho."[1] Other tactics used by staff members include promises to be careful, to minimize the potential pain, and to relieve it as speedily as possible. Patients often attempt to elicit such promises when they are not made initially.

A patient not familiar with the properties of the upcoming pain should be *alerted* to it, and the conscientious staff member will essentially specify those properties, telling the anticipated intensity of pain, how long it will last, and when it will actually appear during the course of the proceedings. Wary or frightened patients may demand a great deal of such specific information.

When the action begins, the tactics and countertactics designed to *minimize* the pain tend to become more varied and complex. Aside from purely technical or experiential expertise, the inflicter may use certain interactional tactics. Physical therapists, for instance, tell a patient to help "set the pace," that is, if the pain peaks, the regimen can be slowed down or temporarily halted. Nurses debriding burn wounds will work rapidly, assuring the patient that the faster they go the sooner the inevitably painful procedure will be over. In some kinds of painful regimens or diagnostic procedures when the personnel are not on crowded schedules, they can delegate responsibility to the patient: "Tell me if it hurts, and I will stop for a while."

With regard to keeping the intensity and duration of pain minimal, the patient's tactics are probably more varied, and certainly more urgent. Patients may not only beg staff to be careful, but they may warn that they will "cut out" or not go through the procedure again if it hurts too much (not, however, if they, themselves, define the procedure as absolutely necessary). They may warn implicitly, by pointing to a black-and-blue arm left by a preceding technician. They will also protest verbally, or *pretend* that it hurts in order to make the inflicter proceed more carefully. They will say sarcastically that they hurt enough already without adding to the suffering. They will draw comparisons between how much it hurts this time as compared to previous times, and other such shaming tactics. Sometimes they even insist on directing the procedure (as in the example given earlier of the cancer patient), insisting or assuming that they know their own bodies better than the personnel, as did a university student who knew that he reacted very slowly to pain killers, but who could not convince the personnel at the dental clinic that they needed to give medication longer in advance than they did ordinarily. Patients will also negotiate to do some part of the painful procedure themselves, knowing their own bodily reactions better, as with burn patients who rub off the ointment themselves during the debridement bath. Their argument is that even the best intentioned and trained nurses "can't feel it" as they can.

The major task, however, is to get the job done, pain or no pain. From the staff's viewpoint, this means there should be minimal interference in the activity itself by the patients. They have to do their part, being quiet, passive, and even inert if the task requires that, or more actively cooperative if necessary. The implicit contract, it will be remembered, involves the patient's additional cooperation in *enduring* pain and in keeping *pain expression* appropriate to the situation. Thus, most of the staff's tactics are devoted to getting the patient to endure and to keep expression from interfering too much.

Staff members will shame, scold, chide, even threaten (especially with children) to "do it anyhow." They will persuade or encourage: "Try to relax, honey, let us look at you—just a little."[2] They will promise that it will soon be over and promise rewards (ice cream to children) for good performance. They will give temporal markers to keep endurance up: "Just two more times" or "just one more minute," or "the worst is over." These tactics are especially effective if there is either great trust or great ignorance of the procedure.

The use of specific tactics is related both to the assessments made of the patient and also to contingencies, such as scheduling, how tired the staff members are, and their relations with the patient (and with each other if more than one is involved).

Use of tactics is also related to each staff member's "style," since each is likely to have developed a generalized manner of handling pain-infliction situations and pain-inflicted patients. One urologist we observed had developed a style of gruffly reassuring each of his pediatric patients that the catheterization wouldn't hurt very much, when in fact it was often quite painful. A different style is illustrated by a nurse's comment about patients' favorable reactions to the technicians who came around to draw blood, "if they are cheerful and have a good approach."

A more subtle tactical mode than style is what might be termed "presence." Some nurses can, with their compassion, their concern, their flow of encouraging language and comforting gestures, their gentle holding of a patient's body during a painful procedure, help the patient find courage and suppress bodily movements and impulses to yell and moan.

Patients too have a range of tactics for controlling their own expressions and for "hanging on." These include self-distraction, or somehow girding oneself for the painful moment or the peak of pain. Many of the tactics used to minimize pain (like bargaining for a slower pace in a painful physical exercise) are also means for enduring the ordeal. There are also many internalized tactics of which observers are not necessarily aware: exhorting oneself to endure, not to make a fool of oneself, to take pride in making no outward sign. Hopefully, the patient and the staff will settle for a noninterfering kind of pain expression, such as sobbing but keeping the body immobile, or swearing but going on with the painful regimen.

TWO ASPECTS OF PAIN EXPRESSION

There are two important aspects of pain expression in relation to task interference that should be specially noted. One aspect pertains to the *mode of expression.* Some modes will not necessarily interfere with the work at hand although the expression is very great (yelling loud and even long). Conversely, the expression may be minimal but interfere greatly with work (slight movements of the body).

A second important aspect of pain expression is the *amount of expression.* There is always an implicit, if rough, *calculus* (a method of measuring, with incremental changes) made by both the staff and the patient concerning how much expression of pain properly goes with how much actual pain. If the expression is defined as excessive by the patients themselves, they are likely to feel ashamed and may even quickly apologize for unseemly behavior. If the expression is defined as excessive by the staff but not by the patients, then the staff will scold, attempt to shame them, warn them that they can be hurt by their movements or by disturbing the proceedings, or even threaten to discontinue the procedure, to the patient's detriment. If the patient is a child, the staff may pin down limbs and continue work despite screaming or other protestations. With young children, such coercion must often take the place of verbal persuasion or negotiation.

In these regards, tubbing and debridement sessions with burn patients are very instructive. Since the pain inflicted is very great and the sessions take some minutes, patients are permitted much leeway in the amount and variety of noises they emit; but they must refrain from interfering with the nurses' teamwork. New patients may need to be taught this, but once taught, they must carry out their part of the bargain. Young children may have to suffer some coercion during painful treatments. It is worth adding that nurses new to such experience have some difficulty both in inflicting the pain and in enduring expressive noise. The more experienced nurses, if not entirely inured, have learned to accept noise as an exchange for technically efficient work.

VARIABLE CONDITIONS AND TACTICS

The preceding discussion of tactics should also have exemplified how different tactics will appear when various organizational, staff, patient, and pain properties are in play. Here are a few additional situations that underline some other conditions for tactical variance.

The "insider" patient   A pediatric nurse brought to the hospital because of an auto accident and about to have her knee x-rayed, reasoned that the procedure was of no clinical value and would add to her pain, so she protested. The technician wished to go ahead, but the nurse negotiated successfully with the radiologist.

The patient's representative   A resident wished to do a procedure but the nurse wished to delay it because the patient was in great pain. The resident resisted her persuasion, so the nurse phoned the chief resident, who backed up her judgment.

A quick, one-shot procedure   The physician essentially says: "This is going to hurt like hell, so just grit your teeth and don't move an inch—you can swear and yell and move around *afterward*."

Pain infliction procedure involving tabooed bodily area or activity   Young male children were catheterized and then asked to urinate while lying flat on the table. The urologist, quite alert to the children's fear of pain, used anticipatory reassuring tactics, but was completely insensitive to the children's reactions to urinating publicly. Furthermore, the pain was sometimes much more than the children felt they were warned against. Here is another variant of basically the same situation: A group of male medical students, interns, and residents were in an examining room at the ob-gyn clinic, watching the chief resident examine a female patient's vaginal tract. Each got a chance to look closely, and the resident also demonstrated a painful procedure, but with only a brief warning word to the woman. Everyone's gaze was narrowly focused on the vaginal area.

A nurse stood at the shoulder of the prone patient squeezing her hand and patting her hair. Between observers and the patient and nurse there was the traditional barrier—the patient's raised, sheet-draped knees. When the examination was over, the professionals filed out. As the door closed, the woman burst into tears. Humiliation? Pain? Or both?

The inexperienced or incompetent staff member and the experienced patient A new physiotherapist arrived and began to go through regimen exercises with a burn patient who had only recently received a new skin graft. The physiotherapist was rather rough and the patient, in danger of a damaged skin graft as well as confronted with intense pain atop her ongoing pain, began to scream but could not get the physiotherapist to stop. The patient finally kicked the therapist hard and persistently, and that was the end of the session.

ACCUSATIONS OF INCOMPETENCE OR NEGLIGENCE

It is easy to see that the implicit (sometimes explicit) contract which allows the accomplishment of the primary task can be violated, either in actuality or in the opinion of one of the contractual agents. The considerable fragility which characterizes the basic contract is suggested by the following fieldnote, which shows both tactical, explicit promising by a physician and the thin ice on which the physician skates in fulfilling promises:

> An M.D. persuades a wary child to sit on a stool, saying: "This won't hurt." The doctor takes out cotton and asks: "That didn't hurt, did it?" The child nods assent. Then the M.D. wants to wipe the bloody nose with cotton, but the child makes a defensive gesture. The M.D. says: "It's soft," and puts a piece in the child's palm. The child holds the cotton, feeling it, while M.D. wipes the nose and probes a bit with another piece of cotton.

Since the obligations of the contract are reciprocal, a patient of course can be reprimanded for breaking his side of the bargain. The stage is set, on both sides, for accusations of bad faith or bad conduct. The blaming, as in any political arena, will often be mutual.

From the staff's viewpoint, the patient can be blamed for failing to endure the pain; after all, it is only a byproduct of a task done for the patient's own good. He can also be blamed for failing to control extreme expressions of displeasure and slowing up accomplishment of the primary tasks.

A number of conditions underlie the possibility that the patient will also make accusations. The most general set of conditions is that the patient, like the staff, makes a distinction between necessary and unnecessary pain. The latter, of course, pertains to pain that is an unanticipated byproduct of the primary task, pain that the patient either has not been told about or has been told would not occur. However, unnecessary pain pertains also to necessary pain when the pain is more intense or of longer duration than expected. The inflicter is usually held responsible for all types of unnecessary pain: unanticipated, overly intense and long-lasting.

As the patient sees it, the unnecessary pain can be caused either by *incompetence* (lack of skill) or *negligence* (carelessness, indifference). The patient may erroneously accuse pain inflicters, believing they have been careless when in fact they are inexperienced or they have made errors involving skill. Or, the patient may think the staff less than competent when in fact there has been some actual negligence displayed. Experienced patients, such as those on extended physiotherapy regimens, are more likely to spot the difference between incompetence and negligence.

Before discussing the conditions and consequences of experience in assigning blame, it will be useful to note some common organizational reasons for a staff member's actual negligence or incompetence. Concerning incompetence: The main fault usually lies with personnel who either are insufficiently skilled at their techniques or at "working on" particular kinds of patients. That deficiency of skill can stem from insufficient basic training; lack of enough in-service training to keep up with advances in technologies; at the very least, inadequate information about types of patients new to the personnel (a newness often caused by such factors as staff rotation).

The organizational conditions fostering negligence are perhaps more complex. To prevent or minimize pain engendered in cardiac patients by postoperative breathing regimens, patients must receive their drugs before doing the breathing, and receive them at exactly the right time. But unfortunately this involves a more complex intermeshing of staff work than is usually accomplished. Hence, this kind of pain infliction through organizational negligence seems fairly frequent on CCUs. Other contributory organizational factors include a staff on a tight schedule, or one with a heavy load of medically difficult patients. A staff focused on technical aspects of care to the almost total exclusion of the humanistic aspects is also likely to be negligent in its infliction of pain during the pursuit of its main tasks.

Hospitals and clinics also seem often to proliferate a tendency to discount the patient's opinions on medical and even procedural mat-

ters, so that when a staff member and patient do not really know
each other, a discounting of the patient's cues or utterances is likely.
The patient is even more likely to be disregarded if he has earned a
negative reputation on the ward or clinic—a frequent phenomenon,
alas, in our health facilities. (Recall Mrs. Abel and the No. 25 needle.
See also Mrs. Noble in Chapter 14.) Quite aside from an actual reputation, however, certain people get additional short shrift, or at least
less concern is shown for them, because they are of "low social
value": for example, some of the drunks, suicide attempts, victims of
knife slashings, "accident cases," and various of the low or socio-
economic or "undesirable" ethnic and racial groups who appear regularly at the emergency rooms of our hospitals.[3]

Now let us return to the differences which a patient's experience
might make in accusations of incompetency or negligence. Even
without experience with specific procedures, treatments, or regimens, laypersons can sometimes recognize lack of skill in the manner, approach, style, or actual words of the pain inflicter. Experience
leaves the patient less at the mercy of such negligence. For instance,
a physician who suffered a bad wound while skiing was brought to
another physician who proceeded to stitch up the wound without using any local anesthetic. As any layperson would, the victim
protested such negligence. The working physician then lightly
sprayed a desensitizing liquid on the wound and proceeded to stitch,
soon asking: "Does it hurt?" He got an angry blast, an accusation of
incompetence right back: "What do you expect when all you did was
spray lightly and not get it in the tissues!"

A patient who time and again goes through the same regimens
or procedures can quickly learn to judge the skill of personnel. Essentially, each new potential pain inflicter is on trial. Patients also
become better at distinguishing between individual reasons (unpleasant person, doesn't like me) and organizational reasons (overworked, not enough staff) for negligence. Such comparisons go hand
in hand with the repeated infliction situation. Also, if a number of
patients know they are undergoing the same treatments, as with
physical therapy, they will share their evaluative comparisons so that
certain staff members, like certain patients, receive reputations. Naturally, if a staff member is viewed as *both* incompetent and
negligent, then patients would rather not have their fate, or at least
their comfort, in such hands.

Patients differ in the manner in which they express themselves
to staff when they believe they have suffered from some degree of incompetence or negligence. Sometimes they can be very direct; at
other times they choose to remain silent. Conditions eliciting direct

comments are fairly obvious: The patient is surprised into angry ex-
clamation, or fears that the same inflicter will return unless somehow
reprimanded. Patients may even be quite fearful of potential damage,
as well as of the pain itself, and command, as one did to a physical
therapist: "Don't touch me again! You obviously don't know what
you're doing." Among the reasons for keeping silent: the pain is insufficient to complain about, or the procedure is only done once, or
the person is shy, does not like to complain, or is simply overawed
by the personnel's authority. Silence can also be a response when the
patient fears, sometimes accurately, that there may be reprisals for
complaining or blaming. An experienced person may recognize the
dangers of being defined as a "bad" patient.

Those accusations which patients do level at a staff member are
often met by two kinds of counterstatements. The first is based,
whether justified or not, on the strategy that the strongest defense is
an offense: "You moved!" or "What do you expect with all that
racket you've been making?" In other words, the staff member
accuses the patient of failing to keep his or her part of the implicit
contract.

The second type of defense is to retort that someone has misread
the situation; the task is very difficult and a certain amount of pain is
inevitable, or what looks like undue and unseemly haste or careless
procedure is really nothing of the sort. In short: signs are at best ambiguous, and only the truly experienced (that is, the professional) can
read them correctly. Both types of counterstatement can be delivered
with a variety of gestural and tonal expression, signifying a range of
disapproval running from reluctant countercomplaint through annoyance, anger, fury, disgust, desperation. After all, the main job simply
must be done, with or without the patient's cooperation. Understandably, such sets of tactics and countertactics may end in an
increasingly vicious spiral of bad feeling, bad temper and bad health
care.

CHRONIC DISEASE AND PAIN INFLICTION

Since chronic illness is the predominant type of disease today, a very
high proportion of the patients seen at the health facilities are suffering from ongoing or periodic flare-ups of pain; but whether or not
this is so, each patient is likely to have a substantial experiential history of contact with health personnel and with their potentially
painful regimens, treatments, and diagnostic procedures. If hospitals
and clinics handled only emergency and infectiously ill patients, then
pain infliction would be less complex. The painful moments or days

are quickly over, and that's that. But with chronically ill persons, transient pain is not so characteristic.

Furthermore, the patient often has some ongoing pain which may not even derive from the condition being treated and of which the staff is unaware. Worse still, the patient will have a "pain biography" associated with previous illnesses and to which he or she will relate the current infliction of pain. One example should suffice. Persons with back pain come to hospitals with pain biographies that often include genuine problems in legitimating their pain to others (as will be seen in Chapter 8), including the current staff. Any *new* infliction of pain is necessarily regarded in relation to experiential history. Thus: "The new pain is nothing much if the procedure may help since I am desperate." or "The new pain is just one more neglectful act on the part of a staff member who doesn't know or believe my story."

The predominance of chronically ill patients, then, can result in two unfortunate sets of consequences. If the patient has had one more bad experience with pain infliction, she carries that in her memory, adding it to her pain biography. It becomes part of her future reactions to personnel at any health facility. As for the personnel, the experiences they have with uncooperative, accusatory patients result in stereotyping or labeling of new patients who remind them of previous offenders. "She's just like Mrs. Abel. Lord help us!" The consequence of this is, quite clearly, that medical, nursing, and rehabilitative care can be less than effective.

ACCOUNTABILITY AND CONTROL

The principal reason for ineffectiveness is that health facilities are organized to deal more with acute than with chronic illnesses. When the disease being treated is acute, a patient's previous experiences with hospitals, health personnel, drugs, regimens, and symptoms—including pain—do not matter so much. The overwhelming prevalence of chronically ill patients, however, means that those matters should be systematically taken into account. Otherwise, treatment will be ineffective.

"Taking into account" means pointed interviews with patients, recording of relevant communicated information on medical charts, communication among the staff, and the reporting back of actions taken in relation to such relevant data. As we have remarked earlier and elsewhere,[4] genuine accountability needs to be established.

With regard to the infliction of pain, this accountability is particularly needed with those services and at those clinics where pain may be inflicted with some regularity. In the emergency room, quick action is so imperative that the staff cannot pause for such accountability. But there is no such imperative in x-ray or physical rehabilitation services, or in surgical wards where a proportion of the patients are chronically ill and not merely there for some special surgery, or medical wards which often have a complement of geriatric patients and other chronic sufferers (see Chapters 5 and 12). Obviously, this kind of accountability cannot be instituted without bringing patients more decisively, openly, and effectively into the organized system of responsibility itself.

Why cannot accountability in pain-infliction situations be instituted without, as some might characterize it, "bowing" to the patient? The answer is that many staff members see the accountability questions as a threat to their control of the work itself—what is done, how it is done, when it is done.

Does this pit staff and patient in a never-ending contest which nobody can truly "win?" We need not be nearly that pessimistic. After all, much necessary pain is inflicted during activities where both parties share equivalent goals as well as evaluations of each other's reciprocal jobs. Whether implicit or explicit, the contract is taken up and acted upon in good faith. In countless other situations, patients suffer silently or complain only mildly, yielding to what seems the inevitability of the staff's control of the work situations. At the other extreme, open warfare erupts during which patients attempt to obtain some measure of control over the work being done "on," and presumably "for" and "with" them. We have touched upon some consequences of that warfare. This entire range of unfortunate consequences might be largely eliminated if health facilities would undertake to design a genuine system of accountability with regard to those tasks which might induce pain. In short, the basic principles of cooperative activity must be made explicit and more total, rather than implicit and more segmented.

That goal does not promise complete harmony by any means, since cooperation always involves some measure of tension, some conflict, and in the instance of pain infliction, some effective persuasion, tough negotiation, and occasionally the use of negotiation with more than a hint of threat built into it.

REFERENCES

1. Cooper, I. 1973. *The victim is always the same.* New York: Harper and Row, p. 63.
2. Ibid., p. 31.

3. Glaser, B., and Strauss, A. 1964. Social loss of dying patients. *American Journal of Nursing* 64:119–121.

4. Strauss, A.; Glaser, B.; and Quint, J. 1964. The non-account-ability of terminal care. *Hospitals* 38:73–87.

Pain Expression and Control: Burn Care Unit*

7

I never imagined anything could be so painful.

I thought the pain would never end.

I don't know how I tolerated the pain.

I always thought of myself as strong about tolerating pain. I was a dentist's delight, but this pain is indescribably terrible.

This are typical statements made by patients on an intensive burn care unit, most of whom suffered intense and persistent pain. Yet their expression of the pain was not at all equal to their description of it. In fact, the relative absence of pain expression on this ward was not only striking, but somewhat unreal. The relative absence of expression in spite of the severe pain becomes understandable, however, when viewed in terms of (1) the organizational and interactional features of the intensive burn unit, and (2) the nature of burn pain and the burn regimen. On the burn unit, as will be evident, the salient pain tasks, both for patients and staff, are the *enduring of pain* and the *controlling of pain expression*.

*Originally published in slightly altered form. Copyright © October 1974, The American Journal of Nursing Company. Reproduced, with permission, from *Nursing Outlook*.

BURN UNIT CHARACTERISTICS

Intensive burn care units are highly specialized and isolated. Space is organized around not only the management of the critically ill patient and the treatment of burns, but also the prevention of complicating infections. The unit which we studied had its own special operating, treatment, and tub rooms. Special barrier techniques of gowning, masking, and capping were required of everyone entering the unit. Visitors were limited to the patients' immediate families. As on other critical care units, the acutely ill patient had little privacy and was in open view of the staff to allow constant monitoring.[1]

In addition—and here the burn unit differs from other types of intensive care facilities—patients remain well beyond the critical stage. Sometimes weeks or even months of hospitalization are necessary to take them from the acute through the skin reconstruction phase. The openness of the unit and the long stay in an enclosed and isolated space have a tremendous effect on the patients' pain expression.

Burn care is highly complex, intense, and technical, requiring great staff expertise. The responsibilities are major ones, including those related to survival care, the treatment of burn wounds, prevention of complications, and skin reconstruction. As in other intensive care units, the staff's focus is narrowly and intensely on the medical aspect of care, as opposed to the "whole patient."

BURN PAIN

The outstanding features of burn pain are its intensity and long duration. In addition, recovery requires the performance of many painful treatments. The degree and duration of pain suffered by an individual patient will, of course, depend on the extent and location of the burn and on such other important factors as anxiety level, pain tolerance, and age.

In a typical burn pain trajectory, barring complications, the base line or primary pain from the burn itself is very high in the initial, acute postburn phase. The primary pain gradually subsides but for weeks thereafter, until the skin heals or skin grafts are applied and take, the pain level will peak above the base line because of secondary pain, that is, pain inflicted by treatment. These peaks of pain are very intense because the treatment—tubbing, dressing changes, debridement, and physiotherapy—are often simultaneously or serially inflicted.

In the daily tubbing, for example, where the patient is immersed in a tub to remove encrusted medication, adhering dressing, exudates, and necrotic tissues, simultaneous massive pain is brought about because three or four nurses are scrubbing and treating different parts of the burned surface. This regimen is then followed by the application of medications (some cause pain and burning), possible further debridement, and the application of dressings. Several times a day additional pain peaks may occur because of physiotherapy, dressing changes, and other treatments.

In the second stage, involving skin grafts, pain is often noticeably reduced. However, there is now pain from the donor skin site until it heals, with lesser pain accompanying the dressing changes.

Throughout all these phases there are also lesser pains and discomforts associated with immobilization, mobilization, and the itching and tingling from tissue regeneration. When the burns are extensive, the patient will require many serial skin-reconstruction surgeries, with accompanying peaks of pain from treatments that stretch over many months. In the final phase there is a dull chronic pain, with lesser peaks of pain associated with nerve regeneration, as well as the discomforts of stretching muscles and joints from vigorous physiotherapy.

As in any illness there are degrees to which health professionals can prevent, minimize, or control pain. But this pain management must be balanced against other priorities and concerns, and there are many special problems with burns. For example, patients must not be completely "knocked out" by analgesics or narcotics, for they must be able to cooperate with the treatments. They must also be alert enough to assure a food and fluid intake adequate for tissue healing, yet the pain must not be so intense that it causes loss of appetite. Moreover, because of the long duration of pain, the staff must prevent not only loss of drug effectiveness, but also the development of drug dependency. Thus, staff must constantly assess the patients' pain levels, pain tolerances, and anxiety levels in order to juggle the drugs and tranquilizers used throughout the illness.

BURN PAIN EXPRESSION AND CONTROL

Controlling *treatment-inflicted* pain poses very special problems because, short of complete anesthesia, drugs cannot adequately control that pain, particularly during the tubbing treatment. Under these conditions, the effort is primarily directed toward reducing the degree of pain through the administration of narcotics before the treatments, or by reducing the duration of the pain by working swiftly, deftly, and in teams.

Staff members are constantly saying to a patient, "It will be over soon." "Just a bit longer." Patients are constantly crying out, "For God's sake, hurry!" They soon learn that the relief gained by temporarily stopping the treatment will merely prolong their agony.

Among the main characteristics of an intensive burn care unit, then, are that it is populated primarily by patients whose pain is of long duration and whose treatments necessitate numerous inflictions of pain. The staff members are unavoidably the inflicting agents; the pain they induce is irreducible and is simultaneously, serially, and repeatedly inflicted. It becomes essential that pain expression be kept within reasonable limits. A patient who, without inhibition, cries, screams, moans, groans, and constantly complains of pain is intolerable and devastating, both for the staff and the other patients.

Under the conditions just described, a process occurs whereby the unit's organization and the staff's work focus will shape the nature of pain expression management. In addition to controlling the patients' pain expression, staff members need also control their own response to pain and its expression, and they must do this in the midst of overwhelming agony and misery and in a situation where they themselves are the major agents for increasing patients' pain.

MANAGEMENT OF BURN PAIN EXPRESSION

As indicated earlier, the staff's focus is intensely and narrowly on the medical, as opposed to the psychosocial, components of care. High priority and prestige are accorded to technical competence. Also the temporal focus is upon the "here and now"—to carry the patient through the acute illness—with less emphasis on the posthospital phase of care. This narrow focus is understandable because of the immense responsibilities associated with survival and burn care and the large numbers of acutely ill patients who are totally dependent upon the staff.

The intense and immediate focus also makes easier a most difficult situation for the staff members; it prevents them from thinking about the patient's possibly tragic future, one which may well cast doubt on the value of their efforts. Thus, patients are discouraged from expressing anxieties about their social and psychological futures, while much effort is directed toward socializing them to accept the painful treatments as absolutely necessary for recovery.

Where pain is inevitable and irreducible, there is a tendency for staff to focus on other concerns. The literature on the medical management of burns, for instance, indicates primary concern with the complexities of technical treatment. Pain management and psychosocial aspects receive only fleeting attention. This is completely understandable; although the staff members are immersed in and surrounded by pain, they are limited in their capacity to relieve it, and besides, they have more pressing priorities.

In our study, staff generally tended to assess pain as less severe than the patient indicated it was. Most staff thought pain expression, especially complaints of pain and requests for pain relief, stemmed largely from anxiety. In fact, some even thought that burn pain was more "discomfort" than pain, but they did concede that treatments were painful. This accords with Artz and Moncrief, who believe that physical pain is considerably less severe than is generally supposed and that emotionally induced pain is a serious problem.[2]

The more experienced nurses tended to control pain with smaller doses of drugs than did the less experienced. Nurses told us that when they first came to the unit they gave narcotics rather frequently and were overly concerned about hurting patients during the treatments. As time went on, however, they gave smaller amounts of drugs and were less concerned with inflicting pain, because they knew the treatments were crucial to recovery. In fact, some nurses can become so inured to pain that they may hum while giving a painful tubbing, much as they might while engaged in any other serious but not crisis-laden work.

Important influences in controlling the patient's general behavior as well as pain expression were the staff's technical competence, along with the unit's outstanding reputation for burn care. Many patients, when transferred from other facilities, learned from staff and other patients that only this unit had the facilities and expertise to cope with major burns and was the "best place for burns." Thus the unit's reputation and the assured and competent mien of the staff members helped to reduce anxiety and encouraged patients to feel confidence and trust in them, plus a sense of gratitude and indebtedness. In addition, many patients with major burns were completely helpless and totally dependent on the staff and were, therefore, willing to follow the latter's dictates.

Understandable, too, was the staff members' manipulation of their expertise—creating the image that they "know what's best" for the patient. This allowed them to control the patient under circumstances of irreducible and unavoidable pain. This manipulation was justified by the high priority and prestige accorded technical competence, but it further reduced any focus on psychosocial competence. Such manipulation of professional medical competence to calm and control patients, it should be pointed out, is an effective and useful approach in many professional–client encounters.

LEARNING AND ENDURING

The patients on a burn unit are always in various stages of the burn
and pain trajectories, in open view of each other, and spend a rather
long period together in an enclosed space. These conditions give the
patients a chance to rehearse and interpret their own illnesses and
pain trajectories and to compare them with those of others.[3] Through
these activities they learn the norms and limits of pain expression
and relief associated with the various phases of illness; the probable
duration of the various phases; the various methods of tolerating
pain; and the complications that may alter pain trajectory.

The rate of learning will differ in accordance with a number of
contingencies, one of which is the physical placement of the patient
on the unit. In the unit that we studied, patients in the early, acute
phase were usually placed in a two-bed room and later transferred to
the large ward. Sometimes, however, because of a lack of space, they
were immediately placed in the large ward. When this happened,
they learned about the temporal phases of pain earlier than would
otherwise be the case.

For example, a man with burns on his face, chest, arms, and
hand was placed in a two-bed room next to a patient suffering severe
70% body surface burns and whose condition was very unstable.
Although the less seriously burned patient was responding satisfactorily to therapy, he had difficulty in believing it until he was moved
to the large ward. He had been unduly concerned with dying and
had expressed these fears. In contrast, another patient with equally
severe burns was admitted directly to the large ward and was able to
look around and make comparisons. This patient tended to accept the
staff's reassurances and was less concerned with dying.

PATIENT GROUP SUPPORT

Another important contingency is the composition of the patient
group at any given time—for instance, a group with similar burns
enabling comparison of progress, or the presence or lack of presence
of an articulate and experienced patient willing to play supporter and
interpreter to a newer patient. Also important is the willingness or
unwillingness of staff, according to their individual or group philosophies, to apprise patients of their physical status. Furthermore, the
patients' belief in the information provided will depend upon
whether the information is from a doctor or nurse, or from a new or
experienced staff member.

Patients learn the various calculi of experienced pain and pain
expression: the duration and intensity of pain accompanying each

phase of illness, the mode of pain, its location, and how it may be appropriately expressed. They learn, for instance, that the greater the degree and extent of burns, the longer the illness and pain trajectory; the greatest pain is in the early acute phase with the tubbing and other treatments; skin graft greatly reduces the pain; anxiety increases pain perception but can be controlled by a positive attitude and the use of tranquilizers.

In the early, acute phase, patients learn, no amount of drug will completely control the pain, and so it must be endured. They also learn that some moaning, groaning, and yelling are acceptable during treatments, but not if continued for a long time because of the demoralizing effects on other patients. A great deal of pain expression after the grafting is not only unacceptable, it is not understandable.

In the early phase, a patient's toleration of pain and control of its expression are accomplished primarily by learning that eventually it will end and that others have suffered similarly. Patient after patient told us how comforting it was to know that others also moaned, groaned, and screamed during the painful treatment. Those past the acute phase frequently told the newcomers: "You think the tubbing is never going to end and you can't bear another day of pain, but it will come to an end." "We all went through it." "Once the graft is on, it won't be so bad."

Or they told patients who constantly complained of pain and asked for relief: "No shot will completely stop the pain. It has to run its course. You've got to learn to tolerate it. Distract yourself. Watch TV. Walk around. Do anything to stop thinking about the pain." One patient who could not tolerate the treatment threatened to walk out of the hospital, but was dissuaded by other patients who used themselves as examples of having suffered and passed the acute phase.

In contrast, a burn patient who was treated on a general surgical unit in another hospital could not be persuaded to continue the painful therapy. Another patient treated in a similar facility said that she was anxious throughout her hospitalization, because there were no other patients with whom she could compare her progress.

Patients learn that pain medications are dispensed only at prescribed intervals and over certain phases and periods. They are told, and overhear the staff telling other patients: "It's too early for another shot." "If you take the pain shots too frequently, they lose their effectiveness and won't hold you when you really need it." "With the graft there's less pain. A pill should hold you instead of a shot." "Do you want to get addicted?"

Patients also learn from each other about pacing drugs by asking for tranquilizers between pain drugs to take the edge off the pain.

They learn the various ways to control pain expression during painful treatments: distracting themselves by turning up the volume on
radio earphones, watching television intently, stuffing something in
their mouths to bite on, using self-hypnosis by loudly yelling, "It
doesn't hurt. It doesn't hurt." Religious patients will often urge others to pray.

GRADIENTS OF BURN PAIN AND ITS EXPRESSION

Patients constantly make comparisons among themselves, not only to
locate themselves along the illness and pain trajectory, but also to
measure how much pain expression is legitimate and allowable. The
comparisons are in terms of the extent and location of burns, the different amounts of pain experienced in the phases of the illness, and
the rate of recovery—whether they are on schedule or not. Patients
with less severe and extensive burns told us they had less "right" to
complain of pain than those with more extensive burns. They felt,
too, that those with facial and hand involvement had more cause for
anxiety and, therefore, more right to have and express pain.

The most severe treatment pains were used as a measure of the
lesser pains. "Nothing is worse than the tubbing pain," the patients
constantly remarked. Having tolerated the intolerable with an injection, then they learned to tolerate lesser pains with less potent oral
medication.

When patients felt that staff negligence had increased their pain
—poor timing of the pretreatment medication, for instance, or no
premedication at all—they felt justified in increasing their pain expression. They not only moaned and groaned more than usual, but
they felt justified in saying to the staff: "Easy there. Gentle now. After all, the premedication is about worn off." Or "Take it easy. I
didn't get a shot before, you know." They also learned to rate staff
members on their sympathy, roughness, or gentleness. When treatments themselves were rated as rough, then a patient felt justified in
being more expressive of pain; other patients also believed such expression was more justified.

Patients told us that when they had exerted tremendous effort to
control their own expressions of both pain and anxiety, then excessive or inappropriate expression on the part of other patients was demoralizing. Hence, as a group they tried to help—often, literally, to
teach—the newer patients to control their expressiveness. Their approaches to assessment and methods of handling the overly
expressive patient were quite sophisticated and not dissimilar to
those of the professional staff. They located the patient on a general

illness and pain continuum to determine if the pain expression was within reasonable limits. They tried to learn the personal history in order to gain insight into the cause and level of anxiety.

A CASE IN POINT

Both Tom and Jerry were similarly injured, with burns on the face, arms, and hand, but Tom was more severely burned than Jerry. Also, Tom was further along than Jerry in his illness and pain phases and, at the time of Jerry's admission, was in the large ward, eagerly awaiting his skin grafts.

Jerry had been transferred from a general hospital to a two-bed room on the burn unit. While at the general hospital his pain had been controlled by 100 to 150 mg of Demerol, but staff on the burn unit considered this dosage unnecessarily high and reduced it, an action that Jerry thought indicated lack of sympathy. For days he complained constantly of pain and requested medication, only to be told that more frequent shots could not be given.

On the fifth day Jerry was moved to the large ward next to Tom, who found it strange that Jerry complained so much about pain when Jerry had less extensive burns than he did. Jerry was not consoled by pep talks from Tom and other patients who told him that the pain would soon end, that they all went through it, and that this unit was the "best damn place to be."

Tom had discovered a few weeks earlier that anxiety had much to do with increase of pain, so he told Jerry this and advised him to ask for an increase in tranquilizers. Tranquilizers were increased, but without noticeable decrease in Jerry's pain expression. Tom then tried shaming Jerry by comparing him with another patient who had more extensive burns but managed pain expression well. Jerry was chagrined about his behavior, but he could not figure out the discrepancy.

Another patient discovered that Jerry was very concerned with finances and was also upset that his doctor hadn't visited him for several days. He advised Jerry to contact the social worker and also told him that although his doctor had not visited him, he was daily apprised of his progress. Jerry then admitted that anxiety had a great deal to do with his low toleration of pain.

Meanwhile Tom had skin grafting on his hand and arms and, although uncomfortable, he assessed his pain as "nothing compared to the tubbing" and was therefore willing to endure his pain with less potent drugs. At the same time Jerry discovered that some patients were not recovering on schedule because of complications. Jerry complained to the researcher that he was not satisfied with the information given by staff.

Even after Jerry had skin grafts on his hands, he continued to be overly expressive when undergoing dressing changes and other treatments. Tom couldn't comprehend Jerry's pain—and told him so—since Jerry had been assigned to the gentlest and most skilled nurse. But when Tom's successful skin graft finally was unveiled and he had use of his hands, Jerry's pain expression was markedly reduced! He apologized to other patients for having been unduly expressive and justified his behavior as stemming from anxiety: he had not been properly apprised by staff about his progress, he had never before been sick and didn't know what to expect, and so on.

OTHER VARIABLES

Burned children present special difficulties that stem from the unit's organizational and interactional limitations. Young children with limited ability to reason, or with limited or distorted time sense, cannot be as easily consoled as older children and adults when told about the need for treatment or that intense pain will last only a few days or weeks. In fact, two children we observed cried harder and longer as their stay extended.[4] Adult patients on the unit felt frustrated because the usual socializing approaches to help the patient tolerate pain did not work with children. After living through days of a child's constant crying, the adult patients tended to lose their patience and sympathy, resorting to punitive methods in controlling the child's pain expression.

A significant organizational factor in this situation is that caring for children is *not* the salient focus on a burn unit. In contrast, burn management on a pediatric unit would include staff who, by virtue of their specialized interest and training, not only possess wider interactional approaches to manage children, but also have greater resources such as a playroom, play therapist, and child psychologist. Then, of course, working with burned children is very difficult for the staff members, because they must cope with their own feelings as agents of intense and protracted assault on a helpless and pitiful child.[5]

By and large, though, the support and pressure of the patient group, together with the staff's socialization of the patients, controlled pain expression within reasonable limits; however, the situation changed at one time when an articulate and medically sophisticated patient was admitted. He contested not only the staff's medical management but its pain-management approaches as well, backing up many of his arguments with seemingly logical reasons.

This patient's attacks on staff members encouraged other patients to express their doubts, anxieties, and disgruntlement about their care. An increase in their general expressiveness tended to upset the "sentimental order" of the unit—i.e., the collective mood, composure, and morale necessary to maintain order—and to frustrate the staff's usual method of encouraging patients to cooperate with the treatment and care.[6]

We observed that in addition to control of pain expression, controls were also placed on patients' expressions of anxiety concerning their social futures. Patients learned that such expression was not only frowned upon by the staff, but reasoned that it could be devastating for other patients. It is significant that those who discussed such anxieties with the researcher stated that they had not discussed them with others. Several patients commented about another: "I know so-and-so is very upset because I hear him crying quietly during the night. It really makes me feel bad."

The patients making these statements were similarly described by other patients. It was not unusual to find patient after patient preoccupied with his or her own gloomy thoughts. We need only add that understandings about not expressing anxiety about the future can be relevant to experience with pain during the hospital stay.

IMPLICATIONS FOR PATIENT CARE

In burn units, where staff has certain pressing priorities and is limited as to how much it can relieve pain, endurance of pain and patient–patient support pertaining to that task are understandably crucial. All patients interviewed stated that other patients were their greatest source of support. It would appear, then, that burn workers might more deliberately and more effectively utilize the patients as a resource. To do so would require further information about patient–patient pain talk and patient–staff pain talk during the hospitalization, and interviews with patients about the kinds of approaches which were helpful or not helpful.

For example, the patients we interviewed stated that being informed about the temporal phases and what to expect during these phases helped reduce their pain by reducing their anxiety. They commented, too, that the staff needed to take many variables into consideration in deciding when and how much information might be given to patients. Patients' discussion of pain management was sophisticated. They were aware that pain assessment was indeed a complex problem, and that staff faced a difficult pain-management situation in view of its many priority problems.

It follows logically that any better utilization of the patient group as a resource in pain management would call for some reshaping of the unit's *organization*. This might not require additional staff, but it would require more *communication* to and from patients, genuine *staff focus on pain work* other than the obvious inflicted pain and its limited relief, and somewhat the same administrative *accountability* that is demanded for medical and procedural matters.

REFERENCES

1.   Strauss, A. 1968. Intensive care unit: its characteristics and social relationships. *Nursing Clinics of North America* 3:7–15.

2.   Artz, C. P., and Moncrief, J. A. 1969. *The treatment of burns*. 2d ed. Philadelphia: W. B. Saunders, p. 285.

3.   Glaser, B., and Strauss, A. 1971. *Status passage*. Chicago: Aldine, pp. 116–141.

4.   Kueffner, M. 1973. A qualitative study of the passage through hospitalization of severely burned isolated school-age children. Unpublished doctoral dissertation, University of California, San Francisco.

5.   Quinby, S. V., and Bernstein, N. R. 1971. Identity problems and the adaptation of nurses to severely burned children. *American Journal of Psychiatry* 128:58–63.

6.   Glaser, B., and Strauss, A. 1965. *Awareness of dying*. Chicago: Aldine, pp. 226–228.

Part 4

Assessment, Legitimation, and Relief

Assessment and Legitimation on an Orthopedic Ward*

8

One of the most complicated of pain tasks is the relieving of pain, although it seems relatively straightforward. Of course its technical aspects can be difficult, since the countering of pain with the proper measures of relief can present great and sometimes insuperable problems. By contrast, the moral and social aspects of relieving pain may, at first, appear essentially nonproblematic; after all, most people in pain who request relief get it without much difficulty. Is it not their right? At home they dose themselves; in the hospital the staff is obligated to relieve them of pain if that help does not impede recovery from illness. Yet, as we have seen in the case of Mrs. Abel, relief is not necessarily given quickly, efficiently, pleasantly, or willingly. Indeed, the related acts of requesting and giving relief can give rise to complicated and anguished dramas.

One of the major issues for the potential reliever of pain is that of properly assessing the amount, indeed the very pres-

*This chapter by Carolyn Wiener was originally published under the title "Pain Assessment and Legitimation on an Orthopedic Ward." Its form has been somewhat altered. Copyright © 1975, The American Journal of Nursing Company. Reproduced, with permission, from *Nursing Outlook*.

ence, of pain. The person who claims to have pain must legitimate
it. In Chapter 8, we describe and analyze characteristic events
which occur on an orthopedic ward when patients claim to have back
pain. The major issues are those of assessment and legitimation. (In
Chapter 9, we shall discuss in considerable detail the principal elements involved in that complicated task called "relieving pain" and
some of the consequential issues to which those elements give rise
on hospital wards.)

INTRODUCTION

Conditions of ambiguity arise when the staff acknowledges the existence of pain and attempts to relieve it, but the degree of pain remains in doubt. Such conditions generate the twin problems of *staff
assessment* and *patient legitimation*. What are the consequences for patient care, interaction, and work when patient and staff assessment
differ and the patient fails to legitimate pain?

   On orthopedic wards such as the one we observed, the salient
dimensions of pain work are likely to be the handling of pain *expression* and the work attendant on the patient's *endurance*. Where
there is good cooperation, the assessment of pain by both parties is
reasonably close and the accompanying pain tasks are facilitated; the
patient need not legitimate.

   But let us assume that assessment (for whatever reason) is quite
difficult. Let us assume also a tendency for staff to underestimate or
disbelieve the degree of pain expressed by the patient. Then there remains a legitimating job to be done by the patient—provided she
recognizes the staff's different assessment of pain. Trouble arises if
she is unaware of this discrepancy, has inaccurate knowledge of or
disagrees with the staff's assessment of her pain, and objects rather
than complies. Then in attempting to "convince" the staff, she is perceived as "noncooperative" in her pain tasks.

   Not all of the patients on an orthopedic ward present management problems; many present no problem at all. Some may disagree
with but play according to staff's interactional rules or, for various
reasons, their legitimation problems are not especially severe. Nevertheless, the burden of "difficult" cases is a common and understandable complaint from staff (including physiotherapeutic personnel). This chapter is therefore concerned with events that occur when
pain expression is assessed as disproportionate and when the staff
remains unconvinced that the patient has reached the limit of endurance. It illuminates the manner in which the perspectives of both
staff and patient inadvertently generate a cycle of increased pain

work. Notice also that we are discussing *chronic* pain—or chronic illness with accompanying pain. One should also keep in mind that although this chapter is about orthopedic pain, it might apply with a bit of qualification to any other severe chronic pain which staff finds difficult to assess.

DISCREPANT PERSPECTIVES AND THEIR SOURCES

With low-back pain, the discrepant perspectives of staff and patient pertain basically to staff's actual inability to diagnose accurately. Although "bad back" ranks third among chronic conditions that limit the activities of Americans, back pain remains exceedingly difficult to diagnose. As Wiles has said, "There is little agreement as to the etiology, which is often speculative, and as to treatment, which is usually empirical."[1] Diagnostic problems stem partially from the unreliability of clinical findings. Neither x-rays nor myelograms are always conclusive and, as Inman and Saunders have said, "Too often we are compelled in low-back syndromes to rely on the sole subjective reaction of the patient, always unsatisfactory as a guide to definite and rational therapy."[2]

The patients referred to in this chapter were all diagnosed as having disk or vertebral problems. Some conditions clearly had started with an injury; in other cases the etiology was ambiguous and onset gradual. Treatment had included bed rest, traction, ultrasound treatments, bracing, or surgery.

Most of these patients had long medical biographies. Some had returned to the hospital because fusions did not "take"; one had had a period of relief, but the deep-seated remainder of an operated disk was shedding disk matter and there was new pressure on a nerve; some now had new herniated disks. In some cases the back disease had progressed too fast or for too long, and there was permanent damage to nerve roots. Many patients had had suspicions or verifications of previous medical mismanagement and were, therefore, often mistrustful and sometimes angry, still looking for a miracle. Others were hoping for long-term but not necessarily total relief. Many were guarded in their expectations.

Understandably, the staff does not view such patients as highly desirable. Their course of illness is unpredictable, the difficulties in objectively validating their pain and its source cast suspicion on its degree, and the limited relief options available when pain appears intractable lead to the staff's frustration and helplessness. Herein lies the initial discrepancy in perspective—over the issue of *etiology*.

Staff believes strongly in psychogenic factors as an important source of back pain. Patients, however, while not denying that emotions can intensify the pain, are not willing to accept a totally psychogenic explanation, which would imply that their pain was not "real." Although the staff's different perspective is not explicitly communicated to the patient, it does affect staff's interpretation of patient behavior and the actions taken to deal with it.

A second discrepancy in perspective occurs over the *signs* or *visibility* of pain. Even when x-ray or myelogram clearly indicates some pathology, staff is still not always convinced of the degree of pain that patients claim, for a similar abnormality will distress one person but not another. The patient usually does not know of the staff's skepticism regarding visibility. Persons who have had an unsuccessful medical experience or previous legitimation-of-pain problems feel vindicated when the doctor reports that clinical tests show a substantive basis for their pain. It never occurs to them that the staff's doubt has not been totally dispelled.

A similar misunderstanding occurs with a treatment such as the use of ultrasound. During the treatment, patients not only feel but see their muscles twitching and read this as a sign that the treatment is doing some good. They do not realize that the physiotherapist who is administering the ultrasound may think the treatment is more a placebo than medically therapeutic.

A third discrepancy in perspective occurs over *relief procedures,* whose efficacy is often questioned by the staff. In large teaching centers, the personnel on an orthopedic ward rarely see successful back patients. They are more likely to see those who are returning for a second and third operation, and they have no way of knowing whether those who do not come back are simply "living with it," are shopping elsewhere, or are actually cured.

Many of them, therefore, question why patients expose themselves to surgery when there is such a low rate of success and so high a risk. Patients, on the other hand, have often tried all the options—had no permanent relief after traction, for instance, or found the discomfort of a brace outweighed the potential benefit—and now see the risk as worth taking when weighed against the unrelieved pain and the consequent interference with the normal conduct of their lives.

Yet a fourth discrepancy in perspective relates to the *endurance* of pain. It stems from the failure of patients with low-back pain to realize that they are being compared with other patients who, for one reason or another, might have higher degrees of pain tolerance. On a particular ward, for instance, many longstanding arthritic persons may have had arthroplasty; these patients are often more tolerant than others of postoperative pain because of their long experience with pain and because the surgery frequently brings less pain than the affected joint did previously.

The low-back patients may be unaware of other patients and the comparisons the staff is making. They may be further disadvantaged by not being on a large, open, homogeneous ward where they can compare themselves with others and where there is patient-to-patient pain talk and support.

Considering all the circumstances just described, the staff's assessment of pain is obviously not a simple matter. Although they look for signs by which accurate assessment might be made, they observe these signs in interactional situations that affect their perceptions about the handling of expression and endurance of pain. Patients may be inhibited from natural expression or, in their inability to endure and their zeal to convince, may adopt modes of expression which are unacceptable to staff. This interplay will be examined in this chapter, but first we shall look at the organizational features involved in the assessment of low-back pain.

ASSESSMENT: MINIMAL INFORMATION BASE

An initial problem is that the assessments are based on minimal information. The patient's record will provide information about why he has been hospitalized, drugs to which he is allergic, his weight and vital signs, and previous hospitalizations. This, however, does not provide a composite picture of the "whole person." Many other important aspects of the patient's biography (for instance, his experience with illness, pain, and medical care), while integral to *his* perspective, are not generally known to the staff.

Lacking such information, the staff's knowledge of patient biographies is composed of bits and snatches pieced together from incomplete accounts and, therefore, subject to distortion. Furthermore, the communicated information is highly limited and selective, often obtained when the patient is in distress, crying, or begging for relief.

The staff frequently has the most information about patients with poor reputations. Sometimes, when a patient's back disease has been diagnosed on another ward, he may be transferred to the orthopedic ward along with an already damaged reputation. His reputation and biography may then be further distorted due to inadequate communication among the day, evening, and night shifts.

Most importantly, the biographies rarely contain any acknowledgment that, before entering the hospital, the patient has had pain to manage and relationships to deal with, or has developed his own coping strategies. Thus, a wide discrepancy occurs between how patients see themselves and how they are seen by the staff.

INTERACTIONAL ASSESSMENT

Assessment, for the most part, is based upon the staff's ability to read the signs—in situ and behavioral, sent out by the patient—a reading that is greatly affected by interactional and experiential variables. Behavior (actually, the patient's pain tasks of expressing and enduring) is read in the light of interactional rules of which the patient may be totally unaware, or of which she has inaccurate knowledge, or with which she may overtly disagree. Here cooperation over pain work breaks down, and the discrepancy gap between staff and patient widens further.

For example, when asked about their general discounting of degree of pain in back patients, nurses replied, "They make a lot of fuss that everything hurts when they have visitors, but they can get in all kinds of positions the rest of the time." Or, as a physical therapist explained about one patient, "You can tell by the way she moves around the bed and the room; if you're in a lot of pain you just can't do that. She acts more as though it were a hotel rather than a hospital room."

Most people with chronic disease have learned to keep pain expression as minimal as possible; they develop strategies for covering up.[3] Covering up is not denial in the psychological sense: ". . . it is a rejection by the patient of the handicap as his total identity. In effect, it is the rejection of the social significance of the handicap and not rejection of the handicap per se."[4] However, people with chronic back pain who have developed this coping strategy may not be aware, now that they are hospitalized, that they must modify their behavior to convice others of the reality of their pain.

STATUS-FORCING AND LIMITS

There are social conventions for forcing persons into or for making them accept certain positions, however temporary. This process is called status-forcing.[5] Thus, in addition to deliberate covering up of pain as just described, other persons with low-back problems may be status-forced into keeping their pain expression invisible.

It may be made clear, as one back patient put it, "that they don't want to be around someone who complains all the time." Or others may express disbelief in the pain, especially when they have stakes in the sufferer's remaining active. "My neighbor will ask me to drive him some place and if I say I have to lie down he says, 'Man, you're always lying down. There's nothing wrong with you.' " In either case, failure to convince results in the status-forcing of the person in pain.

As a consequence of such status-forcing, a person with previous negative experiences in regard to pain endurance enters the hospital with an already "spoiled identity."[6] Such people are no longer coping satisfactorily, according to others' definitions, and will have picked up feelings that they are giving in too easily, not making the best of it—that they are deficient in character or weak-willed. In other words, they begin to view themselves as others view them. They know their pain is real but their identity is altered and—more importantly for our purposes—their behavior is altered as well. Consequences run the gamut from stoic teeth-gritters to those who feel driven to employ unacceptable tactics in order to convince.

In the hospital, no one explicitly tells patients of staff policy or of how the staff decides on suitable limits for pain expression. In fact, on wards such as the one we examined, there are differences in these conceptions, both within and between shifts. Patients learn about pain expression from the staff's explicit and implicit cues, cues pertaining to when and how to express pain, as well as to perceptions of pain legitimacy or lack thereof.

THE WHENS AND HOWS OF PAIN EXPRESSION

People with chronic pain learn not to express their pain constantly (cf., Chapter 9), and yet staff members sometimes need an outward manifestation so they can make an accurate assessment. Thus, it is acceptable for the patient to express pain at expected points—ideally, three to four hours after medication—but the rest of the time pain is expected to be endured.

One way that the staff status-forces patients into enduring pain is to place a value on stoicism. The nurse urges: "The doctor says you can have the medication in three hours, but why don't you try to wait awhile?" Or she forces the patient into longer endurance by stretching out the 15-minute promised return. Another tactic is to assign to the "complaining" patient a staff member who is able to "set limits, and treat him firmly, like a child." (Shades of Mrs. Abel!)

Staff members signal to patients by facial expression, body posture, or, when pain expression is excessive, by explicit statement, that expressions like loud moaning or whimpering are not acceptable. Or they simply avoid confrontation ("I get busy with bedpans"). Nurses also signal when they dislike that patient's mode of asking for relief—for instance, asking too often, whining, wheedling, or usurping the nurses' authority by phoning the doctor. Observations about the status of the pain are often explicitly stated. "You should (or shouldn't) be having that much pain." But, as noted earlier, these evaluations are based on comparison with other patients, a comparison of dubious value when dealing with low-back pain.

Nurses will admit that they are more sympathetic with the teeth-gritters than with the overly expressive patients, and that they will ask those who are enduring silently, "Wouldn't you like something?" Obviously, however, this tendency does not cover all passive and stoic patients, or there would not be stories such as the one concerning the woman who suddenly demanded to sign herself out because for three days she had not been given any pain medication, although she had a prn order. The nurse who described the transformation of this initially pleasant, placid patient was perplexed: "We didn't know she was in pain; we were waiting for her to ask."

Some patients never pick up the staff's cues; they are not aware that they have exceeded the limits. Sometimes, however, they know the staff's rules but cannot control their pain expression. An example is the patient (a nurse) whose unsuccessful fourth surgery and intense pain left her totally defenseless: "I hate to cry when someone else is around, but I can't help it."

To summarize the interactional bases for assessment: The patient is expected to take *some but not too much* responsibility in assessment and to cooperate by asking for relief, *at the right time* and *in the right way*. But this general rule may impede accurate pain assessment of patients who have established a pattern of covering up their pain or who feel status-forced into doing so; those who do not know that it is their responsibility to convince or who are not skilled at convincing; or those who cannot control their expression of pain.

EXPERIENTIAL ASSESSMENT

Patients are not the only ones to have biographies; staff members have psychosocial and pain biographies too. A significant component of assessment is the experiential background of the staff member doing the assessing. Thus, nurses and physiotherapists compare complaining back patients with their own experiences with pain. Comparison may also be based on a pain ideology which has been reinforced by experience, as demonstrated in the following quotation from a nurse whose mother was also a nurse: "I have had some back pain but I was brought up to feel if you have pain, bear it. There was not even any aspirin in my house."

Testing Tactics

When staff members are unsure of their assessments, they employ various tactics to test judgment. One tactic is to test for disparities between general behavior and the expression of pain. A nurse who found one patient's mode and frequency of expression unacceptable (the patient always began whimpering one hour after receiving medication) satisfied herself that the expression was disproportionate: "One day I stood outside her door and there was no sound. As soon as my shadow fell across her door, she started to whimper." This patient had employed the wrong strategy; it only proved to the nurse that the pain was really not very great.

Perhaps the best illustration of the influence of discrepant perspectives on assessment is provided by the differing views on distraction. Thus, persons in pain cannot send out pain signals all the time, if only because of the pure exhaustion of constantly focusing on pain. Yet, one can both be distracted and distract himself from pain. Under such circumstances one will feel it less and consequently express it less.

Patients acknowledge this of course. "When I was busy, I didn't think about the pain. Even if I didn't feel like getting up in the morning, once I got into the office I would be distracted from the pain." They know, however, that a price is often pain once the distraction is over: an increased awareness of the pain, fatigue, and irritability. Further, they know that when pain intensifies, nothing distracts them, and then they avoid being with others. To them, the potential of distraction is definitely no criterion for judging the legitimacy of their pain.

In the hospital, there is not only less to distract patients, but also they have an increased anxiety and focus on the pain, a fear of the unknown, and are continually reassessing their condition. (Am I improving? Am I developing a resistance to the medication?) Some personnel do recognize that if distraction were used as a strategy there might be greater endurance of pain. "Maybe if we took the time to talk to patients, they wouldn't need the medication." Others view distractability as proof, at least with certain patients, that the pain is not as intense as the patient would have them believe.

Stereotyping

Patients who send out the wrong behavioral cues or employ unfavorable tactics come to be stereotyped, which makes their job of convincing all the harder. (Stereotyping is a justificatory device for categorical acceptance or rejection of a group and as a screening or rationalizing device to maintain simplicity in perception and thinking.[7]) Stereotyping on an orthopedic ward derives, in large measure, from the staff's difficulty in coping with infinite pain. They would prefer a patient who presents the ideal surgical model of finite pain, who is relieved with Demerol the first few days, Percodan the next, aspirin thereafter, and finally sent happily home. In contrast, the staff feels much helplessness and frustration in dealing with unpredictable pain and illness, and this is compounded by patient behavior which, albeit unwittingly, reinforces the staff's frustration and helplessness. One way to cope with "difficult" or "demanding" patients is to see them as types. "Clock-watchers," "crocks," "malingerers," and "manipulators" are some of the labels. Let us look at each type, as it appears on this ward.

ADDICTION AND CLOCK WATCHING

Some people with long pain biographies expect that with hospitalization their pain will be allayed. But staff members expect that patients will necessarily have to suffer to some degree. Since the main form of pain expression in the U.S. is to ask for drugs, and since the main form of relief employed by staff is to administer drugs, the patient, paradoxically, is using the mode of expression expected to be most acceptable to staff, and yet it leads to a discounting type of assessment. "He's addicted" is uttered with varying degrees of contempt.

Staff attitudes on addiction apparently are quite typically American, as described by Lindesmith, who comments skeptically, "The conventional [American] view of addiction is that is is an escape mechanism for defective persons, variously characterized as 'inadequate,' 'inferior,' 'frustrated,' or 'psychopathic.' "[8] Hence, the patient's use of a supposedly unobjectionable avenue of relief may further taint an already spoiled identity and a questionable reputation.

Here, different views among the total staff are quite relevant. Some doctors feel the back cannot be treated before pain is somewhat relieved and the patient relaxed—thus the heavy use of drugs. Nurses, on the other hand, tend to be concerned not only because the patient will need more and more medication due to the unpredictable course of illness, but also because complicity has been forced upon them. "The doctor prescribed the drug, but we have to administer it."

Many nurses on the ward we observed saw "weaning" from drugs as an essential part of their job. The extent of their responsibility tied in with one of the structural conditions of the ward: unlike physicians on some other wards, orthopedic surgeons are not around very much. Nurses were particularly critical of a doctor when they felt that he had not confronted a patient with the intractability of the pain, so that the patient might "face up" to the dangers of addiction and endure the pain properly.

The problem may at times also be associated with the difficulty of coordinating the work shifts. "Sometimes you get a doctor who wants to cooperate in weaning a patient. You can agree, but there are all those shifts and someone is bound to view matters differently. Too many feel they would rather shut the patient up and have a quiet ward." Often, each professional plays it his or her own way. One nurse described the resident writing a weaker order than that prescribed by the doctor, the patient then complaining to the doctor, the doctor then changing the order, the resident changing it again— and all the while the nurse taking as much leeway as possible.

Patients, too, worry about addiction, but their resolve has often been lowered by experienced pain and the constant specter of increased pain. If one has a long biography of chronic pain, one has also a ritualized drug regimen based on previous trial and error. Such people must cede *control* of their drugs to the staff when they enter the hospital, but they are not ready to cede *use* of their drugs until they are certain that the recommended therapy has worked. The nursing staff is not infrequently ready to wean them from medication before they are ready to be weaned.

In addition, people with chronic pain know that if they wait until the pain reaches a high peak, the normal dosage will not relieve it. They know that when pain is extremely intense, the muscles tense and pain increases. They have, therefore, developed a pattern of anticipating their pain needs. Though an order has been left for medication every three to four hours, their pain peak may return long before that, and they are concerned that there be no mistiming. They are also concerned lest their peak conflict with the staff's schedule— that is, come at a time when the nurses are busy with other patients or during the change shifts. To the patient, a short wait may seem like an eternity.

Add to this at least one previous bad experience with hospital mistiming, and you have patients "anticipating," "on the buzzer early," and stereotyped as a clock watcher. Their desperate behavior —keeping a time sheet on the tissue box, begging for drugs before the allotted interval has passed—reinforces the previous assessment that they are addicted. Such patients believe they have learned the rules of the hospital game, but from the nurses' perspective they have learned the wrong rules. Their behavior reaffirms the clock-watcher stereotype.

PSYCHOGENIC STEREOTYPING AND "CROCKS"

A very great impediment to the patient's successful convincing of staff members is the widespread psychogenic stereotyping that is

associated with low-back pain. With the popularization of psycho-
analytic concepts, people are all too ready to use them, pejoratively,
as a means of labeling. Staff are no more immune to this temptation
than anyone else, and terms like "paranoid" and "schizophrenic"
were liberally used on this as on many other wards. One patient, for
instance, was characterized as a masochist because he always wanted
a shot instead of pills.

The literature frequently refers to the back with such meta-
phorical phrases as "an emotional weather vane." As Berland and
Addison explain: "Probably the overwhelming emotion provoked by
the sharp pain and by the serious disability that comes with a back
attack is fear."[9] There is a circuitous quality to pain—worry and tension increase pain, which further increases worry and tension—and
low-back pain is especially vulnerable to this phenomenon.

Psychogenic assessment, however, goes far beyond this acknowledged reciprocal relationship between back pain and emotions.
Psychiatrist Thomas Szasz has developed the concept of "painful persons" who produce undiagnosable pain in order to create meaning in
their lives and who crave medical and surgical intervention to legitimate their role as sick persons.[10] An indication of the widespread
acceptance of this concept lies in the fact that a name has been de-
vised to stereotype it. Patients who have vague and untreatable
psychosomatic complaints (including pain) but no discernible physical pathology are often called "crocks" by hospital personnel.

Opinions and authorities differ, however. For every proponent
of psychiatric evaluation prior to lengthy exploration for organic
causation in the treatment of low-back pain, one can find a coun-
terpart warning that "unfamiliarity and inexplicability far too often
tempt the physician to brand the symptoms as psychogenic."[11-12]
(The mind–body dualism really works overtime on issues like "intractable" chronic pain.)

Additional complicating factors intervene. Patients who have
suffered prolonged pain are quite likely to manifest signs of depression, making it difficult to determine which occurred first, the pain
or the depression. Too often their biographies will reveal evidence of
psychic stress, making psychogenic evaluation a convenient catchall.

There is no definitive answer to the chicken-and-egg question of
low-back pain and emotions, but it is important to consider the consequences of doubts raised through general acceptance of the linkage.
Sometimes the staff's psychogenic stereotyping is aggravated by the
patient's behavior. A patient may appear to be a crock when either
inarticulate or overly articulate, or when seemingly not very intelligent. Persons are also labeled because they have characteristics

that remind staff of other crocks, or because they have fallen into a pattern of overacting to legitimate their pain. Assessment may also be related to the drugs that patients are taking; if the drugs affect their rationality, the psychotic image is compounded.

Psychogenic assessment leads quite naturally to the assumption that since back pain cannot always be verified clinically, it can be "used." "It is filling a need; if they didn't have back surgery they would have something else." "These people want an operation for sympathy. There's nothing like an operation for sympathy." Judgments regarding pain as a secondary gain are not so much a denial of pain as they are assessments about "giving in," and they tie in with feelings (regarding addiction) that patients should face up to their pain.

In part, too, this particular stereotyping can be associated with the interlocking of patient reputation with physician reputation. For instance, a number of back patients we observed were patients of one physician, whose unorthodoxy was an annoyance to the nursing staff. His heavy use of drugs (he believed strong medication was necessary for relaxation of muscles) conflicted with their anxiety regarding addiction. His hours for rounds (between midnight and 2:00 A.M.) conflicted with normal hospital schedule. Also, controversy surrounded his surgical methods, since he had pioneered new procedures. The staff was convinced that this physician attracted a certain type of undesirable patient, a type referred by doctors who were fed up with their complaints. These patients were labeled from the moment they arrived. Ironically, not only were they unaware that they should be working their way out of this "crock" assessment, but they referred to their doctor as a "miracle man."

Malingerers and Uses of Pain

Suspicion of the use of pain as an "out" is manifested in yet another stereotype, that of the malingerer. This is seen particularly, but not exclusively in industrial accident cases or in those with pending litigation. As one orthopedic surgeon said: "There are people who love to be disabled. I've seen thousands of people over the years, and half of them hate their work. Unconsciously they are looking for a way out."

Surely, the relationship of low-back pain to opting out of work is related to the type of work a person does. Back pain has a different meaning for the professional who can pace his work and get off his feet than it does for the hod carrier or the telephone repairperson. The staff may be correct in regarding some patients as malingerers,

but they are just as surely stereotyping many who are expressing
genuine pain.

Negotiators and Manipulators

The generally unequal division of power between staff and patient
adds, because of the stereotyping of patients as "manipulators," to
the staff's problem of making accurate pain assessments and the patient's task of legitimating pain.

In these days of increased "people power," it is noteworthy that
hospitals and clinics are not at all organized around patients' rights.
One might reason, for instance, that people have a right to express
their pain, and a right to have it relieved. The staff has a comparable
right (given adequate reasons) to give relief, deny it, or "wait it out."
However logical this reasoning may appear on paper, it is not represented in the actual distribution of power. Patients may make
requests, but power and authority fall on the side of the staff. When
a patient makes too many demands or appears too knowledgeable,
staff members may read this as a sign that they are losing control.
Seen as stepping on the exclusive domain of the staff, such a patient
is often stereotyped as a manipulator, with the result that both patient and staff begin to think of themselves as adversaries.

The patient is also hampered because there is no one person
with whom to negotiate and requests must be made of a variety of
health care persons. The patient sees them on a one-to-one basis, but
these individuals have the advantage of coming together at some
point and sharing information regarding the patient. Our colleague,
Marcella Davis, remarked in one of her fieldnotes:

> One hears staff members say, "Well, he told me so and so," and
> others say, "He told me something quite different." The point is that
> the patient may be trying to locate whom to address his statements
> to . . . if he is not socialized to what to do and how to behave but
> must find out through trial and error, it is not unusual for him to be
> asking his questions a bit differently from each different staff person.
> Also, he may be asking each at a different time so the situation may
> have changed or his perception of it may have changed so that his
> request becomes altered according to this perceived or actual
> change. . . . Rather than exploring with the patient what the sit-
> uation is all about, a more economical means is adopted by the staff
> and the patient is promptly labeled a "manipulator."

A source of frustration for some patients is their expectation that,
once hospitalized, they will see more of their doctors and learn more

about their back disease than they actually do. Yet, as previously pointed out, surgeons may be on the ward only infrequently. Add to this a doctor who makes his rounds at midnight, when a drugged patient cannot remember the most pressing questions, and the problem is further exacerbated. Or add a third party, a healthy member of the patient's family, who is going to be assertive on the patient's behalf, and there is further trouble. Just as clock watchers have learned the wrong rules of the hospital game, so too have the manipulators.

VARIATIONS AND IMPLICATIONS

Obviously, there is wide variation in the staff's reading of behavioral signs, just as there is variety in the choice of indicators upon which judgments about both pain and patient adherence to the unwritten interactional rules are made. Similarly variable is the extent of patients' awareness of the discrepancies between their own and the staff's perspectives on their pain. Those being judged may not know what judgments are being made; if they do know, they may not know on what criteria or they may disagree with the verdict.

The importance for pain work lies in the relationship between the way staff members read the signs and the resulting assessment and relief, and in the fact that any tension produced by conflicting perspectives further tightens muscles and increases pain. As noted earlier, many pass through their hospitalization with only minor or no legitimating problems. Many are aware of the organizational conditions and accept the distribution of power with as much equanimity as they can muster: "I know the nurses are not going to deviate from written instructions, so I don't ask." And many, if unhappy during their hospital stay, quickly put unhappiness aside when they are home, particularly if they are at last relieved of pain.

The problems attendant on assessment and legitimating are by no means confined to orthopedic patients. The ambiguity surrounding low-back pain has to do with its etiology and visibility, relief procedures, and degree of endurance. These and other dimensions of ambiguity may vary from ward to ward, but where ambiguity of pain is salient (whether orthopedic or not), the discrepant staff–patient perspectives will result in similar assessment and legitimating problems.

Other organizational features of the ward—minimal information for assessment, nonaccountability for psychosocial factors, experiential assessment based on personal ideology, the interlocking of patient and doctor reputation, rotating shifts, the inaccessibility of doctors and the concomitant increased responsibility of nurses, the unequal distribution of power and diminished negotiative rights for patients—also vary in salience from ward to ward.

The main point is that when the organizational features of a particular ward are disregarded, interactional consequences will circle back and result in increased pain work. If the staff members do not think organizationally and interactionally about their pain work—do not see it as a cooperative venture in which the patient is actively involved—they will continue to be less understanding of patient behavior and to rely on the simplification provided by stereotyping.

Staff members must then attend not only to the management of patients' pain expression but also to the management of their own reactions to that expression. Otherwise, the consequences can be low expression and less work for staff, but increased strain on patients, with profound effects upon their abilities to live with their illnesses and upon their attitudes toward future hospitalizations.

REFERENCES

1. Wiles, P. 1959. *Essentials of orthopaedics.* 3d ed. Boston: Little, Brown, p. 52.

2. Inman, V. T., and Saunders, J. B. 1947. Anatomico-physiological aspects of injuries of the intervertebral disc. *Journal of Bone and Joint Surgery* 29:641.

3. Wiener, C. L. 1975. The burden of rheumatoid arthritis: tolerating the uncertainty. *Social Science and Medicine* 9:97–104.

4. Davis, M. Z. 1973. *Living with multiple sclerosis: a social psychological analysis.* Springfield, Ill.: Charles C Thomas, p. 18.

5. Strauss, A. L. 1969. *Mirrors and masks.* San Francisco: Sociology Press, pp. 77–84.

6. Goffman, E. 1963. *Stigma: notes on the management of spoiled identity.* Englewood Cliffs, N.J.: Prentice-Hall, p. 4.

7. Allport, G. W. 1954. *The nature of prejudice.* Cambridge, Mass.: Addison-Wesley, pp. 189–204.

8. Lindesmith, A. R. 1968. *Addiction and opiates.* Chicago: Aldine, p. 17.

9. Berland, T., and Addison, R. G. 1973. *Living with your bad back.* New York: Bantam Books, p. 32, 141.

10. Szasz, T. S. 1968. The psychology of persistent pain. A portrait of l'homme douloureux. In *Pain,* proceedings of the International Symposium on Pain, organized by the Laboratory of Psy-

chophysiology, Faculty of Sciences, University of Paris, eds. A. Soulairac et al. . . New York: Academic Press, pp. 111–112.

11.   Engle, G. L. 1959. Psychogenic pain and the pain-prone patient. *American Journal of Medicine* 26:899–918.

12.   Hanraets, R. R. M. J. 1957. *The degenerative back and its differential diagnosis.* Translated by M. E. Hollander. Princeton, N.J.: Van Nostrand, p. 649.

The Relieving of Pain

9

The relieving of pain is one of the principal pain tasks in hospitals. This would seem to be a relatively straightforward task, complicated only by technical, physiologic, or pharmacologic difficulties. But the job can often become quite complicated, as the foregoing chapters illustrate. Readers will find that the guidelines offered here can be applied to virtually all situations involving the relief of pain.

MAIN-JOB BALANCING

Let us begin with a simple case. We all know what it's like to wake up in the morning with a headache. Without much internal debate about the desirability of swallowing aspirin or some other painkiller, most of us readily reach for it. Some, however, would rather suffer the pain because of previous experiences with side effects, whether slight or severe, from palliative drugs. These people are explicitly balancing those side effects against either the inconvenience of the pain itself or an estimation of how it might affect their day. Those who reach unhesitatingly for the aspirin do not need to balance, or are doing it implicitly ("the pain is not worth bearing all day," or "it's worth going upstairs for the aspirin since the pain's not disappearing").

Within the hospital, a major balancing occurs between the two analytically distinguishable activities of relieving the patient's pain and doing the main job. Sometimes the main job pertains to diagnosis, surgery, or treatment and may involve doing a procedure "on" a particular patient, monitoring a machine to which the patient is hooked up, giving a test, making the patient breathe deeply, or cleaning a wound. These are important jobs, they may indeed be vital jobs, and they are almost always associated with the patient's primary trajectory—that is, with the patient's illness.

Sometimes the main job itself is to relieve pain, as with the chronic back pain sufferers discussed in the preceding chapter. At other times, the main job and pain relief are so closely related that they cannot be separated. A patient with a coronary condition may be given medication immediately on request because the pain may be an indication of potential coronary danger. Similarly, the alleviation of pain experienced by patients with kidney transplants has high priority because the greater a patient's anxiety, the greater the chance the transplant will be rejected.

It is possible that pain may be so closely associated with a main job—say, with proper diagnosis—that the physician must pay a great deal of attention to the pain itself. She may not want to relieve it until she has had a chance to observe, for that observation might give her valuable diagnostic cues. In this case the patient, if the pain is not extremely severe, will have to experience some discomfort until the main job—diagnosis—is done.

It is clear that decisions involving "pain interference" must follow a balancing of priorities. Does the pain itself interfere with the main job? If not, then unless it's quite severe, staff will wait to give relief. One obstetric nurse sternly instructed a complaining mother-to-be: "You're just going to have to cope. You're the only one who can do it. I can't do it for you. They will give you what you need after you have dilated enough, but if it's too soon, it will slow the labor and eventually will just hurt again. So you will just have to learn to cope." In short, do your immediate job, an essential part of the larger job, and then if necessary you will get the pain medication.

If the pain interferes very much—as when a child is screaming and squirming—then pain is relieved even if work on the main job must wait; otherwise it may not get done or may have to be redone. These are judgments made by the potential reliever, and they may be contested by patients who think differently or who are angry during and after procedures. The reliever may also change his mind and cease doing a procedure when he sees how much pain the patient is enduring, especially if there is infliction of pain in addition to on-going pain. Affecting that judgment, of course, are organizational considerations such as his relationship with the particular patient , and the amount of competition for his time and energy there is from other patients.

Complicating the interference calculus, then, is another that pertains to the degree of urgency of the main task. If something is judged as "needs to be done quickly," then relief is likely to be put off until the urgent job is done. A medically vital job, such as one involving lifesaving measures, will take precedence. In emergency rooms a combination of tight time budgets and pressing measures means that patients may have to endure pain until later. Conversely, even in emergency rooms, if the medical job is not pressing and the flow of work is slow, then the patient is more likely to receive a painkiller immediately and even be allowed time for it to take effect before being "worked on."

Because these delicate balances are judgmental in character, they may cause debate not only between patient and staff but among the staff itself. For instance, we once observed a sharp disagreement between a neurosurgeon and a consulting psychiatrist about giving pain relief. The surgeon was quite willing to put a dorsal stimulator "in" the patient in order to relieve her tremendous pain. He could see no reason to forego this procedure: however, the psychiatrist believed the patient's pain was symptomatic of deeper psychic processes and that its relief would not get at the basic problem; furthermore, he was balancing his recommendation about relief against the difficulty of removing the dorsal stimulator if it did not, as he predicted, actually relieve the patient. Such staff disagreements grow, of course, when patients have long hospitalizations with difficult illness and pain trajectories or when they develop negative reputations among the staff. In either case (as with Mrs. Abel, and as we shall see with Mrs. Price later), there will be intense and frequent staff dissension over the issue of relief.

On the other hand, common ideologies or relatively routine pain situations virtually insure a fair degree of staff unanimity. On a cardiac pulmonary unit we observed, the staff generally agreed that postoperative pain, highly intense and added to by frequent daily regimens involving inflicted pain, ought to be continually relieved and minimized by properly timed medication. (In fact, it was only the researcher who disagreed somewhat with the staff, for she perceived there could be more efficient relief on this ward if certain organizational conditions were changed, since the existing ones frequently led to mistiming so that the patient did not get medication soon enough.)

RECIPROCAL EXPECTATIONS CONCERNING RELIEF WORK

Relieving pain may seem to be a task only for the staff, but it is one which is shared with the patient. Whether agreement about this is explicit or implicit, there is work for each to do. Since the patient's tasks are less obvious, let us look first at the following typical set of expectations.

For one thing, the patient must sensibly balance the need for pain relief against the main job itself—"sensibly" meaning that the staff's judgment has to be trusted to a certain extent. If it is judged necessary that a patient wait for relief, then the patient must endure properly. "Enduring properly" has at least three components. First, the amount and kind of expression of pain should be appropriate to the amount and kind of pain that actually exists. Second, the patient must try to wait until the designated time for relief rather than rushing the staff as it carries on other business. Third, expression of pain should not interfere with any main task being performed in the patient's behalf.

The staff members also expect that they, *not* the patient, will do the relieving; that is their job. So the patient is supposed to surrender all pain medications on entry to the ward and not hoard or stockpile as did Mrs. Abel. In order that staff can do its relief work successfully, it needs the patient's cooperation in properly flashing cues for pain and in making explicit requests for relief. How else can a busy staff relieve pain efficiently and successfully? (One sees this expectation that patients will cooperate, will take some responsibility in obtaining relief when surgical nurses tell patients to ask for medications if and when they hurt or ask: "Do you need a pain shot?") Of course the patient's requests should be honest, or else they will confuse or even play havoc with the staff's assessments concerning the need for relief.

That is true not only of requesting too much, but of requesting too little. For instance, a prospective mother who has her own extreme standards of "all pain possible, no relief while delivering" can prove bothersome to staff members: possibly because they simply don't agree and are frustrated at not being able to carry out their duty when the patient is so obviously in great pain; possibly because the patient endures just so far and then breaks down at an inopportune time and requires medication. The frequently encountered stoics can also present problems, since pain can be an important indicator, but mostly since there really seems to be no need for them to suffer so much. A friend of ours who underwent surgery waved aside the prescribed medication for her postoperative pain, requesting only aspirin, for she neither wanted side effects from the medication nor felt she would buckle under her pain. The nurses were very upset, since they were primed for her postop pain with the doctor's medication order. She upset them further by finally asking her physician to prescribe only aspirin after despairing of convincing them that her request was legitimate.

When a patient makes requests for relief, the staff expects that he will not play one staff member against another. This amounts to assuming that the patient will make an honest request of the appropriate relief agent and accept his or her judgment on the proper kind and amount of relief. No turning to a second or third staff member when not satisfied with the first. No going "upstairs" either.

There are other implicit rules, or assumptions, behind the expectation that patients will properly make their requests. For instance, concerning style: ordinary rules of politeness and tact certainly govern the way patients should ask for relief. The rules of politeness include not asking too demandingly or nastily and not screaming or shouting. Of course, a patient who is on the ragged edge from intractable pain, anxiety, or fear of dying is more likely to be allowed some latitude, but the rules are only relaxed, not abolished. (Mrs. Abel broke those rules and was punished for doing so, though some staff members finally came to realize that her pain was genuine and great.)

Besides style, there are also considerations of time—when relief should and should not be requested. However reasonable it may seem that someone should ask for pain relief, there are certain times when answering the request can be very difficult. These times include during a change of shift or directly thereafter when the personnel are just getting underway with high-priority jobs. Another time would be when it's obvious that a staff member is engaged in an emergency duty or is attending busily to a roommate's needs. Patients who ask for relief directly after arriving on the ward, while other procedures are underway, sometimes evoke annoyance because staff feels their pain is not so great that they cannot wait a bit. On a ward filled with patients hospitalized for neurological disorders, those who asked for pain medications during the admission process tended to be defined as potentially "demanding." Thus, the building of a reputation begins early and often negatively.

The places where patients ask for relief can also make a difference. While at x-ray, they should not *unduly* indicate pain or otherwise request relief, but they should wait until they are back on the ward. The implicit rules of this game also require that a patient refrain from requesting higher quantities of painkillers than he knows have been ordered by the physician, or at shorter intervals than they have been prescribed, unless there is very good justification for such requests.

How do staff members teach these rules to patients? Because the rules are mainly implicit, the teaching also tends to be implicit: by the tone of voice, use of one's body as an indicator of "not now, too busy," and so on. Teaching can be more explicit, however: "I've told you before, don't ask before your next medication is due!" Or staff simply ignores the patient's light when it's been on too often before the scheduled time for medication. Sometimes a nurse angrily scolds the patient for breaking a rule, a rule sometimes so implicit that the patient hasn't yet realized it existed.

How and when do patients learn the rules? Presumably they learn by being sensitive, or at least not too insensitive, to the staff's cues and explicit directives. They also learn as on the intensive burn unit, through the coaching of other patients. Remember, too, that many patients, ill from chronic diseases, have had repeated hospitalizations. However, whether or not a patient chooses to abide by a given rule is quite another matter.

The staff's side of pain-relieving tasks is characterized by certain expectations that are easily comprehended. The patient has the right to have pain relief ("other things being equal") and the staff's job is to do that appropriately, with knowledgeability and proper timing. If a staff member cannot do this, or has not the legal right to do so, then he or she should manage to appoint the proper agent to do the job. Relief should be given in an appropriate style: that is, willingly, cooperatively, and politely—not grudgingly, reluctantly, or nastily. Potential side effects should be managed efficiently. If relief is delayed or foregone, then there should be adequate reason for that.

When staff members unaccountably deny these expectations, and break these implicit rules, then a patient might accuse them of negligence or incompetence, although the accusations are not always made aloud. But when someone is really angry or outraged:

> *That night I had a cramp in my stomach and asked the nurse for some kind of pain medicine. Since the Demerol had been discontinued, she called the intern. I told him I had a cramp in my stomach. He asked if I was getting my period! I pointed out to him*

that my stomach was nowhere near my reproductive system, so that
I could hardly mistake a stomach cramp for menstrual cramps.

In its turn, the staff can accuse the patient of breaking rules pertaining to relief. The woman just quoted recounts that she went over the head of the ward's resident by telephone to get stronger pain medication: "He was furious with me."

ASSESSING THE PAIN

The phenomenon of pain assessment is not new to readers of this book. They have seen it in full-blown form in the previous chapter, have witnessed some anguishing scenes involving staff assessment of Mrs. Abel's pains, and perhaps have even noted its implicit presence in our discussions of inflicted pain and surgical pain. We shall draw on all those discussions here as we address the more general issues surrounding the related activities of assessing and relieving pain.

We begin with a note written after observing at a clinic conference involving an arthritic patient. It illustrates several themes that will appear prominently in the following pages.

> When I spotted a woman and her husband sitting outside the room, I took a guess that she was to be presented. She is 56 years old, and worked in a bed spring factory. Pain started in her knees; she continued to work but complained to fellow workers. It got increasingly worse, but she had two weeks until vacation and was pushing to make it, but couldn't: "The last day I went in I knew I couldn't go on working . . ."[11] Since then she has gotten much worse. Pain in shoulders, hip. Till December, she was going out. Now she doesn't go out at all, except to come to clinic. Can't get comfortable at home; moves around from chair to chair. Up at night. Has a terrible time getting into bathtub; bathed that day on her knees. Takes only aspirin: "They don't want me to take anything else until they find out what's causing it."
>
> The staff was assembling inside the room. The doctor who was presenting the patient gave a quick rundown, varying from what she herself had told me, as follows: said it started in the hip (she said knees) and her knees hurt slightly (she didn't sound to me as if anything was "slightly"). The doctor added she had a lot of stiffness, and had told him it took a long time to get out of bed. She had been coming to the clinic for two months: "Pain has gotten worse all the time." I jotted down a couple of comments: "Whether it is true pain or weakness is almost impossible to document," and "There is no way we can move her that she doesn't have pain." He suggested the group watch her walk and try to get up from a chair, then: "Maybe some of you can decide if it

is pain or weakness." She was told to walk back and forth, and to get up and down from the chair. She was wearing a heavy leather coat, and Dr. Smith said it was too hard to see anything and would she mind putting on a gown. Then they decided she should lie on the table. Another doctor then tried manipulating her in all kinds of positions, holding her leg and having her push, saying: "Don't let me bend it." No one asked about pain at this point. She showed nothing on her face, and I was struck by the contrast between what she had clearly communicated to me less than ten minutes ago, and how impersonal it became when reported by the doctor. The physical therapist sitting next to me said: "She couldn't do that well when I saw her for the first time." Shortly later: "She's having less pain." I said: "She told me she's having more pain." The physical therapist asked: "Mrs. Smith, are you having more or less pain than when you first came in?" The patient answered: "More."

After the manipulation, they started to question her, and she was very articulate. "Sometimes it hurts so bad in the shoulders that it seems like my nightgown or housecoat irritates it more. Sometimes I can't even wear a bra." Someone asked: "When the shoulders hurt, do the hips hurt too?" "Maybe the shoulders are so bad that I'm not concentrating on my hips. But when I sit for awhile, I can't get up." There were further questions like "Do you have more trouble going up stairs than down?" Then she was ushered out to await the verdict.

The doctor who had done the manipulating said the muscles appeared strong. "I don't understand even after examining her. We have to assume, if she's honest, it must be pain and not weakness." There was further discussion along these lines until another physician said: "I don't see the problem. It can be both. I don't know why we have to belabor the difference." Someone started a discussion of possible polymyositis. Part of the question pertained to whether such a disease could exist with the primary symptom being pain.

The manipulating doctor said at one point: "I certainly have the feeling that she is not psychoneurotic," to which another said quietly: "I'm not so sure." The presenting physician said: "I've seen her four times and she doesn't seem overwhelmed by emotional problems. She would like to work." Someone said: "It may be subconscious, but at least it is not conscious. She tried to overcome everything we did here."

They decided to do a muscle biopsy, and then one physician cited a study showing such a test was the least positive diagnostic tool for this disease. He got them to agree that if it was positive then that was clear, but if negative they shouldn't believe that proved anything. Dr. Jones: "That's true of a lot of our tests," but another doctor reviewed her other abnormalities, saying: "She has signs of polymyositis and we have to ask why." When he was reviewing those abnormalities, the doubter: "*I'd*

like to have a nickle for every time that's true of other inpatients." There
was some talk of putting her on a low dose of Prednisone as a therapeutic test, but it was decided that was "not fair to do."

They agreed finally on a muscle biopsy, which they wanted to do on her
as an outpatient to the clinic. Three physicians went to talk to her and
her husband. The main problem was arranging a date—the husband
had taken so much time off work he could take no more. They agreed to
do it the following Tuesday; one week away. I asked her later if the
conference had been rough on her. She was noncommital but her
husband said: "She'd do anything to get over the pain." I asked if there
was any talk of relief while she awaited the test, and she replied no,
other than what I heard in the examining room, when they asked her if
she took aspirin. "So I guess that's all they want me to take."

In the preceding study we have seen staff discussions and disagreements about *how much,* if any, pain there is; *what kind* of pain
it is (psychological or organic); questions of the patient's *credibility;*
the issue of which indicators might reflect the pain, including the patient's *pain expression;* and, hovering over this discussion, the issue
of relief measures appropriate to the particular pain. In the next
pages, we shall see how these issues are related to larger aspects of
assessing and relieving pain.

CREDIBILITY: CONDITIONS AND CALCULUS

Pain has one quite peculiar property: "Only the person who is experiencing (feeling) pain can directly perceive it."[1] This means that
other people must rely upon the verbal report of the person who is
claiming that he is in pain, or they must interpret his gestures as
indicators of pain. "When onlookers expect pain, then crying,
groaning, grimacing, wincing, perspiring, or the clenching of teeth
may easily convince them. If they do not expect him to have pain,
then he must make his pain plausible,"[1] that is, manage to legitimate
its existence. There is, then, an issue of credibility—either of the
claim to pain, or of the person as a believable individual.

Of course, there are countless instances when the question of
credibility does not arise, as when someone simply announces he has
developed a slight headache, or turns an ankle and later grimaces as
he walks. Even if he says his headache is killing him, or remarks as
he hobbles along that his ankle now hurts like crazy, we do not usually doubt him. At the other extreme, people like Mrs. Abel or the
back-pain "complainers" encounter genuine difficulties in legitimating their pains to others who are skeptical. These contrasting

situations already suggest different conditions of ease and difficulty in establishing (or assuming) credibility.

Among the conditions making for ease of credibility are the following: (1) when the pain situation seems so clear that ordinarily one does not even think of raising the issue of credibility, or when there are visible indicators which others can read, like facial swelling or a bump on the head. In these cases claims of pain are unlikely to be contested. In short, there is what we might term a calculus which involves an equivalence of claimed pain and illness.

In hospitals, the patient's credibility—insofar as it rests on this kind of calculus—is strengthened by at least two other conditions. First, if the claimed pain matches the expected illness trajectory, then staff is very unlikely to doubt the self-assessment. In some instances, as we have seen, even if the pain is more or different from what is expected, an experienced staff may suspect complications. Staff members, of course, need to be experienced in that trajectory. Otherwise they don't know what to expect. A second condition pertaining to this calculus is the degree of trust which the staff places in the patient. If they believe the patient to be honest, credible, and generally cooperative, then a report about pain is likely to seem plausible. Of course, if all the preceding conditions obtain (trust, expected trajectory, visible indicators), there is virtually no likelihood that the staff will be skeptical about a patient's claims.

Before examining the conditions which mitigate against such accommodating reception of patients' claims, we might pause to contrast a few conditions under which the staff may wonder about how to judge a pain when the issue of credibility does not arise. With very young children it sometimes is most difficult to tell how much actual pain they may be experiencing, or whether they are just lonely, anxious, or frightened. The same is true when a patient is partly disoriented or speaks a foreign language that no staff member understands. Personnel sometimes wonder, too, about patients who are almost completely nonsentient. Do they feel pain? Once on a kidney transplant unit, we observed that the staff was probably underestimating the amount of pain, indeed sometimes missing the pain altogether, because the pain was masked by other discomforting symptoms and complications. Staff members sometimes also recognize difficulty in assessing pain when a patient is very stoic and tightly controls pain expression.

The interesting thing about the stoic is that he stands the credibility issue on its head. Because he makes little or no claim to pain, the staff is likely to underestimate his pain. Experienced nurses, or those who know the particular patient, may, of course, be suspicious

of small claims or lack of pain expression and use tactics to get him
to admit to the truth. They will try to persuade him that it is all right
to express pain in appropriate measure. They are essentially relief
prompters, prompting the patient to speak his rightful lines. There
is, in other words, another important calculus, touched on earlier.
This involves an equivalence between the actual amount of pain and
the amount or kind of expression deemed appropriate. Mark Zborowski has reported that Americans of Italian descent customarily
express their pain so loudly and broadly—at least it seems so to staff
members of other ethnic backgrounds—that questions about using
the expression as an accurate indicator of pain are raised among the
hospital staff.[2] As we have seen, when personnel begin to doubt the
credibility of a patient or begin to regard him as a demanding, uncooperative person, then that affects their judgments about what his
expressions really mean. Also, if a downward cycle of poor and even
hostile relationships develops between patient and staff, then patient
credibility sinks correspondingly. If the illness trajectory seems pretty
much on course, then the expression calculus will seem even more
out of alignment.

CREDIBILITY: TACTICS AND COUNTERTACTICS

When nurses and other staff members are dubious about a claim to
pain, they talk among themselves about the physical signs that the
patient exhibits, and also about the pain expression and even the
person's character. Their observations can lead to a discounting of
claims concerning the amount of pain or even its presence. Said one
nurse about orthopedic patients: "They make a lot of fuss that everything hurts when they have visitors, but they can get into all
kinds of positions the rest of the time." If nurses are dubious or uncertain about a claim, they will use standard tactics to "test." "I hate
to go into the room, but the patient is moaning. What do I do? I tell
her she is doing fine, and leave the room. When I come back if she is
still moaning and asking for medication, I give her something." This
nurse added that it is difficult, with this kind of patient, "to tell if
she's playacting." Her tactic is interesting because it is based on the
assumption that the patient—if she has no real pain—will reduce or
stop claiming pain providing one waits long enough. Of course the
patient might just give up trying to persuade this potential relief
agent!

Another tactic is to space out the scheduling of a medication. If
the patient doesn't notice or complain, the pain must be less than
claimed. Nurses also engage in sleuthing; they observe the patient

when she's not noticing to see if her crying stops or her body position or other physical signs indicate less pain than claimed. The use of placebos is also a tool in this game of maybe yes/maybe no. If the claimed pain is reduced after the use of a placebo, then the claim was too strong or should never have been considered. The placebo need not even consist of a false medication. One physical therapist thought of ultrasonic treatments given to orthopedic patients as placebos; these are not genuine relievers of pain. Hence, when a patient after a treatment said, "That's great!" the therapist simply discounted in her own mind the patient's claim to pain. Even physical signs, however, can be discredited, as when a psychologist who had tested a patient on a rehabilitation ward wrote his own assessment: She was "monumentally dependent, exhibiting an exaggerated inability to do things . . . a chance to use her disability."

Most often, of course, patients need not legitimate their pain. However, when personnel show skepticism toward self-assessments and requests for relief, or when proper relief is not forthcoming, then patients may lose patience, grow angry, and make demands. Even the staff's use of placebos, when recognized or revealed, can be countered. One nurse told the researcher that patients say: "Look I know I've had placebos in the hospital and I know they work for me, but I know they won't work at home when I have to take care of my family and face all the problems of daily living. I will feel the pain if I need my medication."

A patient's redoubling of effort, especially when accompanied by angry responses to the staff's actions, can quickly bring about the downward interactional spiral which is difficult indeed for anyone to reverse. We have seen this process in Mrs. Abel's case. When she began her attempts to convince the staff that she really did have considerable pain by crying and complaining, she only managed to persuade them that she had very little pain or at least much less than she "pretended." The more she attempted to legitimate her pain during the first months of hospitalization, the more she gave the impression of being "overdemanding," of not being honest about her assertions. After her readmission, when she insisted on even greater pain, the nurses discounted this claim because she would sleep right through the night or would forget her so-called pain when she became engrossed in conversation. Like many patients, then, Mrs. Abel adopted tactics designed to insure that her own assessment of pain would receive proper credence. Her tactics sometimes worked, but they often irritated and finally angered the staff. The staff, too, used standard countertactics—routine modes of dealing with patients like Mrs. Abel. They finally discounted her assessments almost entirely, turned a deaf ear to criticisms, gave her drugs at longer intervals than she imagined the physician had ordered, spelled each other in the onerous task of ministering to her needs and demands, and ended by almost completely withdrawing from her. This entire course of events also vividly illustrates how the staff members' daily assessments of pain can be profoundly affected by the snowballing of collective judgments. The daily assessment does not stand on its own.

Apropos of collective judgments, whenever the staff members are doubtful or skeptical about a patient's claims to pain (especially when the claiming tactics have misfired), there is likely to be lively discussion of the situation. Personnel feed information to each other about observed behavior and other physical indicators, concurring or disagreeing in their estimations and evaluations. Earlier we over-heard one of those discussions in the form of a diagnostic confer-ence, but there are also the more run-of-the-mill ward conferences and the many informal discussions at the nursing stations and in the halls. Judgments are not fixed for all time and reassessments are con-tinuously made. Nor are estimations of pain always revised downward, since staff often does discover its misestimations and misreadings, or the patient becomes better at persuading the staff that new conditions have developed. ("When we first saw [an ampu-tee] she was complaining so much, we . . . didn't know that she had an infection in the stump." Or in the instance of a kidney transplant patient mentioned earlier who had a vague complaint of discomfort which was treated with back rubs, she was later discovered to have an advanced infection which fulminated into septicemia.)

RELIEF WORK: DIMENSIONS AND COMPLEXITIES

Just as there is an assessment task there is also a relief task, which, to be done properly, depends of course on the proper assessment of pain. Specific relief jobs can be very simple, but some turn out to be very complicated. Aside from difficulties in assessing pain and dif-ficulties that sometimes occur in finding a relief measure that will really work with particular pains, the complexities of relieving are re-lated to the fact that it is being done not by the patient or his family at home, but by a group of strangers (the staff) in an organization (hospital or clinic).

Furthermore, if we think of relieving only in terms of matching a medication to a pain, we tremendously oversimplify what is in-volved. There is a question of what kind of relief measure is to be carried out. If medication is required, then in what amounts? How frequently? In what combinations? There is even the question of who is legitimately to prescribe the relief measure. Also, who is to be the actual agent of relief? Considering that there can be disagreement not only between the patient and the staff but also among the staff itself on any of those issues, we can only marvel that there aren't more battles and emotional outbursts over relief than there are.

Mode of Relief: Availability, Knowledge, Choice

One of our primary questions involves the specific mode of relief to be used. Drugs? Surgery? A dorsal stimulator? Body positioning? Psychotherapy? Distraction? Immediately relevant to answering that question is whether or not a given relief measure is actually available. For instance, in some countries, certain drugs often are unavailable or are too expensive for everyday use. And even in industrialized countries, surgical techniques that might relieve pain are not always available at every hospital. Experience and knowledge-ability are also relevant to what is "available" since a combination of drugs may actually be within reach, but the physician may be unaware that this combination is effective for relieving a particular kind of pain.

Legitimacy or legality can also be involved in the availability of a relief measure, as when a nurse on the night shift knows which medication might ease a patient's pain but cannot reach a physician to sanction its use. Or a person in pain may know from experience what drug will relieve the pain but be unable to reach a physician for the necessary prescription. On one cancer ward we observed, the head nurse carefully negotiated with each new rotating resident so she would never lack for medication to relieve patients' pains. Occasionally an incoming resident would disagree, so she would have to appeal to the chief of service.

How desperate the availability situation can become is illustrated by the following account of a woman who had just returned from having a set of x-rays taken for what would later be diagnosed as a severe gall bladder infection:

> *About an hour later I was overcome by the most horrible pains I have ever experienced. . . . I remember I wished I was dead. I was vomiting and doubled over in a gripping pain and was sweating profusely. I didn't see how I could wait another week and a half for my appointment with the physician to find out what to do about my condition so I called his office. He was not in and the secretary told me that he was all booked up for the day. I told her that something*

had to be done as I was in unbearable pain—much worse than any-
thing I had had before. One of his associates got on the phone and
by this time I was quite upset about the casualness with which my
pains were being treated. With a great deal of effort, I gasped into
the phone that I was in terrible pain, to which the doctor replied
that it wouldn't help me to act like an hysterical woman. I slammed
the phone down. I was lying in a heap on my bed, alternating be-
tween crying in pain and crying in frustration, when the nurse
called back and said my physician could see me at 1:45 if I could get
to the office.

Availability aside, the mode of relief utilized is closely related to the particular experiences of the person or persons making the decision to use it. Since so many patients are chronically ill, they are likely to be relatively experienced in relieving their own pains. An arthritic learns experientially that a warm house and a blanket over the legs will relieve pain somewhat. Or someone with an esophageal hernia learns that a particular position will get rid of painful gas. In contrast, those having pain from acute illness are less likely to know what will relieve their pain, and if they do not discover a proper mode by accident or by experimentation (with drugs or body positioning), they are entirely dependent upon expert counsel or prescription.

A vivid illustration of a combination of experience and lack of experience is given by Mrs. Wertenbaker's account of her husband's decision to die from his cancer at home.[3] He received expert advice concerning which drugs to use and was aided in getting adequate supplies (even of morphine, illegal in France where he was living). On the whole, he managed to keep his pain within endurable bounds, but as his symptoms worsened, Mrs. Wertenbaker described that "when the *crisis* came then he would sit on the edge of something so as to touch a surface with as little of his body as possible."[3] He had learned proper body positioning. He had also learned from experience that sometimes medication in liquid form was more effective than pills. On the other hand, he suffered more pain as he neared death than he might have under the care of an experienced hospital staff because his illness trajectory, along with its associated pain, took some unexpected turns. So much so that his wife, experienced as she had become, during some crises when his pain got out of control went into a kind of fugue from which she did not emerge until the crisis was over.

In hospitals, staff members utilize not only painkillers but other modes of relief. When the pain is assessed as "functional," then they agree to try distraction, or tranquilizers, or in desperation to call in the consulting psychiatrist. When the pain is assessed as "real," then medication may be combined with, or substituted for, proper body positioning, as well as distraction or just spending more time with the patient. What may be termed "presence" is also utilized; some staff members are able to help lessen pain simply by acting in reassuring ways—by generally effective styles of being "there" and being "around." Touching, hand holding, and other nonverbal gestures are essential to this kind of relieving. (Presence is *not* equivalent to merely being in the same room. It means some kind of action which is significant to the person in pain; however, just being in the patient's room may sometimes be helpful.)

Since presence, distraction, and the teaching or arranging of body positioning take time and tolerance, there is a distinct tendency on the wards to utilize medications as the primary mode of relief. Relief work is only of many other kinds of work in which the staff is engaged, and it must balance work priorities. A general reliance on the technology of medication, plus actual or perceived shortages of time, result in insuring that drugs become the principal mode of relieving pain.

It is illuminating to contrast this conventional and widespread situation with that obtaining in a special British hospital (St. Joseph's Hospice in London), administered and described by Dr. Cicely Saunders.[4] She has a carefully formulated philosophy (we shall discuss it more fully in the chapter on intractable pain) about the care of dying patients, most of them dying from cancer, and an associated operational philosophy which includes the minimizing and relieving of pain. She believes it is important that "drugs must be given regularly" and no patient allowed to wait in fear or anxiety "until the 'proper' time." Also it is part of her philosophy that the staff members do "all that we can do to enable patients to *live* until they die . . . and includes the care of the family, the mind, and the spirit as well as the care of the body." The staff attempts to help "mobilize the patient's own resources" and allow him to "come to his own personal victory." If medically possible, the staff promises permanent relief and builds trust in its capacity to carry out that promise.

In the more usual hospital setting, when staff draws away as it sometimes does from the bedsides of dying patients who have raised considerable work problems or created emotional difficulties, presence, distraction, body positioning, and other nonmedication modes of relief tend to be disregarded.

> *One woman . . . behaved so "badly" for so many weeks that the nurses gradually took to spending as little time with her as possible. Shortly before she died, the chaplain entered her room and found her*

in considerable pain. She said, "I'm looking for the nurses." The
chaplain, when later describing the scene, remarked that "I'd been
pushing the nurses on this just as hard as I could and was wondering
how far I could go." He helped to rearrange the patient's body on
the bed so as to reduce her pain. Then he and she prayed together.
As he left the room, he asked: "Is there something else you would
like the nurses to do for you?" She said: "Yes, see that one comes
immediately." The chaplain thought to himself that he wasn't sure
he could manage that particular feat. In the hallway he found a
nurse and, putting his arm around her, he asked: "How about doing
me a favor? Would you go in and take care of Mrs. Plum immediat-
ely?" She answered: "Yes, I'll do it for you as a favor."[5]

When even massive doses of medications don't seem to work,
the staff may turn in desperation to a mode of relief like the experimental surgery used with Mrs. Abel. An unusual but perfectly
understandable instance of desperate choice of relief mode was given
to us by a sociologist, Sheldon Messinger, who has done research in
a mental hospital: "I remember an M.D. at Napa (state mental hospital) telling me that she used EST (electric shock therapy) in a
particular case, not because she thought it likely to do any good in
the long run, but because 'the patient was in pain and I'm trained to
help. I had to do something. What else was there to do?' "

Although frequently the physician does not give the patient any
choice of relief mode, sometimes he or she will talk over the options.
Then they will negotiate or choose together the preferred one. When
patients are not offered options, the staff runs the risk of discovering
that the patient has previously experienced adverse side effects from
certain drugs and would have warned staff members if he had
known what they were using. Sometimes the patient *has* advised
them but they disregarded the warning. The consequence is annoyance or anger, and the staff members run the additional risk of being
blamed for negligence or incompetence. The patient's reaction is
likely to be even stronger if he, as with many of the chronically ill,
has had previous experiences of this kind. Such experienced patients
will even refuse certain drugs prescribed for relief—codeine, Demerol, morphine—declaring that such painkillers are ineffective for them.

The doctor insists that a cancer patient be on LevoDromoran. She
knows Levo doesn't work any more for her, but she can't convince
him that methadone will do it. Despite the assistant chief's support,
the doctor insists on Levo. She has a terrible night, hanging on to
the bed to prevent herself from groaning and moaning. The next day
she regains control over her relief because the nurse realizes Levo is

not working by itself, and the patient is able to explain to the resi-dent the efficacy of a combination of Percodan with morphine plus aspirin. The next day the physician still insists on Levo, but the resi-dent adds morphine.

Regarding such experienced patients, one nurse stated: "They have hardened attitudes" and can't be "brought around." Sometimes the staff tries the countertactic of using a placebo. As with any mode of relief which actually inflicts further pain before it relieves, this might arouse the patient's anger if used without warning, so it must be considered by the patient before use.

Drugs: Amounts, Frequencies, Combinations

When at home, a person in pain can decide what medication to take (if it is already in the medicine cabinet) and can even improvise with the prescribed dosages. The chronically ill with lengthy biographies are likely to have experimented in order to get better control over their daily, weekly, or occasional pain.

When hospitalized, at least in the United States, patients cede that control to the staff, except insofar as they can hoard drugs or persuade or negotiate in accordance with their perceptions of drug effectiveness. An extreme degree of this ceding of control is illustra-ted when patients hospitalized for respiratory diseases must yield all their medications, including the aspirin they take for arthritic aches or occasional eyestrain. Since some disagreement between the patient and staff over amount and frequency of medication is likely, and each (especially the patient) does not always win the negotiative rounds, the tension between them sometimes becomes intense. Even when both more or less agree, relationships can become acrimonious because organizational conditions interfere with effective carrying out of those agreements.

Amount of medication   Although a patient and physician may agree on assessment of pain, the physician can still underestimate the amount of drug necessary for adequate relief. On one cardiac pul-monary unit a very large patient received insufficient medication to relieve his postoperative pain. In such a situation, the patient has no need to legitimate the extent of his pain; he needs only to request additional medication. Of course, physicians can also overestimate. We must not, however, mistake *deliberate* overdosing for over-estimation, as in the instance of an intern who, before leaving the ward for the night, increased the medication for a "neurotic" patient so that nobody, least of all he, would be disturbed during the night. Similarly, a resident remarked that sometimes when a patient keeps "bugging you" for more pain medication, you give a larger dose than needed just to get him "off your back."

In American hospitals, only the physician can legally prescribe both the drugs and the amounts to be used for a patient's relief. The actual relieving through "giving the drug" is delegated to the nursing personnel. When the physician orders drugs, then, the nurses have little official discretionary power unless that is delegated to them. But because they spend much more time with or around the patient, they are, or think they are, in a better position to assess (or reassess) pain and to make suggestions about maintaining or changing prescribed medications and their dosages. Under relatively routine conditions, as with straightforward postoperative care, and especially where trustful relations exist between nurse and physician, the latter will accept suggested revisions. Under other conditions, the physician is reluctant or unwilling to follow the nurses' counsel. Understandably, these conditions include: when lack of trust exists, when the physician believes the nurses are inexperienced, and when angry with or biased against the patient. (In Mrs. Abel's case, the physician hewed pretty much to his own evaluations since he not only continued to make his own assessments of pain but also grew to mistrust the nurses' feelings about the patient.) Sometimes a physician will increase medication, believing the patient's assessment of pain rather than trusting the nurses' judgment, thus adding to the tension between them.

An illuminating instance of how a nurse will avoid doing what a physician has ordered is afforded by the following field observation of a neurological ward:

> The physician left an order for a large pain dosage for the patient, who was responding with "no effect, absolutely no effect" according to the nurse. After another visit to the ward by the physician, the nurse turned to the evening nurse who was just coming on: "You give. I'm not giving any more to her. Do you realize she weighs only 85 pounds?" Asked whether she questioned orders much, the nurse said no but it happened occasionally. Once there was a very slight young girl, unconscious from drugs, "wiped out," and the nurse thereafter refused to give the medications. The physician had to come and do it himself, she said.

By passing on the job to the evening nurse, the day nurse was saying, without directly confronting the physician, she wanted no part in it. By saying "no" directly to the physician, she would have been more openly challenging the legitimacy of his prescribed dosage.

Do nurses sometimes disobey physicians' orders and alter their dosages? We have no direct evidence on this question. It seems unlikely that nurses would increase the amount of medication; it seems far more likely that they might decrease it. (One way the amount can be reduced is by stretching out the intervals of time between which the medication is offered to the patient.) However, it *is* common practice to interpret the physician's standing orders so as to give the lowest amounts permitted, for often the physician will write the orders simply giving the personnel a dosage range. This may lead to a conflict between a nurse and a patient who thinks an effective agreement has been reached with the physician and then discovers it has not.

The nursing personnel's actual errors—giving too much or too little medication—are another topic entirely. Medication errors have been much referred to in the literature.[6-11] For our purposes, it is only necessary to note that these may be due to organizational variables such as a very busy staff or an inexperienced medication nurse. In addition, there can be some real differences between what the physician orders and what the patient receives, especially when the physician has written orders giving minimum and maximum options. The day shift may understand that the maximum should be given today, but the night shift does not receive this information and runs into trouble with the patient by giving minimum dosages.

One area of potentially serious conflict among the staff involves "addiction." As remarked earlier, American attitudes toward addiction pervade the staff; hence the stands that staff members take toward the possibility of a patient becoming "hooked" are not necessarily professional in character. When nurses believe a physician has been ordering too much of an addictive drug, they may do two things. They may persuade the patient to endure more pain and take less medication, explaining the possibility of addiction, and/or they may attempt to persuade the physician and the supporting housestaff to decrease the dosages. As we shall see in the next chapter, nurses may continue to worry about addiction after the physician and even the patient have given up all hope of the patient's surviving.

Another area of frequent conflict between the patient and the nursing personnel is over the amounts of medication being given. The patient believes either that the physician has underestimated the amount of painkiller necessary or that the pain has increased sufficiently to allow the dosage to be increased. (If a patient requests that dosages be lowered, the staff usually accedes with alacrity.) If a patient requests that dosages be raised, the nurse must act as a messenger, carrying the request upward either to the head nurse, who relays it to the physician, or to the physician herself. A shy or more "cooperative" patient will wait longer to make such a request. Sometimes these patients are helped out by other patients, who act in the ailing patient's behalf and relay the message. In contrast, a patient who is too "demanding" may have the request ignored or delayed in its upward course. Impatient or desperate patients, of course, become their own pain messengers, attempting to reach the physician on their own.

The potential staff messenger who has denied a previous request is likely to respond with anger or at least annoyance both to the "going upstairs" tactic and to the patient's accusation of negligence. Here is a vivid illustration of this kind of interaction:

> Finally, I couldn't stand the pain any more, and I figured I should get some Demerol and atropine, but I didn't know if it would interfere with the surgery which was to be done the next day. Clearly, I couldn't trust this jackass of a resident who hadn't even bothered to ask me why I was moaning and running in and out of the bathroom, so I went out into the hall and told the nurse that I wanted her to call Dr. X. She told me to get right back into bed, and I told her I wouldn't until I had spoken with him. (I know I sound positively obnoxious, which I suppose I was, but it was the only way to make sure . . .). The nurse called the resident and told him that I didn't want to get back into bed. He started saying he would be giving the medical orders around here, and I said that I didn't wish to deal with him. If he wanted me to get back into bed he could call Dr. X so that I could find out what drugs to take for my pain. I thought he was going to hit me. He was furious but started to dial. . . . Finally he got Dr. X on the phone and said . . . "Your patient, Ms. Y, is having bad pains in her belly." Then he cupped his hand over the phone and said to me: "Now will you go back to your bed so I can talk with your doctor." Now I had really had it! So I snatched the phone from him and said: "Oh, why don't you go to bed yourself. I don't need you to talk to my doctor. I want to talk to him myself." I spoke to Dr. X who told me that I could indeed have Demerol and atropine, and that it would not interfere with the surgery. . . . Without another word, I went back to bed, pleased with myself. . . . The resident was so furious with me. . . .

To avoid scenes like this, personnel sometimes attempt to fool the patient by using placebos; they use them because they judge it unwise or unnecessary to increase the medication. A placebo can also be used as an element in a graded series of efforts to stem the tide of increased medication. For instance, on the burn unit described earlier, when a patient asks for increased medication after a skin graft the staff often gives a placebo. If that doesn't work, they give or increase tranquilizing drugs; if that doesn't work, they use more potent drugs. When painkillers and placebos are given in combination with other types of medication, the juggling can be quite complicated—so much so that the personnel's focus on pain, potential addiction, and weaning can lead to their ignoring the side effects of other drugs. One nursing team leader said that the staff members were so concentrated on pain and narcotics that they didn't notice side effects ("a dry tongue") from atropine being given for intestinal muscle spasms.

Frequency of medication Tension between patient and staff is perhaps even more noticeable when disputes arise over how frequently medication is given for relief. Associated with this issue are patients "leaning on the buzzer," "putting on their lights," "stockpiling," and "going upstairs" to rectify what they consider the staff's negligence or even cruelty. The following issues are what is basically involved, aside from the deteriorating interactional cycles.

First, for various reasons, the personnel may fail to give medication at the scheduled time or fail to respond to requests to speed up the schedule. They may be busy and forget. Even when there is an urgent reminder from a patient, staff may be very busy or even involved with emergency care. (As one patient said about his roommate: "Suddenly the pain was so bad that he couldn't talk—lay there wincing in agony. I went to his physical therapist who was helping another move a paralyzed man . . . and couldn't very well drop him, so some time elapsed." Sometimes the physician cannot be reached by the nurse, so that she can get the order changed, and in the meantime the nurse is subject to bitter complaints; sometimes the medication will hold for only one hour. Organizational features do little to alleviate the nurses' difficulties in reaching the physicians —sometimes surgeons are busy operating for long hours during the day. When a patient's pain is unexpectedly great but no leeway is written into the order, the nurses' hands are tied both as to speeding up the medication schedule and as to increasing the dosage.

Sometimes, also, day nurses forget to get a renewal order from the physician, and the night nurses must bear the brunt of the patient's anger because he needs relief now, not later! During the night, the nurses may attempt other modes of relief, like distraction and spending time with the patient, rather than bothering the physician. Or they stall: "You wouldn't necessarily call the house physician unless pain was very severe." Night nurses have been known to use old orders, the next morning reminding the day staff to get a retroactive renewal order.

A second general reason for tension between patients and the nursing staff arises when nurses believe that the physician is over-medicating the patient. When this is the case, they will give the pain reliever "every four hours on the dot" and not a minute sooner. They also do this when the physician has written a flexible order, "give every three or four hours," even if the patient insists that there is considerable pain. (As one patient impatiently asked us: "Why do nurses think that four-hour rule is so sacrosanct?") Here is a vivid instance recorded by one researcher after an operation. After being wheeled from the recovery room into the surgical ward at night:

> I was feeling dazed with pain after about an hour. I called the nurse and asked for something for the pain. She looked at me . . . then left the room without saying anything. After about ten minutes I buzzed again, and she came in, and seemed to be irritated. I asked for Demerol. She said it wasn't time yet. I had to wait for an hour and a half.

Later this patient had an opportunity to check the records:

> There were orders for IV fluids, etc. Then, under medications, were directions to administer Demerol, dosage 75 to 100 mg every 3 to 4 hours, at patient's request. . . . The records of the nurse indicate that I was given the smallest dosage, in the largest time interval— 75 mg every 4 hours. . . . The next day, when I saw Dr. P., he mentioned he understood I had been complaining about the pain, so he was telling the nurses to give me 100 mg every 3 hours.

A third general reason for tension between patient and staff over scheduling results when the patient does not trust personnel to bring the medication on time. Like Mrs. Abel, the patient will remind the nurses ahead of time that "it's almost time" or put on the room light to remind them that it is time. In anticipation of a careless or dis-senting staff member, a patient may stockpile drugs for those bad moments when the medication is really needed. Nurses get upset and frustrated by, or angry at, these overanxious patients who, de-spite the considerable time spent giving them care and reassurance, put on their lights just five minutes after the nurses have turned to other work. Patients, especially those experienced in the vagaries of pain peaks, may become tense about potential mistiming if the medication does not arrive precisely on time, and this tenseness can intensify the pain.

In any event, continued tension over scheduling—especially when abetted by conflict over increasing the dosages or by discrepancies between staff's and patient's assessment of the pain itself—leads to vicious spirals of bad feeling and staff withdrawals. When trust is mutual, when the nurse can convince the patient to "hang on" and not take so much medication for his own welfare, then such downward interactional spirals are much less probable. Unfortunately, worsening illness trajectories with increasing pain do not help to generate mutual trust and from time to time result in mutual desperation. (Our case histories illustrate all too vividly such desperation and spirals.)

REFERENCES

1.   Glaser, B., and Strauss, A. 1970. *Anguish*. San Francisco: Sociology Press, p. 106.

2.   Zborowski, M. 1969. *People in pain*. San Francisco: Jossey-Bass, pp. 137–149.

3.   Wertenbaker, L. 1957. *Death of a man*. New York: Random House.

4.   Saunders, C. 1965. The last stages of life. *American Journal of Nursing* 65:70–75.

5.   Glaser, B., and Strauss, A. 1965. *Awareness of dying*. Chicago: Aldine, p. 96.

6.   Anderson, R. D. 1971. The physician's contribution to hospital medication errors. *American Journal of Hospital Pharmacy* 28:18–25.

7.   Byrne, A. K. 1953. Errors in giving medications. *American Journal of Nursing* 53:829–831.

8.   Hershey, N. 1963. Question the drug order . . . the courts lay down the law. *American Journal of Nursing* 63:96–97.

9.   Hershey, N. 1964. The apparent erroneous order. *American Journal of Nursing* 64:111–112.

10.   Kron, N. 1962. Stepping beyond the five rights of administering drugs. *American Journal of Nursing* 62:62–63.

11.   Satren, M. A., and Chapanis, A. 1960. A critical incident study of hospital medication errors. *Hospitals* 34:32 passim, May 1, 1960, 34:53 passim, May 16, 1960.

Dying and Painless Comfort*

10

A special phase of the illness trajectory begins when a hospitalized patient is defined as dying. There is a shift to "comfort care," and the nurse tends to "take over as the main custodian of [the] care."[1] Relief work and the minimization of pain become tasks of primary importance. The major dimensions of relieving appear again, albeit in forms characteristic of this phase of the illness trajectory.

PAINLESS COMFORT

Most of the nurse's energy is concentrated on maintaining *painless* comfort for the patient. While painlessness is a goal that is desirable for all patients, it takes on added importance for a patient who has only that left to hope for. For such a patient, lethal risks to insure painlessness through narcotics are legitimate, though they would never be taken for patients who can be expected to bear pain in the service of recovery. (The possibility of addiction

---

*This chapter is reproduced, in slightly altered form, from *Awareness of Dying* by Barney Glaser and Anselm Strauss (Chicago, Aldine, 1965, pp. 208–225). Copyright © 1965 by Anselm Strauss. Reprinted by permission.

is now irrelevant because the dying patient can *never* be taken off the narcotics.)

Painless comfort is a goal strongly emphasized by doctors, family, nurses and other patients (as well as the patient himself), for few people can stand another's pain. If a patient is in too much pain, everyone is upset by the "scream at the end of the hall," which threatens to disrupt the routine work as well as the sentimental order of the ward. Thus, the nurse is under considerable social pressure to successfully control the patient's pain.

Differential Death Expectations

To accomplish this task, a nurse must have adequate sedation orders from the doctor. How adequate the doctor's instructions appear to the nurse depends on their differential appraisal of the patient's stage of dying. If both doctor and nurse are aware that the patient is in the "nothing-more-to-do" phase, then the doctor's instructions are very likely to allow the nurse to use her own discretion in the dosage necessary to keep the patient free of pain. She may even risk lethal dosages. "None of the nurses believe in euthanasia, but it's just that as you give these heavy doses of narcotics you think that this may be the last one he can take." One nurse reported that her instructions gave her a leeway that would allow the patient to die in the line of *her* duty. The implicit instruction was: "Give [this degree of medication] to the patient every ⸺ hours until dead."

If the doctor is aware that there is nothing more to do for the patient and gives very loose instructions to a nurse who is unaware of the patient's condition, she may be frightened by so much discretionary power. She will "cover" herself by phoning the doctor to check dosages or to request lower dosage orders, checking with the head nurse, sticking as close to the order as its looseness permits, and so on. She fears that if anything happens to the patient she could be accused of negligence in her interpretation of the loose orders. She also fears loss of self-control when faced with pain that she knows she can, within the limits of her orders, blot out with a heavy but potentially lethal dose.

A nurse who realizes somewhat before the doctor does that the patient is either in, or soon will be in, the "nothing-more-to-do" phase, faces other interaction problems. If the doctor, in preparing to leave the ward, has not given her sufficiently loose instructions to ensure painless comfort, she must act fast. She will have to corner the doctor and either remind him that he has left no instructions or suggest to him possible changes in old or current instructions. Say-

ing she might need them and asking what she should do, she prods
the doctor into giving leeway. If this tactic fails, or if she is too shy
to try it, two alternatives remain. One is to engage in "invisible acts"
of increased dosage; some nurses, particularly private nurses, do take
matters into their own hands. The other alternative is to try to reach
the doctor by phone when the patient's pain becomes uncontrollable
under present orders. This is one condition under which the nurse
and her supervisor will make every effort to reach the doctor, no
matter where he is, what he is doing, or what time it is. Having
reached him, she tries to bring the doctor's awareness into line with
hers by pointing out changes in physical condition, indicating that
there is nothing left to do but insure painlessness. Then she requests
a change in sedation orders.

Patient's Awareness

The patient's part in how the nurse insures his comfort depends on
the awareness context. A nurse may ease the transition to an open
awareness context by promising painless comfort until death. A typical sequence of interaction is the following: The doctor tells the dying
patient that there is basically not much more to do for him medically
except to control the pain. This announcement immediately leads the
patient to develop tactics for securing sedation. Normally, a patient
in this stage does not worry about becoming an addict, or about becoming immune to any one painkiller. He is concerned only with
minimizing the pain, and he starts by trying, by various interaction
tactics, to control the nurse's management of it. The pressure of this
attempt often makes a nurse wish she were maintaining comfort under the cover of a closed awareness context; then the patient, still
motivated to recover, will put up with some pain—and leave it up to
her to manage it.

Furthermore, the announcement by the doctor usually leaves the
patient very depressed. To cope with this initial response, the nurses
stand by with medication to relieve emotional as well as physical
pain. As one nurse put it: "If no one had helped him that day I think
he might have committed suicide; he was in an awful state. We gave
him medication." And thus he was immediately introduced to the
looser regulations surrounding sedation. He would no longer have to
put up with as much pain; he could depend fairly well on the nurses
to insure comfort.

Most often, the patient wants the nurse to increase dosage; and a
common tactic is using verbal indicators of pain such as moans and
complaints. The nurse must judge whether the patient is in physical
pain and, if so, to what degree. This task is difficult since the indi-

cators of pain are often poor or unreliable; a patient who says he or
she is in pain may be expressing, to one degree or another, only
emotional pain. Although a disturbed patient may have to be tran-
quilized, a narcotic should not be wasted on emotional pain, because
its effectiveness, which declines with tolerance, must be reserved for
physical pain often over a long period of time. Thus, when a patient
uses "moaning and groaning" tactics to obtain more sedation than
ordered, the nurse must use countertactics to test if there is reason to
doubt the physical origin of the pain. She may give a placebo or
tranquilizer; she may walk past the room a few times to see whether
the "moaning and groaning" occurs only when her footsteps are au-
dible, and so on.

Maneuvering of this kind tends to result in irregular dosages and
fluctuating levels of pain for the patient, which in turn may make
him wish to control the scheduling of injections and dosages. Some
patients dispense with manipulation of verbal indicators and proceed
directly to try to establish control over schedules. The patient on a
periodic (rather than demand) schedule may concentrate on trying to
shorten the time between injections. He may act confused in his time
perspective, ringing for the nurse at the three-and-a-half-hour point
and asking for another shot on the grounds that his four-hour interval is up. Or he rings for the nurse after two hours to say: "You'll be
sure to be on time for my next injection, won't you?" thus trying to
control the schedule by enforcing it. He may also get family members
to keep close watch for transgressions. Patients also try to negotiate
for a different schedule on the grounds that the regular one is not
adequate.

Patients on demand schedules depend primarily on their handling of indicators of pain, since "demand" means when the nurse
judges the patient needs it. Such a patient may also stick his hand
out for medication every time a nurse passes. If these tactics do not
work, he may threaten suicide or try to negotiate for a regular schedule, or he may go through other staff members to put pressure on the
nurse. He can ask the doctor to order the nurse to give him regular
or more frequent sedation, or he can enlist the aid of family members. A family member can create a status-forcing scene, saying it is
the nurse's job to relieve the patient's pain, but she is, it appears,
negligent in this duty. (Needless to say, anxious family members often do this without prompting.) Lastly, a chaplain may be asked, as a
neutral, to institute a conference of patient, nurse, doctor, and family
to arrange a sedation schedule that is satisfactory to all.

The demand schedule can be very demoralizing to the aware
patient, since it necessarily means more pain. Because the nurse is

watching for symptoms, the patient must withstand some pain before it is reduced by her action. This pain may make the patient
think: "I am surely going this time." On the other hand, a patient
who finds himself supporting longer and longer periods without sedation may feel hopeful and think he is improving, though he is
experiencing only a temporary reprieve. His pressuring the nurse to
increase or reduce sedation will be guided by these conditions linked
with the demand schedule.

We have described the typical situation but not the infrequent
patient who is aware that death is certain but refuses narcotics, perhaps to keep clear-headed enough to arrange his affairs before the
family takes over, or perhaps merely to demonstrate his prowess.
(These patients too, however, are often given narcotics in spite of
their wishes, if their pain disturbs others, for the nurses' job is to
protect the sentimental order of the ward as well as to preserve the
hospital routine. This is one instance in which patients are not allowed to manage their own dying—when it interferes with the social
organization of the hospital.)

To reduce dosage, patients may use a "no complaining" tactic.
Then the nurse must watch for other indicators of pain since, in the
interests of others on the ward, she cannot let the patient support so
much pain that he breaks down or sets a "bad" example of nursing
care for other more fearful patients. The goal of painless comfort
must be pursued, but under these conditions it is very difficult to
achieve, for when a patient says very little it is hard to ascertain how
much a given dosage reduces his pain.

"Can't Talk"

A patient on a demand schedule increases the pressure on the nurse
if his physical condition deteriorates to the point where he can no
longer ask for sedation because he is "snowed" by sedation. This
problem applies particularly to research patients who, to minimize
narcotics interference with the study drug, are kept on a demand
schedule for painkillers. As one nurse said, "They are kept under sedation, but there is this carelessness. They don't give medication
unless it's asked for and these patients often aren't in a condition to
ask, yet I am sure they are in pain." Nurses use several methods to
establish degree of pain: turning the patient to watch his response or
asking him to blink or move his hand if he is in pain. Sometimes the
nurse talks with the patient about this stage of dying before it arrives, either on her own initiative or because the patient negotiates

with her. In one nurse's words, the response is: "We always reassure them that we will give them whatever they need to keep the pain under control." This promise, however, ignores the fact that when verbal contact with the patient is lost, indicators of pain are harder to read and verify. Thus, "We sedate heavily in the end," a nurse told us. This is one way of playing it safe.

Under this "can't talk" condition, before death, the nurse is relieved of several pressures from the patient. She no longer needs to "explain," or to parry the patient's request for an explanation, every time she changes a periodic schedule or after each demand-schedule injection. As he approaches death, a patient on a periodic schedule puts less and less pressure on the nurse, when a regular increase in dosage is built into the periodic schedule. This causes the patient at this stage to be either too "snowed" by narcotics to talk effectively, or to not be able to talk at all. Thus, the nurse no longer has to worry about avoiding talk of death, nor does she have to listen to "Why don't you let me die?" or "For God's sake, let me die," or "Don't let me die," nor must she handle his negotiation for more narcotics. In the last phase of dying, nurses are particularly vulnerable to the patient who begs for help, especially for painkillers. They want to provide more sedation as a way of "doing something" within their power in order to relieve their own feelings of medical helplessness.

Some of the benefits otherwise inherent in the open awareness context are lost when the patient can no longer talk. From the patient's point of view, he loses whatever control he had established over insuring painless comfort, and over management of his dying when he loses the ability to negotiate for more narcotics. One advantage of open awareness is that the patient can take leave of his family, but when he is heavily sedated this advantage is lost too. Even if the patient can communicate, heavy sedation makes him mentally vague, which tends to disturb relatives who wish to make final farewells. Patients in this condition are also unable to sustain useful relations with a chaplain or social worker. In short, the aware patient who cannot talk cannot interact very well even on the basis of open awareness.

"LET THE PATIENT DIE"

When painless comfort is no longer possible for the dying patient, nurses are reduced to a state of helplessness, which one nurse expressed as follows: "You can't do anything, even to relieve the pain in the end, sometimes, and the patients keep wanting things done

for them." They can no longer achieve the only goal of patient care
that remained to work for. As they watch a patient lingering pain-
fully, a collective mood develops among the nurses—an urgent wish
to "let him die." This is their most frequent response to their inability to provide comfort. (A less preferred alternative is to put the
patient into living sleep with drugs—a social death.) One nurse
stated this "let die" alternative to painless comfort explicitly: "We
can't relieve her pain, everybody wants her to die for her sake,
meaning her suffering, we can't even help her. Once we can't help
her, let her die for God's sake, for our sakes as well as theirs."

Other nurses are just as direct: "The quicker she dies, the better
without suffering." "Why should he be saved to go on living like a
vegetable?" "Why should he be saved for a life of continual suffering?" "Maybe it is for the best, maybe it is a blessing if he goes."
And in reference to research patients, "I think a man should be left
to die in peace with plenty of narcotics." When the patient does die,
the collective mood of the nurses changes to one of great relief. No
longer must they be frustrated by their inability to provide comfort
and by the "waste and senselessness" of undue lingering or
prolonging.

To be sure, this collective mood runs counter to the medical ideal
of prolonging life. A student nurse displayed clear recognition of this
ambivalence: "We had a patient, a cancer patient, who wanted to
come to the hospital. Everything was done for him, even if he didn't
want it. They gave him everything to prolong, to save this person, if
that is what you want to call it. This isn't actually saving, but once
you come to the hospital everyone is concerned to preserve your life,
the person has no choice; well, it is just a question of ethics." She realized that in the nothing-more-to-do phase, prolonging is *not* saving
and can only be justified in terms of an "ethic," which is weak support indeed in these cases. Thus, most nurses feel that "let him die"
is the best alternative to painful prolonging, though some remain
ambivalent. One nurse, evidently wanting to support the ideal, questioned her judgment that the patient was really in the "nothing more
to do" phase: "How do I really know he is going to die; how do I really know; therefore, how can I possibly let him die?" Another nurse
resolved her ambivalence by means of unquestioning compliance
with the ideal. She registered annoyance, indignation and irritation
at the thought of *not* prolonging at all costs as well as at the thought
of actually helping the patient die. Other nurses regard the ideal as a
public shield over the invisible acts, or system of acts, by which they
let the patient die.[1]

Patients and Open Awareness

In the closed awareness context the collective mood of "let him die" develops spontaneously among the nurses, regardless of the patient's overt demands. In the open awareness context, however, this mood may be supported and even initiated by the patient's requests to be allowed to die. A patient's longing to die—"Please God let me go"— is reciprocated by the nurses' "It's a blessing if he goes." Just as a patient's struggle to live encourages nurses to help him, his struggle to die may arouse their sympathy and prompt them to help him attain his objective. One nurse stood by for a patient's request to die, so that she could step in and ask the doctor to "let him die."

"Request" is too mild a way to describe this behavior: many patients actually beg and plead to be allowed to die. A doctor has lucidly described this patient, covering the two essential conditions of nothing-more-to-do and too much pain: "A cancer patient for whom every conceivable avenue of treatment has been explored with total failure, and this patient moreover is suffering from excruciating pain and is pleading for release."[2] Patients who say, "Please leave me alone, I want to die, I don't want any tests like this," or "Why don't you let me die?" confirm the nurses' conviction that the best way out is death. Statements like "I'm dying right now, get me out of my misery," may express a transition from a closed awareness context to an open one; the patient registers a "let me die" mood as he registers realization of his change of status. Such a quick change in awareness context can bring into the open the nurses' collective hidden desire to let him die, and prompt their active assistance in achieving the mutual goal. Too quick a transition, however, may cause an unaware nurse to doubt the patient's reading of his own condition and consider him morbid.

Sedation Tactics

When doctor and nurse *agree* that the best course is to let the patient die, the doctor may order cessation of most or all equipment in use and give the nurse loose sedation orders to insure painless comfort until the end. These sedation orders allow the nurse much discretion and therefore encourage her to use active tactics to help the patient die (as opposed to the more passive nonrescue tactics). Under these conditions she can manipulate sedation with little or no fear that she will be accused of negligence. By manipulating sedation, or its counteractants, she can ease the patient to death when adverse conditions multiply and become too much for all concerned: the patient is begging for death, he is deteriorating physically, pain cannot be controlled, the family is going through an ordeal that is pushing it to the breaking point.

Loose sedation orders give the nurse enough latitude to administer potentially lethal doses in the hope of achieving painless comfort. In this way she can help the patient die. One nurse said, "It may kill her, but why not let her go free of pain?" If the dose does turn out to be fatal, then the nurse can withhold the counteracting stimulant. If it is not fatal, then she can increase the dosage next time. And since she is following—or stretching—the orders of a doctor who agrees with her assessment of the patient's fate, she need not fear accusations of negligence from him, and she can be confident that he will protect her should others raise questions about her "interpretation of orders." Another factor encouraging this strategy is the patient's attempt to control or increase sedation. The nurse can purposefully yield to a patient's "moaning and groaning" or distorted time perspectives so that eventually she is giving sedation oftener.

Nonrescue tactics depend on whether the nurse's inactivity during a crisis can be observed by others, but sedation tactics are not nearly so contingent on visibility. A nurse can apply the needle or give the pill in the presence of others, since it is part of her job, and the patient need not be in an obviously critical condition. Any adverse effects are too subtle for most observers to distinguish from those of routine medication. When charting what has happened, however, the nurse generally must be backed up by a doctor's orders. Thus, a nurse who *disagrees* with a doctor about the patient's fate takes quite a risk in manipulating sedation. She must falsify or avoid recording her "invisible act," and usually this is too drastic a deviation from professional standards for her to contemplate. Normally, as we have indicated, a nurse in this situation will first try to convince the doctor that the patient's case is hopeless and that letting him die is the sensible thing to do. They may also talk with a relative to obtain the family's consent and support.

When a nurse *disagrees* with a doctor who is certain there is nothing more to do and accordingly gives flexible sedation orders, she may be alarmed, as we noted before, by the responsibility implicitly given her for the patient's survival. Her tendency then is to seek more control in her orders, to prevent her from going too far in striving for the patient's comfort. Of course, this is a problem only for a nurse who still believes that the patient *can* survive.

Several structural conditions inhibit use of sedation tactics to let the patient die. If the patient is a research subject, even a doctor who

agrees that he is in the nothing-more-to-do stage may not give sufficiently flexible orders to allow the nurse much latitude. She is
supposed to minimize sedation, so that it does not interfere with a
clinical experiment, and if she gives overdoses on her own, the doctor is not likely to back her up. She is expected to keep the patient
going until the end of the study.

   In a closed awareness context, the patient may beg not for death
but for a reduction in narcotics, because he is afraid of addiction.
Sometimes unaware family members have the same concern. If social
and family affairs are still unsettled, use of sedation tactics is often
precluded by patient or family request. And if a family member is
traveling from afar for a last visit with the patient, sedation can be
manipulated only to prolong life while keeping the patient conscious.

Open Awareness and Autoeuthanasia.

Another tactic for letting the patient die, which is possible in the
open awareness context, is to permit autoeuthanasia. The prelude is
a distressing scene in which a pain-ridden patient begs to die, while
the nurse has no way to help or cannot bring herself to help him. But
she may tacitly agree to let the patient take his own life. She may
even provide him with a "setup" for his suicide by leaving pills at
his bedside, removing his constraints, or leaving him alone in his
room or in a bathroom. Autoeuthanasia is, of course, also attempted
by patients without a nurse's surreptitious assistance. Sometimes the
ward arrangements are such that patients are put in a separate
"dying" room (which is a more convenient place for the patient to attempt autoeuthanasia), and left unwatched for comparatively long
periods of time. Even when autoeuthanasia is anticipated the ward
may have no room available with barred windows, for example, or
staff shortages may preclude adequate surveillance.

   Nurses often understand and even sympathize with patients in
great pain who attempt autoeuthanasia, when it is consistent with
their own collective desire to "let him die." Their collective reaction
is usually relief, not moral indignation or feelings of professional
incompetence. Just as letting the patient die seems a realistic alternative for them, autoeuthanasia seems a realistic alternative for the
patient, as far as they are concerned. The patient's awareness of this
alternative is a basic turning-point in his passage toward death. The
essential idea behind "turning points" is the awareness that "I am
not the same as I was, as I used to be."[3] At this point he grasps the
most important implication of his condition—that there is nothing

more to do—and realizes that the medical staff is merely managing this last phase of his dying as best they can. When he also realizes that his physical condition will soon prevent him from trying to manage his own dying, as well as the staff's managing of it, he recognizes autoeuthanasia as the only alternative to giving the staff complete control over his fate.

Nurses are trained to motivate patients to recover, and patients soon learn, if they do not know already, that they are supposed to be willing to get well. But this goal, like many other medical ideals, is inappropriate for a patient in the nothing-more-to-do phase. It makes more sense to motivate him to die; that is, to get him to accept his impending death and prepare for it. A nurse who is able to help motivate the patient to die (most nurses we met were not, however) can teach him how to die "gracefully." And this tactic may abet the tacit permission for autoeuthanasia, for he may also learn that it may be best, in the end, for him to manage his own death, to arrange a painless, easy departure and forestall an indefinite prolonging which, toward the end, he may be powerless to prevent. In this way he can insure a shorter ordeal for his family and a more presentable, undeteriorated physical condition for the last farewells. Indeed, we have known active people in the prime of life, many years before this stressful turning point, to contemplate just such a plan when they ask themselves, "What would I do?"

REFERENCES

1. Strauss, A.; Glaser, B.; and Quint, J. 1964. The non-accountability of terminal care—an aspect of hospital organization. *Hospitals* 36:73–87.

2. *San Francisco Chronicle*, June 1963.

3. Strauss, A. 1959. *Mirrors and masks*. New York: Free Press of Glencoe.

Tractable and Intractable Pain

11

IDEOLOGICAL AND ORGANIZATIONAL CONSIDERATIONS

Organizational and ideological considerations certainly affect how, how much, how well, and even when pain is relieved. With the aim of bringing those considerations to the foreground, we shall contrast two organizational situations. The first is quite unusual: it involves a special ideology pertaining to giving comfort care to the dying in a setting specifically designed for that purpose. Pain among these patients is an ever-present threat, and it is to be minimized and relieved. Although "medical," the style of pain management and the organization of work are very different from that reflected in the foregoing chapter on terminal care. The second situation involves intractable pain and the contemporary effort to combat it through special clinics or special modes of treatment carried out within conventional hospitals. We shall see that in the latter instance the customary organization of medical care profoundly impinges upon and affects the newer, more compassionate and humanistic modes of pain management.

IDEOLOGY AND INSTITUTIONALIZED DYING*

Among the best-known institutions where special ideologies guide terminal care is St. Joseph's Hospice in London, about which Dr. Cicely Saunders has written extensively.[1-5] Dr. Saunders worked out, at this hospital, her ideology and its associated operational philosophy of terminal care. The heart of her rationale is that St. Joseph's, as a specialized unit for terminal patients, "does not have the challenge of diagnoses nor the difficult decisions concerning treatment . . . those stages of their illnesses are now over."[6]

It follows that the staff is to look at these incurable patients (virtually all at St. Joseph's are incurable) as "persons in distress" and to "concentrate on giving them relief."[6] Relief—in our terms, comfort care—consists of several elements. First of all, since "at this stage of illness, pain is nearly always continuous," a program of "continuous control is called for." (Dr. Saunders has written in some detail about the pharmacological aspects of her program.) A most important dictum is that "drugs must be given regularly" and no patient kept waiting in fear or anxiety "until the 'proper' time." Dr. Saunders emphasizes the importance not only of carefully tailored pain control itself, but also of establishing and maintaining the patient's trust in the staff's ability to keep him or her reasonably free from pain, until death if necessary. The philsophy is that the "care of the dying demands all that we can do to enable patients to *live* until they die . . . and includes the care of the family, the mind, and the spirit as well as the care of the body."[7]

The establishment of the patient's trust involves the willingness to openly discuss dying with him if he himself recognizes he is dying and chooses to talk of it, as well as the obligation to respond appropriately to indirect and even nonverbal approaches to the topic. Staff response to a patient should be guided by the situation, allowing him to "come to the insight in his own way and time." Above all, staff members' responses must reflect due regard for the patient's own requirements and dignity. The objective is to help "mobilize the patient's own resources" and allow him to "come to his own personal victory." Dr. Saunders offers convincing evidence that this philosophy works with many patients, and she notes that they "have handed on strength and confidence to the others and to all who had the privilege of knowing them."

---

*This section is reproduced, in slightly altered form, from *Time for Dying* by Barney Glaser and Anselm Strauss (Chicago: Aldine, 1968, pp. 67–71). Copyright © 1968 by Anselm Strauss. Reprinted by permission.

Care at St. Joseph's is organized around several structural conditions. Of a total of 150 beds, "forty to fifty are kept for patients with terminal malignant disease who are sent by other hospitals or by family physicians with a prognosis of three months or less; only 10% live longer than that time. The remaining beds . . . are for the frail with no homes and for patients with long-term illness who are not suited for more active units (not for patients needing rehabilitation)."[8] Patients are housed in six-bed units. Nursing personnel are not given unusual training. (There are also nuns at this hospital.) Patients are not moved to separate rooms when near death.

St. Joseph's believes in keeping patients free from pain and helping them achieve a corresponding freedom from fear by sustaining open awareness when needed. This ideology is highly relevant to shaping lingering trajectories. The staff's basic strategy involves shaping each trajectory in conjunction with the patient's own conceptions of how it should be shaped. Primary in cancer is the fear— sometimes all too justified—of dying in constant, severe pain. For a patient, the ideal trajectory will have little or no pain. If this is medically possible, the staff members promise permanent relief, build trust in their capacity to carry out that promise, and point to the patients who are further along in dying (or who may already have died) as examples of their ability to control pain. The patients' stories are the staff's "success stories" and the staff can point to many such stories.

Another key structural condition in this hospital is the personal activity of Dr. Saunders, both as a reliever of pain and as a psychologist who sustains her patients. The latter role is especially called for when patients are aware of their own approaching demise, as most at this hospital are. Patients' awareness relates, in turn, to the staff's ability to "deliver." They are able to help the patient lose undue anxiety about dying itself and come to terms with past life, if need be, precisely because the patient *is aware* of approaching death. It is also important for the patient to have sufficient *time* to come to terms with death; quick death might leave her dying in psychological agony and with many unresolved life problems, whereas a lingering dying without pain, aided by her ability to trust the staff to help her, allows the patient to prepare adequately for a peaceful death.

Another important condition for the effective operation of the sustaining ideology is the absence of families or the presence of only fully cooperative ones. Without this condition, difficulties are encountered. As Dr. Saunders notes, apropos of what we have termed "open" and "closed" awareness about dying:

Relatives vary as patients do in their desire for the truth and many
ask that the patient should not be told and prefer to try to keep up
normal relationships. Some do this successfully to the end. Others
may need to be restrained from overacting or helped to see when the
patient really wants to be honest with them. One patient was
greatly distressed because as she gradually realized she was dying
her husband remained apparently cheerful and oblivious.

However, the guiding philosophy of the staff members in this case
enabled them to tell this husband "what was happening and [he]
was able at last to show her how much he cared."[9]

That the sentimental order may also be disrupted by patients
who respond negatively or not at all to the prevailing ideology is
suggested by the case of a patient described as "difficult to help."
This unmarried, middle-aged German expatriate was a very isolated
and withdrawn woman, despite her fair knowledge of English. "Her
mental suffering was all too apparent. She was extremely difficult to
help and comfort because her whole experience and personality made
such an illness and the publicity of a general ward well nigh intolerable to her. The nursing staff found her difficult to handle and
she found them hard to understand." She repeatedly refused medicines. She complained that the staff members were doing nothing for
her or "were making her worse by what we gave her." She also
"clutched so hard at any sign of improvement that it seemed wrong
to be frank with her." In short, she played havoc with the sentimental order, if not with the work order of the ward. The situation
was saved, almost miraculously, when Dr. Saunders asked a German
friend, a trained psychiatric nurse, to talk with the patient. Although
the patient died without awareness of her own dying, the psychiatric
nurse was able to talk deeply enough with her to get her to express
various fears and troubles, so that she "seemed comforted and peaceful at last" before becoming comatose and dying quickly.

Two additional structural conditions apparently exist in the
wards under Dr. Saunders' direction. Each is crucial to the success of
terminal care there. One has been implied in discussing the "difficult
case" just described: a patient must willingly delegate care to the
staff. As we shall see later, some patients in all countries, and many
patients in some countries, do not delegate care to professionals
when near death. In fact, it is useful to draw a distinction between
the willingness to delegate partial control to the hospital and the willingness to delegate virtually total control. The difficult woman just
discussed was willing to go to the hospital but made plain by various
actions, some highly dramatic (*e.g.*, bursting into tears at one point

and complaining about English doctors), that she was not ceding
much control over her life to the hospital staff. The other structural
condition demands that the staff be able to fulfill promises about
keeping pain under control. The staff at St. Joseph's is extremely conscientious about this. Patients in Asian or African countries, where
drugs tend to be both scarce and expensive, cannot always be promised freedom from their pain. This single structural difference—the
relative availability of pain-control drugs—can make a crucial difference in the interaction between the staff and the patients under their
care.

One final point: At St. Joseph's, the satisfactions that patients
and staff derive from their joint management of the lingering trajectory are undeniable. If such management works well, pain and
anxiety are minimized and acceptance of death is maximized. The
patient can live with dignity and even some pleasure while dying
gracefully. Staff need not cope with unpleasant "scenes" and are able
to take satisfaction in contributing to courageous and relatively
peaceful deaths. For Dr. Saunders and the institution, each "success
story" contributes to strengthening the ideology, and it often also
adds to medicine's knowledge of pain control in terminal cancer
cases.

INTRACTABLE PAIN: THE INTERACTION OF
NEW AND OLD MODES

It is generally believed in hospitals that most if not all pain is tractable—is manageable providing the proper resources are available
and provided nothing and nobody (including an uncooperative patient) interferes with the use of those resources. But a contrary belief
has taken hold in some circles that some pain is relatively intractable
but that innovative, imaginative management might make some of it
at least bearable. In consequence, this decade has seen a growth in
the United States of "pain clinics," as well as the use of various combinations of relief modes within regular hospitals. Intractable pain
can often be rendered tractable, given proper approaches to both the
patient and the pain, whether the pain is rooted in physiology or
psychology. The ideological thrust behind these new clinics and
modes of management is still predominantly medical (or why give
treatment in clinics and hospitals?), but expanded to give greater
weight to psychological and psychiatric perspectives and to treatments perilously close to what many health practitioners might deem
quackery.

The patients who come into these programs and clinics have

chronic illnesses with accompanying chronic pain. They come in last-ditch attempts to get relief from unbearable pains. In a later chapter on arthritics, we shall discuss their daily struggle at home with pain; arthritics typify the kinds of patients and pains dealt with in these pain clinics and pain programs. Most have shopped around, trying various potential solutions to their problems with pain; now they are trying out one more place—one more medical facility.

A notable characteristic of these programs and clinics is their great variability. They differ considerably in prevailing treatment ideologies and how they make them operational, in their screening mechanisms, in their manner of organizing relief tasks, and even in how they organize their divisions of labor. Their variability is doubtless related both to the difficulty of giving genuine and permanent relief to these chronic invalids and to the fact that the professionalized movement to conquer, in its early stages, pain previously defined as intractable. One characteristic of these early stages is the strikingly evident dispute surrounding them, with different opinions and approaches put forth by the medical and nonmedical worlds, the latter populated by academic psychologists, group therapists, advocates of body expression or transcendental meditation or Zen relaxation. To some of these methods are added more conventional styles of clinical psychology, psychiatry, physical therapy, nursing, and medicine.

The intractable pain wards and clinics currently being developed are, of course, added services or research programs, fitted into already existing medical and hospital organizations. Generally these innovations occur in the highly complex organizations of large medical centers. Therefore, among the major factors influencing the institutionalized forms of these new services, are: (1) the resources available, (2) the pain-treatment ideologies of the staffs involved, and (3) the organizational and interactional consequences for the existing organizations into which they are fitted.

As in any new service being developed, the chief of the pain-treatment and service team, usually a physician, must gather a staff and obtain space and equipment, often in an institution already short of space. Work arrangements must be made with a variety of hospital services and personnel. These arrangements may require new kinds of professional–professional and professional–patient relationships. Also there is need for staff training or retraining. The professional staff, including the chief, may be full-time to the new endeavor, or it may be borrowed part-time from another service (social service, psychiatry, neurology, occupational therapy). These numerous professionals will have varying understandings of, and commitments to, the new endeavor. In addition, the new responsibilities will necessarily impinge on each professional's ongoing work. Thus, even in purely medical services, the division of labor within the health team, the breadth of its services, and the institutional form of the particular treatment service will show wide variability from hospital to hospital. As will be discussed later, in the case of intractable-pain treatment services it can be anticipated that the institutional forms will show even greater variabilities, and there is likely to be an extended period of development for such services.

When the new intractable-pain ward or clinic is generously funded so that it can command optimum personnel, space, and equipment, and when it is also headed by a chief who has a definite treatment ideology along with an operational philosophy, then the functioning and development of the service is likely to have fewer discontinuities and ambiguities than might be otherwise expected. In general, one can anticipate that the new service will be in an extended state of "becoming" rather than "being."[10] The extended state of becoming is due in part to the newness of the service—particularly for pain wards which utilize both nonmedical (psychosocial) and medical modes of treatments, with an emphasis on the nonmedical. These wards typically call for psychosocial treatment modes such as milieu therapy and group therapy. Such a ward requires a new kind of organization; that is, a ward organized less on a medical model and more on a psychosocial model. Also, this new ward must usually emerge in a hospital which is already organized along medical lines. Discontinuities and ambiguities of professional roles and relationships can be anticipated. The psychosocial model will require new kinds of professionals, and the professional–professional relationships will be vastly different from those in an acute-care setting. For example, the clinical psychologist, the psychiatric nurse, or the social worker may figure prominently in determining the treatment mode and the ward operation, with the chief (often a neurologist) taking a secondary role—a departure from the usual pecking order in medical acute-care situations. Then too, the kinds of treatment modes required from other services, for example occupational therapy, may be quite different from those customarily provided for acutely ill patients. Not only may these other service personnel have varying understandings of and commitments to the new endeavor, but the new tasks may also impinge on their ongoing work in varying ways.

Relevant to the establishment of a nonmedically oriented pain ward is the requirement for a new kind of professional who has both knowledge of medical pain management and expertise in psychosocial treatment approaches. Such professionals are difficult to find because the training and practice of medicine and psychiatry are traditionally given in two different subworlds of medicine. Given this fact, the selection of professionals may be a "make do" situation. The person selected to manage the ward, usually a nurse, tends to be psychiatrically trained but given specialized training in medical pain management, or a medically specialized "pain" nurse who is taught psychosocial skills.

Decisions about what kinds of psychosocial modes of treatment will be used may be difficult to reach because of the wide diversity of psychiatric ideologies and treatment philosophies.[11, 12] Then too, the training and treatment approaches of clinical psychologists generally are quite different from those of psychiatrists. Thus, such questions as the following are debatable and debated. What kind of milieu therapy is to be used? What will be the nature and substance of group therapy discussions? Who is to lead the discussions? How do we reduce the patients' dependence on pain drugs? On the issue of reducing the patients' dependence on pain narcotics, for example, some are strongly oriented to an operant-conditioning approach while others hold it to be "cruel and authoritarian."

Then, of course, there are disagreements about the criteria for patient selection. Will they all be intractable pain patients, all low-back pain patients, or only certain low-back pain patients? The criteria for patient selection will influence the kind of personnel and the hospital services required, as well as the kinds of relationships which evolve among professionals.

The division of labor (who, what, and how) can be anticipated to develop slowly. A treatment team must be forged from an aggregate of professionals with various approaches, philosophies, and skills. Considerable time is required for team members to understand each other's treatment orientations, identify the areas of needed training, and establish new kinds of professional–professional and professional–patient relationships. Also, those professionals and paraprofessionals who are unsophisticated about the psychiatric world may not realize the varieties of psychiatric ideologies, so they may simply not comprehend the related debates about treatment. "We're feeling our way," is a commonly heard statement by professionals in the evolving pain clinics.

Previous arrangements within the treatment team, as well as with other services and personnel in the hospital, will require renegotiation as conditions change within the team and in other services.[13] Of course, constant negotiations occur in any hospital situation, but the requirements for constant renegotiation increase in this instance, because the ambiguities and discontinuities are likely to be greater in a situation where a nonmedical mode of treatment is introduced into an acute-care setting. The "feeling of the way" is not soon over.

For example, a research diagnostic clinic for intractable pain was established in a large medical center. The diagnostic team consisted of the usual medical group of neurologist, internist, psychologist, psychiatrist, and other appropriate medical specialists. Since the service was a new endeavor, a limited number of patients were accepted into the program. The patients were hospitalized for a few days on a specified ward—an active medical–surgical unit—while they underwent intensive diagnostic tests and interviews. Following the tests and interviews, the total team conferred and made decisions about the kinds of treatment appropriate for each patient.

The nursing staff members were given a few didactic lectures on the phenomenon of pain; the goal of the research was explained and a "pain interview" was developed. This was administered by nurses when new patients were admitted to the unit. The medical team was informed that each patient would be assigned to a "primary nurse," who would be responsible for the patient's total hospital stay and co-ordinate activities so that the patient could have "continuity of care." The primary nurse's observations would be included in the final conference. The assumption of the physicians, of course, was that the primary nurse would resolve many of the problems associated with fragmented care, and that observations about patients would be more consistent. The physicians were not aware that the concept of primary nurse was relatively new and much debated within nursing.[13]

The nursing staff faced difficulties when instituting the new approach, and much of the care was no different from before, for it embodied a division of labor based on usual tasks. More important, the nurses were interacting with patients in terms of their own pain philosophies rather them communicating with each other. Faced with many acutely ill patients, the staff members tended to interact with intractable pain patients only when they complained of pain or when they asked for pain medications. Their perceptions of a patient and his pain remained narrow. Thus, when nurses participated in the final conference, they had made only limited observations of each patient. An hour before the conference they would attempt to talk to other staff members who might have some different observations on a given patient.

The nurses—without sufficient help in coping and interacting with patients who had intractable pain—were often frustrated and even irritated by them. Some nurses openly admitted that increased encounters with them, particularly with the low-back ones, made them become more unsympathetic. "And you know," they added,

"the study is showing that most of the low-back patients' pain is
more psychological than physiological." The new service, then, did
not result in nurses developing greater sensitivity to the problems of
intractable pain patients or more effective ways of interacting with
the patients; instead it furthered their stereotyping them.

When an innovation that is primarily medical has such consequences as the ones just described, then the interactional and
organizational consequences can be anticipated to be even greater
when a nonmedical treatment mode is introduced. And if the resources are far from optimum, the program may be doomed for
failure, or at least have disappointing results. A neurologist, a medically specialized "pain" nurse, and a clinical psychologist were able
to persuade the hospital administration to establish a pain ward in a
large medical research center. The three key professionals were only
part-time to the new endeavor. With the limited resources, they
could only command partial space (eight beds) on a chemotherapy
cancer ward. The psychosocial approach selected was a modified operant-conditioning one—in part because this was familiar both to the
pain nurse and the psychologist—and also a modified milieu therapy
which could be fitted into an acute-care setting. The field of selection
from which they could draw a nurse to administer the ward was
limited, not only because someone skilled both in medical pain management and psychosocial approaches was difficult to find, but also
because the selection entailed drawing from the available nursing
staff of the acute-care hospital. The head nurse, although very interested in the pain ward, felt inadequate in using psychosocial
treatment modalities. Moreover, because the number of patients was
limited and they were not acutely ill, they could not justify supplying
nurses for all three daily shifts. This meant that during the evening
and night shifts, the patients were cared for by the cancer nursing
staff who had limited understanding of the pain program; thus the
staff interacted with the pain patients much as it did with the cancer
patients. Although diversional therapy was a part of the treatment
program, the pain-treatment team could not command an optimum
program from the occupational and recreational services since these
personnel had other work demands.

With the personnel limited both in number and expertise, the
day-to-day operations of the ward fell on the pain-specialist nurse
who had other responsibilities. She had little time to spare to
adequately train the head nurse who felt increasingly incompetent
and frustrated. When the former moved out of the state, the pain
ward simply folded. In the last report, it was noted that a new pain
ward was established with a psychiatrically trained nurse supervisor

who had boned up on the literature related to psychosocial aspects of pain and to the medical management of pain. Because of the lack of space in the medical center, the new ward was housed in a nonacute hospital setting. The staff members here were also "feeling their way."

In any ward situation, personnel turnover affects the shape of the team and its work. On pain wards, the arrival and departure of psychologically trained professionals will alter the team and its work more than in a medical situation. On medical wards the tasks and division of labor are fairly well defined, but that is not so for psychological tasks because of the wide variations in psychiatric and treatment philosophies.

On the current scene, many evolving pain wards seem oriented to an operant-conditioning approach. That is because a preponderant number of the intractable pain patients suffer from back pain and operant-conditioning seems, to the practitioners, to be potentially effective for them. With the growing interest in intractable pain, professionals with different orientations will become involved. Hence, debates over what kind of treatment is appropriate, and claims about who can "treat," can be anticipated.

In summary, great variations on institutional organization among pain clinics and wards can be anticipated given: (1) the varieties of personnel drawn from subworlds within the medical world and also from nonmedical world (psychology, social work), all of whom must together fashion the treatment teams and (2) the necessary attempts to articulate the new organizational arrangements within ongoing, standard, medical organizations. As with any new social movement, it is difficult to predict what form the new organizations, evolving out of the intractable-pain-treatment movement, will take. We would hazard a guess that even an extensive study of these new pain services would not greatly qualify the picture drawn here, but rather illuminate with greater detail and depth the evolving organizational variability, as well as the consequences of that evolution for patients, staffs, and organizations themselves.

REFERENCES

1. Saunders, C. 1965. The last stages of life. *American Journal of Nursing* 65:70–75.

2. Saunders, C. 1959. Care of dying. *Nursing Times* reprint. London: Macmillan.

3. Saunders, C. 1960. The need for institutional care for the patient

with advanced cancer. Paper written for the Cancer Institute, Madras.

4. Saunders, C. 1960. *Care of the dying.* London: Macmillan.

5. Saunders, C. 1964. The symptomatic treatment of incurable malignant disease. *Prescriber's Journal* 4:68–74.

6. Op. cit. The last stages of life, p. 1.

7. Ibid., p. 2.

8. Op. cit. *Care of the dying*, p. 8.

9. Strauss, A. et al. 1964. *Psychiatric ideologies and institutions.* New York: Free Press of Glencoe, pp. 125–126.

10. Ibid., pp. 8–10.

11. Strauss, A. et al. 1963. The hospital and its negotiated order. In *The hospital in modern society*, ed. E. Friedson, pp. 147–169. New York: Free Press of Glencoe.

12. Bucher, R., and Schatzman, L. 1964. Negotiating a division of labor among professionals in the state mental hospital. *Psychiatry* 27:266–277.

13. Manthey, M., and Kramer, M. 1970. A dialogue on primary nursing. *Nursing Forum* 9:356–380.

Part 5

Living with Incurable Pain

Inattentiveness to Chronic Pain: Geriatric Wards

12

We begin this chapter with two rather typical statements made by nurses who work at a large, public, metropolitan, extended-care facility for the chronically ill.

> It's curious, but we have relatively few pain problems with our patients. Most of our patients' pains can be controlled by aspirin, or aspirinlike drugs.

> The families of patients find it strange that at home, they constantly complained about pain, but since coming here complain noticeably less.

In a similar vein, the patients, including those who obviously did have pain (severe arthritis, for instance) would tend to disregard our questions about pain. They preferred to talk about their pasts, their families, or to ask questions about our lives. Not uncommonly, a patient would answer our questions about pain with: "My dear, I always have pain. I can't be thinking about it all the time."

The paradox of patients' inattentiveness to their pain, and their reluctance to express it despite its persistence and lengthy duration, along with the staff's noting of its existence, becomes understandable when viewed from four standpoints: (1) the relationships among illness, pain, and social trajectories; (2) the actuality and threat of the social isolation experienced by patients; (3) the organizational and work features of such extended-care facilities as the one studied; (4) the biographies of both patients and staff members.

ILLNESS, PAIN, AND SOCIAL TRAJECTORIES: GERIATRIC WARDS

A typical geriatric institution is populated by elderly patients institutionalized because (1) they lack or have depleted their financial resources and cannot afford private care, (2) their care is too difficult or complex to manage at home, or (3) they have no reliable family or friends to accept the burden of their care.[1]

Although efforts are made to rehabilitate and relocate them outside the institution, and although some wards inside are organized for rehabilitative purposes, most patients are considered "unrehabilitatable" and "unrelocatable."[2, 3] They have "flunked out" of rehabilitation programs, either at the extended-care facility itself or at other rehabilitation or acute-care hospitals. Having had numerous medical treatments designed to effect a reversal or retardation of their disease processes, they are now in a phase of illness when such treatments are deemed futile. Thus the purpose of their care is to keep an unstable and downward course of illness as stable as possible and without medical crises. Much of the care is related to sheer physical maintenance, or it merges closely with efforts at medical stabilization. Also, the typical patient is in a final downward phase of the social trajectory; this involves partial or total rejection by family and friends.

As for the illness trajectory, its downward progress varies with the severity, length, and kind of illness. Some patients may be institutionalized when in the terminal phases of their illness, as are those with cancer. Others, such as those who suffer from arthritis, stroke, and neurological disorders, may spend many years in such an institution. Regardless of the rates of their downward trajectories, most foresee spending the remainder of their lives there. They see the situation as one of "no exit" except through death.

The pains which may accompany the illness are also of a chronic nature. These people often have much experience with pain, having undergone a variety of treatments and drugs for controlling and minimizing it. Quite often, long before admission to the facility, they have come to terms with living with chronic pain. Over the years they have come to realize that no treatment or drug will reverse the disease process or control their pain. They have learned not only that constant attention to pain is emotionally exhausting but also that their continued expression of pain can disrupt social interaction and result in social isolation: "People don't like to be around people who talk about pain all the time."

Those who previously had relied upon narcotics for relief eventually realize, either on their own or through efforts of the health professionals, that no narcotic can completely relieve their pain and that addiction has its dangers. Their decision not to rely on narcotics is based upon a weighing and balancing of various considerations: pain control versus sociability; pain control versus the drug's side effects; or pain relief versus staff–patient interaction. One patient who had severe arthritis, and who had received an astonishing array of treatments over the years, including twenty surgeries and a wide variety of pain-controlling drugs, had this to say:

> When I arrived here, I was taking codeine for pain every three hours. At the same time, the codeine was getting less and less effective in controlling the pain as I became more and more addicted. My whole life revolved around pain and waiting for the pain drugs. I'd recite poetry to get my mind off the pain. There would be exquisite relief after taking the drug, but these relief periods were getting shorter and shorter, and I was reciting more and more often. Finally I decided this was a stupid way to live. The ward staff didn't want to be around me, and friends didn't want to visit because all I could think about was pain. Then too, the narcotics caused constipation which means suffering taking enemas and laxatives, not to mention the discomforts of getting on and off the bedpan.

> As my body begins to deteriorate more and more, and there is no treatment to stop the deterioration, the only thing I have left is my mind. As long as I was on so much narcotics I couldn't think straight, and couldn't relate to people as I would like. So, I decided to get off the narcotics. It was hard, but I did it "cold turkey." It's amazing how much the mind can control pain. Now an aspirinlike drug controls most of the pain, although I have a dull pain all the time. On rare occasions I'll take codeine. I read more now, and I have wonderful conversations with my friends and family.

In the final phases of social and illness trajectories, separated from family and isolated from the outside world, these people are

faced with coming to terms with their circumstances. When the
downward spiral continues for some years, that task includes the tolerating and enduring of pain as best they can, even though it may
increase in severity. Often it does.

SOCIAL CONTACT: A FIRST PRIORITY

Throughout the wards of such institutions, loneliness and social isolation are pervasive. Quite often the process of isolation precedes the
actual institutionalization, which may not take place until after a long
and isolating illness. The institutionalization heightens the separation from friends, family, even from spouses. In the words of one
nurse: "They are simply abandoned, many of them." Then too, over
the years, their social contacts have tended to dwindle or vanish because of their lessened energy, impaired mobility, and speech,
hearing, or bodily disfigurement. Visitors at the institution are few,
either because no family members or friends live nearby, or because
they have become caught up in their own lives and worlds, or perhaps because their own families and other friends have become
severely ill.

For many patients in these institutions, social contact with the
outside world is limited to the personnel. Patients hunger for contact.
They clutch and hold an interviewer's hands and maneuver conversation to prolong that contact. Without exception, they thanked us
profusely for "visiting." These expressions of gratitude were touching and pathetic. The frequency and numbers of their visitors were
extremely important to them. With continued institutionalization, social contact understandably becomes a first priority. As another nurse
succinctly phrased it: "We have not so much physical pain as the
pain of loneliness." This priority, as we shall see, greatly affects the
relationships between personnel and patients, as well as the way patients manage to endure their pains.

WARD ORGANIZATION AND PAIN WORK

The extended-care facilities share some features of total institutions.[4]
("Total institutions" are usually conceived of as places of residence
where large numbers of men or women, cut off from the wider society, lead an enclosed and formally administered type of life. The
needs of the residents are handled "bureaucratically" rather than in
terms of humane, individualistic considerations.) Despite the top ad-
ministrations' great efforts to individualize and humanize care, the

work of caring for such chronically ill patients tends to become
highly routine.

Relevant to this routinization, of course, is the general societal
neglect of the aged which results in insufficient allocations of funds
and resources to nursing homes and extended-care facilities. Hence
inadequate staffing is a usual feature of such institutions.[5,6] Limited
resources encourage tight scheduling and routinization of work to efficiently accommodate the large numbers of patients. Efficiency is
sought by the sorting and the distributing of patients on the wards,
not so much on the basis of their individual "needs" as in accordance with the amount of work required of the staff.[7] Often the major
criteria for the sorting of patients include their degree of mental al-
ertness and their self-care capabilities. Wards are categorized as
"mentally alert-minimal physical care," "mentally alert-heavy physical care," "semialert-average physical care," and so on. Matched to
these categories are appropriate numbers of staff members.

The management of large numbers of patients by small staffs is
done by organizing the patients' lives into daily and weekly routines.[8] Each ward has hourly, daily, and weekly routines, not only
with respect to patient care but for maintaining the ward itself in a
reasonable state of cleanliness and order. There are times for arising
in the morning, washing for breakfast, feeding, bathing (bed patients
1 through 10 on Monday, bed patients 11 through 20 on Tuesday),
shampooing, cutting toenails, getting into wheelchairs, toileting,
walking, napping, and so on throughout the day.

As we mentioned earlier, the care focus of the personnel is keeping the many unstable illness trajectories as stable as possible. Thus,
the major work revolves around maintaining both hygiene and bodily functioning. There are tasks which pertain to skin and oral
hygiene, adequate nutrition, hydration, elimination, and mobilization. The volume of "body work,"[8] as aptly named by Gubrium, is
very great because many patients are disabled. Also, the work is
physically demanding (patients need moving and lifting, sometimes
even with machinery); therefore much of the body work is carried
out by teams of personnel. This in turn requires further coordination
and the scheduling of work time. Also, the work of preventing bedsores and contractures can be especially difficult when there are large
numbers of helpless and incontinent patients to be serviced. Thus,
there is much routine turning of bodies, handling of bedpans, and
checking of incontinence.

A peculiar characteristic of body work is that it blurs the distinction between medical and physical maintenance. For example, to

prevent muscular atrophy and osteoporotic changes of bone may require therapeutic activities such as passive and active exercise, and teaching or encouraging the patient to be more responsible for his or her own daily care. Efforts are currently being made in extended-care facilities to incorporate rehabilitation concepts (even on custodial wards) into the work of physical maintenance in order both to prevent further deterioration and to further the patient's independence. Yet the blurring of the medical–physical maintenance results in the neglect of "the rehabilitation component."[9] In part the neglect is due to the limited medical understanding of the aides who are largely responsible for the patients' care, and who perceive body maintenance as work rather than as "therapeutic." Also the sheer volume of work mitigates against incorporating the rehabilitation perspective because the work can be done faster when done "for" the patient rather than allowing the patient to carry out the task, especially if one must spend time encouraging the patient. All this routinization of work for the sake of efficiency poses difficulties for individualizing care and may even hasten physical deterioration. It may also adversely affect pain work.

Pain Work

For both patients and staff, pain work is part of the main focus on geriatric wards. The extent to which it is carried on, however, is not readily evident. By contrast, in acute-care hospitals much of the pain work is highly visible, and it is associated with controlling acute pain or minimizing inflicted pain. Staff there relies heavily on drugs to control pain; a patient may endure considerable pain from treatments in order to have a disease reversed, retarded, or cured. However, on extended-care facilities, the pain is mainly chronic, and the inflicted pains are not so much connected with medical treatments as with tasks done to further physical maintenance. Those tasks include moving a painful joint or other part of the body, or insuring that the patient endure the pains deriving from maintenance because bedsores, contractures, or other complications must be prevented.

Patients' requests for relief usually do not get immediate response from the staff because pain and its relief are related to the highly routinized mass work of physical maintenance. For example, a patient may be very uncomfortable from remaining too long in one position or because she was positioned poorly, but staff members, busy with other work, may not immediately attend to pain relief.

More often than not a patient must endure her pain until the next prearranged time for moving her arrives, or until she is moved per schedule from wheelchair back to bed for napping, or she must wait until after everyone's feeding time. Thus, it is not unusual to find patients in wheelchairs attempting to catch the attention of anyone passing in order to be repropped or have a pillow moved back into place or be put back into bed because they are tired and uncomfortable.

Different assessments of the degree of pain suffered by the patient are made, in accordance with their primary work responsibilities, by both nonprofessional and professional nursing personnel. The former, responsible for much of the physical maintenance, generally tend to assess pains as greater than do the professionals. Understandably, they are the major agents of pain infliction, spending more time at the bedside, so, they are more likely to observe grimaces and other pain expressions than the professionals. (Patients' complaints to the researchers were frequently about negligence—an aide or an orderly being too rough in handling them). Since the professional personnel are responsible for the general administration of the ward and for doing the more complex treatments—giving medications and assisting the physicians—their assessments of the pain suffered by a given patient are based to a considerable degree on information provided by the nonprofessionals. Because the latters' focus of work is mainly on getting the body work done, they are not likely to report much about pain. Also, since assessment of pain includes observing such cues as groaning, moaning, crying, and requests for drug relief, and since many patients learn to control their expressions of pain tightly, both professional and nonprofessional personnel probably underestimate the pain. The professionals' assessment is, however, lower than that of the nonprofessionals.

The major pain task faced by all staff members, then, is pain minimization through a gentle handling of the patients' bodies, allowing them to move at their own speeds, and utilizing comfort measures (such as propping pillows here and there). The minimization of pain is largely the nonprofessional staff's responsibility. Much of the work requires intimate knowledge of specific patients—such and such a position is more comfortable than another or moving the body in a particular way is less painful than other ways.

The frequency and kinds of drugs used will vary according to the rate at which the illness trajectories progress. Patients with terminal cancer are given strong narcotics without having to legitimate their pains, and without staff concern about addiction. For patients with slower downward trajectories—that is, for most patients on these wards—there is less reliance on narcotics and greater use of aspirin and other analgesics.

We should add that on these extended-care wards, the patients' main responsibilities concerning pain are, first, to come to terms with living with their chronic pain, even if it is increasing; second, not to be overly expressive about pain (for that might upset the sentimental order of the ward); and third, to learn when and how to ask for drug relief.

Inattention to Pain

There appears to be a process whereby both the staff and patients become, over time, relatively inattentive to pain. The patients learn to endure a continuing, inescapable situation where they have little control over their own lives. They become increasingly dependent on the staff for all aspects of life, as they continue to deteriorate physically and must rely on staff members for a modicum of contact with the outside world.

Where specific organizational features obtain, particularly the presence of a stable staff, individualized pain-minimization tactics may gradually evolve, even though one might assume those are difficult to achieve in these over-populated institutions. There is not only the development of individualized tactics but also, paradoxically, an increased inattentiveness to pain. Contributing to this are (1) the intertwining of the mutual biographies of personnel and patients and (2) their mutual, shared priorities.

MUTUAL BIOGRAPHIES

When the organization is able to maintain a stable staff, then individualized pain-management tactics can evolve. The job stability of the entire staff, together with the extended hospitalization of the typical patient, result in the staff members getting to know each patient rather well and even intimately. They learn a great deal about each patient's social history and about significant details of pain work, such as the right way to prop pillows, the best body positions, or the best ways of interacting with patients to make them more cooperative and seemingly less focused on pain. These details of pain minimization eventually become common knowledge among the personnel. Over time, a tailoring of pain minimization for particular patients develops in what seems otherwise to be a highly standardized institution.

As patients become increasingly isolated from family and friends, they come increasingly to rely on the personnel for social contact and for most aspects of "living." A statement commonly made by staff members is: "We're the only family for him." Over the years, then, the lives of personnel and patients become intertwined. Often the patients live vicariously through the personnel. They are interested in their families, what they do on their days off, etc. In turn, the personnel engage in a number of touching and even compassionate acts designed to brighten the lives of their charges. They bring in favorite dishes cooked at home, wash the patients' personal clothing at home rather than allowing the hospital laundry to ruin it, and shop on their own time for personal items desired by patients.

The patients' complete dependence encourages passivity and compliance with the personnel's dictates and a gratefulness for small favors. Gradually the patients learn to fit into the ward and its routine, becoming socialized to accept their situation by such staff statements as: "We're one big family, and like a family we have to get along with each other. Each of us has to give and take and meet each other half way."

On occasion, the staff may encounter patients who represent great problems in pain management—problems for the whole hospital. For example, one paraplegic became an immense problem not only because she constantly cried about her pain, but because of continued uncooperativeness in failing to endure patiently the pains inflicted during treatments and during physical-maintenance tasks. She was moved from ward to ward, not only to relieve the personnel who had reached their limits of toleration, but because the staff hoped to find a ward whose personnel could work with this woman. Eventually such a ward was found. A concerted effort was made by its staff to individualize the minimization of her pain and socialize her to the ward. Meanwhile—ever so slowly—she came to terms both with her pain and with the prospect of never leaving the institution. Her story is not unusual; indeed it is typical. It suggests that the "one big family" idea helps to persuade patients to endure pain in silence, as they balance covert expression against good relations with the staff. In effect, there is a trade-off in a silent bargain between the two sides.

SOCIAL ISOLATION AND MUTUAL PRIORITY

The bargain is seen even more clearly, perhaps, when one considers the issue of social isolation. As we remarked earlier, the first priority for many, if not most, patients is to have social contact, while the staff members also recognize loneliness and social isolation as a major problem. Thus the hospital as a whole may attempt (as did the one studied) to meet this problem by creating a variety of social activities for patients, including encouraging community groups to visit patients and to organize activities for them. As one patient who went daily to both Catholic and Protestant services explained: she participated in any and all activities offered because they helped her to pass the time, and she needed "not to think about myself so much."

The nurses remarked on a relationship between the patient's perception of pain and his anger and frustration at being "put away" forever in the institution. (This is quite the same as when patients are placed in mental institutions.[10]) They believe that patients complain more about pain when they are first transferred to the extended-care wards, and that patients who are on the admission wards (where they await transfer to an extended-care ward) complain more about pain than those in the extended-care wards. "As long as the patient is angry at the family for placing him here, and so long as the family feels guilty about it, we can't relieve the pains." The nurse who said that attempts indirectly to relieve, or at least minimize, physical pain by helping the family members to relieve their guilt and so ease the patient's transition to the hospital.

> We let the family know that they couldn't possibly manage the patient at home, and we understand the circumstance and there is no alternative . . . that faced with a similar situation I would have to put my mother here. We try to find out from the family about special foods they like, or any special habits so we can, as best we can, fit this into the care, like having wine with their meals, or hot milk before bedtime.

We see then that staff members and patients share a mutual concern with lessening the patients' isolation. There is an implicit trade-off between them; both sides "act right" in handling their respective pain and other tasks. In this fashion, the more or less intractable pain is managed, within a highly politicized context.

THE BURDEN OF CARE

The burden of care and its implied pain tasks are as follows. As long as a chronically ill person is able to care for himself or have someone else share the burden of his care, then he can remain out of an institutionalized setting. At the point when his illness renders his care permanently difficult—even makes it difficult to keep him alive— then his family or other guardians shift the burden of his care to a custodial institution. In addition to custodial care, such institutions may offer their residents excellent medical care which yields them some measure of physical comfort. Yet, since their illnesses are chronic, the perspectives of staff and family alike tend toward fatalism; even the best medical care is unlikely to reverse the sick person's condition sufficiently to allow him to leave the facility. Sometimes relatives are most happy to take him home again, or they are persuaded to do so on a trial basis. We observed one physician who worked immensely hard both to reverse patients' deterioration and to convince their families to accept them at home again.

Most often, however, the geriatric facility represents the end of the road—though the road may still be very long. Until the patient dies, the staff members have accepted the responsibility of keeping him alive and as comfortable as possible. Since they are doing this for many, even a multitude, of sick persons, the custodial problems sometimes take precedence over the purely medical ones. The latter are, anyhow, usually undramatic—comfort care scarcely seems like genuine medical care to enterprising physicians—and they virtually merge with and become indistinguishable from custodial conerns.

Assuming that a patient is still sentient, he will know or eventually learn that the burden of his care—both custodial and medical—has been shifted permanently to these strangers. In accordance, he will learn to express his pain with moderation and feel concern for the reactions of his caretakers. If he does not, he will only add to his discomfort and doubtless, over time, will receive less attention and less adequate care. He may not live as long; and certainly he will be serviced by far less sociable agents. "Carrying on" about pain would only add to the burden of care assumed by the staff members, a burden which in truth is heavy enough or else it would not be shunted to them by his family.

Very little, if any, of all this is said aloud by anyone (except perhaps initially by patients who complain bitterly of having been "dumped.") The bargains are usually silent, and those involving pain seem among the most implicit. While the "better" facilities offer more effective comfort and custodial care, or at least better physical surroundings, the situation there with regard to pain interactions seems not very different. Any change in pain management within these institutions for the chronically ill would require changing the basic conditions under which they operate.

REFERENCES

1.   Calkins, K. 1972. Shouldering the burden. *Omega* 3:23–36.

2. Lieberman, M. A. 1974. Relocation research and social policy. *Gerontologist* 14:494–500.

3. Roth, J., and Eddy, E. 1967. *Rehabilitation for the unwanted*. New York: Atherton.

4. Goffman, I. 1966. *Asylum*. New York: Doubleday-Aldine, p. 6.

5. Subcommittee on Long-Term Care of the Special Committee on Aging, U.S. Senate. 1974–1975. *Nursing homes in the United States: failure and public policy*. 93rd Congress, Report number 93-1420. Washington, D.C.: U.S. Government Printing Office.

6. Townsend, C. 1971. *Old age: the last segregation* (the Nader report). New York: Grossman.

7. Strauss, A. et al. 1964. *Psychiatric ideologies and institutions*. New York: Free Press of Glencoe, pp. 104–124.

8. Gubrium, J. F. 1975. *Living and dying at Murray Manor*. New York: St. Martin's Press, pp. 121–157.

9. Davis, M. Z. 1977. Rehabilitation care in the skilled nursing facilities: the mismatch of organizational structure and patient need. *Journal of Nursing Administration* 7:22–27.

10. Goffman, op. cit., pp. 131–148.

Living with
Rheumatoid Arthritis*

13

In the next pages, we shall look at people who are living as best they can, under ordinary daily circumstances, with incurable, chronic pain. They suffer from rheumatoid arthritis, a systemic disease affecting connective or supporting tissue. Aside from the considerable discomfort, pain, and impairment of mobility and bodily movements stemming from the illness, there can be considerable social impact on arthritics' lives because they live with great uncertainty concerning the coming and going of symptoms. Which ones? Which part of the body? When? For how long? How severe? In what combinations? Consequently, living a normal life is rather difficult. How to achieve the maximum normalization of life and of relations with others while still coping with symptoms—including pain—becomes a major problem.

RESOURCE REDUCTION AND UNCERTAINTY

The etiology of rheumatoid arthritis is unknown, but the result is that the involved tissue becomes inflamed. When the disease at-

This is a modified version of a paper by Carolyn Weiner, "A burden of rheumatoid arthritis: tolerating the uncertainty," *Social Science and Medicine*, 1975.

tacks joint tissue, pain becomes the signal for both patient and physician. In most cases, the onset is insidious, with ill-defined aching and stiffness. In about one-fifth of the cases, severe multiple joint inflammation develops suddenly at onset.[1]

The victim of rheumatoid arthritis is faced with a reduction of personal resources—resources taken for granted by the healthy. More than one kind of resource can be profoundly affected. Mobility may be reduced because of the incapacitating effect of pain, and because weight-bearing joints are so deformed or acutely inflamed as to prevent the arthritic from wearing shoes and to make walking difficult or impossible. A reduction of skill may occur, attributable to increased pain, loss of dexterity, and loss of strength. Joints are not only swollen and painful, but they have limited movement. A progressive disease, it can lead to dislocation of fingers and deformity of hands. A weakening and then wasting of muscle may occur above and below the affected joint, causing a loss of strength. Pots become too heavy to lift, handbags too heavy to carry, doors too heavy to open. Finally, a reduction of energy can occur, caused by the metabolic effect of the disease (its attack on connective tissues) and also by the circuitous quality of pain. (Pain drains energy and fatigue produces more pain.)

Rheumatoid arthritis patients learn, along with their diagnoses, that the disease is not only incurable, but its specific manifestations are unpredictable. Often as not, they hear the physician say: "You're going to have to learn to live with it." The disease imposes a burden which many patients would assess to be a less "livable" condition than merely reduced resources, however, and that is its total absence of predictability. The disease does not often follow a strictly downhill course. Most cases are marked by flare-up and remission. Even in the most hopeful case, bad flare-ups may suddenly occur, just as the most severe case may suddenly and inexplicably become arrested. The disease has been referred to as a "rheumatic iceberg," in that the duration is lifelong even when so quiescent as to be no problem, but quiescence and flare-up are themselves unpredictable.

The variability of progression severity and areas of involvement among these arthritics cannot be stressed enough.[2-4] For example, they may have reduced mobility but no impairment of skill, reduced energy but no interference with mobility, reduced energy one day and renewed energy the next day. Loss of skill will remain fairly constant if it is caused by deformity, but is variable if caused by swelling. The other resources (mobility and energy) can also fluctuate. Thus uncertainty pervades the life of arthritics: on any given day, he does not know beforehand about symptoms: (1) presence (if there will be any pain, swelling or stiffness); (2) place (area of bodily involvement); (3) quantity (degree of disabling intensity); (4) temporality (whether the onset will be gradual or sudden, as well as duration and frequency of flare-ups).

Pressing their claims upon the arthritic in consequence are two imperatives: the inner, or physiological world, monitored for pain and disability readings by the day, sometimes the hour; and the outer world of activity, of maintaining what is perceived as a normal existence. Like two runners in a nightmare race, these two imperatives gain one on the other, only to be overtaken again and again.

When the physiological world gains a lead, the arthritic finds that severe pain is more easily endured by withdrawing from interaction: "I go off by myself . . . to cry, or swear, or both." If these flare-up periods increase, both in duration and frequency, the uncertainty problem will be resolved by the certainty of more bad days than good. The activity world, to extend the metaphor, will have lost the race. The arthritic will have become an invalid and increasingly isolated. But the very uncertainty which makes the disease so intolerable also mitigates against acceptance of invalidism—there is always hope for another remission.

THE HOPE AND THE DREAD

All illnesses provoke theories of causation—circumstantial relationships as discerned by the patient—and rheumatoid arthritis is no exception. Part of the patient's psychological toleration stems from his hope that a remission can be correlated with something he can control, such as diet. Belief in dietary causal linkage may be sustained for a long period, only to be upset by another flare-up.

Hope is primarily directed, however, toward control of symptoms. Uncertainty as to how long a given flare-up will last makes an arthritic vulnerable to folk remedies suggested by friends, kin, other patients, and by the arthritic's own reading of literature. Self-doctoring ranges from ingestion of celery juice or massive doses of vitamin E, to use of plastic bags filled with powdered sulphur and wrapped around the feet at night, or to a poultice of ginger root steeped in vodka and an alloy. The clinic provides a place where such ideas can be exchanged. In addition, there is a trial and error approach to the use of applied heat and change of climate, diet, and appliances.

Even if relieved, arthritics are haunted again by uncertainty, for what they have attributed to a specific relief measure may indeed have been an independent spontaneous remission; but they continue to hope until proven wrong. When a measure is believed to be providing temporary relief, as acupuncture is presently doing for some, the hope becomes extended: "Maybe some week the two days relief I'm getting will become three." The reversal of the hope for remission (i.e. the hope that the arthritis will perform "on cue"), is of course less common. But that this hope can also be felt serves to emphasize the exasperating quality of the uncertainty. One patient reported she waited six weeks for an appointment with an acupuncturist, then was refused treatment because the disease was in remission and might be reactivated by the treatment. Even those whose deformities make their invalidism appear to others as irreversible have so often experienced the oscillations of flare-up and remission that they continue to hope. One man, almost totally incapacitated by his disease, had driven miles to the clinic and waited there four hours for what turned out only to be a refill on his prescription. He explained his patience to the interviewer: "Maybe if you're around when they find something new, they'll try it on you." Similarly, a woman who evinced almost total withdrawal from social contact still hoped to return to adult school "some day."

Countering such psychological tolerance is the fantasy of disease progression. An arthritic may hope for longer and longer remissions, but simultaneously dread the possible course of the disease—the next place it is going to hit. As one expressed it, "I think of my body like a used car, waiting for the next part to go." In a clinic they see others who are worse off and when they say: "I'm lucky it's not in my. . . ." The implication is clear. All this leaves them constantly on the alert. Pain, when it hits in a new place, makes their uncertainty intolerable. Knowing the possibilities is one thing, having them occur is another; the arthritic must wait to see if the pain persists and while waiting his uncertainty is heightened. He begins to worry that the new pain is not really arthritis but something even more serious, requiring professional diagnosis. He is inhibited by a selectivity when reporting symptoms: "If I tell the doctor about all my aches and pains, he won't be listening when it's really important."

The dread of a progressively worsened state brings with it a dread of dependency, expressed frequently as: "I don't want to be a burden." Some fear dependency on kin so much that they will live alone at tremendous sacrifice. To illustrate, one woman, now forty-four, recalled the early onset of her disease, telling of her move then to an apartment and her struggle to continue working:

> It was harrowing. When I got up in the morning my feet were so painful I couldn't stand on them. I would slide out of bed and with my elbow and rump get into the bathroom. I learned to turn the faucets with my elbows.

For her, the activity world pressed on, in spite of the increased pace of her physiological world, and in fact brought her through this early period into a long period of remission.

NORMALIZING IN THE FACE OF UNCERTAINTY

Covering-Up

Arthritics develop a repertoire of strategies to assist in normalizing their lives; i.e., proceeding with the activity imperative *as if* normal. The principal strategy employed is that of "covering-up," concealing the disability and/or pain. Variations of the following quotes appear throughout interviews with them: "If anyone asks me how I am, I say fine," "When I walk I walk as normally as possible—if I walked like I felt like walking, I'd look like I should be in a wheelchair." Covering-up does not constitute a denial of the disease, in the psychological sense of the word. As described by M. Davis: " . . . it is the rejection by the patient of the handicap as if it were his total identity. In effect, it is the rejection of the social significance of the handicap and not rejection of the handicap per se."[5] Unsuccessful covering-up invites the risk of interrupted interaction via offers of help, or questions ("skiing accident?"), or suggestions of home remedies ("Someone at work suggested I try alfalfa. I wanted to tell her I'm not a cow."). Interaction, thus interrupted, impedes the arthritic's ability to view himself as he would prefer to be viewed by others.

There are various conditions under which covering-up is impeded. An arthritic who is subject to sudden attacks, such as freezing of the back with resulting immobility, is a case in point. One woman who had such an attack while visiting her home town found that she could only walk at a creeping pace—some of the time only backwards:

> *People on the street would ask if they could help. . . . the embarrassment was worse than the pain. I thought they would all think I was crazy or drunk.*

Visibility—use of a cane or crutches, wincing when arising from a chair or getting out of a car—is another impediment to covering-up. When the arthritic has the additional problem of deformity, the potential for covering-up is further reduced. Inability to cover-up leads to reactions such as evinced during an interview by a young woman who had struggled to remove coins from her wallet with badly deformed fingers. She said poignantly:

I have just become aware of how uncomfortable people get around
me. They don't want to be reminded of sickness; they are fearful for
themselves, just as young people don't want to be around old people.

If covering-up is successful, a price may be paid, however, because this strategy can drain the person's already depleted energy.
("Do you know the stress you put your body to trying to walk
straight so people won't see you can't walk?") Concomitantly, there
is increased awareness of pain and stiffness once within the confines
of the home. Patients report that after situations in which they
"toughed it out," they give in to their fatigue and nervousness,
dumping their irritability upon close family members.

Keeping-Up

Armed with their strategy for covering-up, and lulled by their good
days, arthritics struggle to keep the activity imperative ahead in the
race, through efforts at "keeping-up"—keeping-up with what they
perceive to be normal activities (preparing a holiday meal for the
family, maintaining a job, participating in a family hike). They may
carry through with an event successfully, then suffer increased pain
and fatigue; but that risk is taken precisely because such payment is
not at all inevitable. Keeping-up efforts may also continue—despite
their seeming irrationality—in order to maintain self-images. To illustrate, one woman, who had a period of relief as the guest of her
daughter, not being allowed to use her hands even to open a car
door, suffered another painful onset the first day home when she
cleaned her sink and bathtub, because "I hate dirt."

Another keeping-up problem occurs for those who have
mastered the art of raising their thresholds of pain toleration. They
may be slow to read the signs of body dysfunction as, for example,
one patient who for a month walked around with a broken leg,
thinking his pain was arthritic.

Some engage in excessive keeping-up—super-normalizing—to
prove a capacity, or to deny incapacity, or to recapture a former identity. Hence pain-free and energetic days invite frenetic activity or
catching-up. The result is often (but again uncertain) that time is
really lost through increased pain or decreased energy the next day.
Super-normalizing further ties in with the uncertainty of ascribing
causes, as with a patient who knows her condition worsens during
the summer, but is unsure about whether it is exacerbated by the
weather or by her increased activities in her garden. Furthermore,
some engage in super-normalizing as a device to distract themselves

from pain. This too may bring increased pain, increased fatigue, and sometimes fever.

Justifying Inaction

Successful covering-up and keeping-up can even turn out to be a mixed blessing. Although relationships generally remain normal when arthritics cannot get by, they then find it harder to justify inaction. Again this is related to the uncertainty of their physical condition—they cannot legitimize their current abnormality because sometimes they are normal; and other times, although hurting, they were covering-up or keeping-up. This difficulty increases when others have stakes in their remaining active, as with a young mother whose condition worsened when she tried to keep up in sports with her husband: "My husband really doesn't understand. He is very healthy and he thinks there is some magic formula that I'm not following—if I would just exercise, or have people over. . . . " Accusations may not always be so overt, but others' stakes are nevertheless troublesome, as with a tennis pro who found it necessary one day to cancel a lesson only to be observed out playing the next; he began to worry that his club members were suspecting him of malingering.

Paradoxically, arthritics who attempt to present a normal image to the world nevertheless are perplexed when they are not taken seriously by others. There is a longing for understanding, for a sensitivity by others, that goes beyond their justifying of inaction. An arthritic may be proud that "nobody knows" and yet wish that "somebody cared." The same person can boast of a mastery of covering-up ("If I went around looking like I feel, no one would want to be with me") and still say, "I don't think anyone has any idea how much pain I have." As expressed by another:

> *Pain is essentially private. Sometimes you wish for someone to understand and be patient with your pain. To allow you to have it!! I do not mean sympathy or pity.*

Pacing

Accompanying the use of the various normalization strategies is the really main one of "pacing"—identifying which activities one is able to do, how often, under what circumstances. Since these activities are what lead one to view oneself as normal, pacing is the arthritic's

means of maintaining an uneasy equilibrium between the
abnormalization and normalization of his life.

Arthritics know it takes them longer to complete daily tasks. For
example, they allow extra time to get dressed, since putting on hose
and tying shoe laces can be agonizingly painful. "I dress a little, lie
down and cry a little, and dress a little more." They decide if they
can work a three day week, or do housework for an hour; they know
if they shop they may not be able to cook. Housework is not spontaneous, but planned around periods of respite. During remission,
the arthritic may have resumed activities or assumed new ones, but
then be forced by a flare-up to cancel some or all of these. Again the
uncertainty factor operates; pacing is not a static decision, but necessarily fluctuates with the monitoring of the physiological imperative.
Along with pacing decisions run all those problems mentioned earlier in relation to justifying inaction.

Decisions on activities (which ones, how often) are also affected
by the time which is lost when resting between activities. Rest is
prescribed, but not always honored, for symptom control; however,
when pain and stiffness are bad, patients find they have no choice
but to lie down. For some, rest becomes a ritualized part of the daily
regimen—an anticipatory device for coping with pain and decreased
energy. Time expended in rest results in a further cut-back of desired
activities. It also may lead to a contingent existence. Since covering-
up and keeping-up have become an integral part of the arthritic's
mechanism for coping, many prefer to rest and then make a fresh assessment of the physiological imperative rather than suffer the
embarrassment of cancelling plans.

RENORMALIZING: THE ADJUSTMENT TO REDUCED ACTIVITY

Renormalizing, i.e. lowering expectations and developing a new set
of norms for action, is directly related to the frequency and duration
of flare-ups. This means, for example, settling for half a window being clean when an arm begins to hurt in the middle of the cleaning,
or, as one put it, "Sometimes I cannot open a jar; I'll bang it on the
sink, and finally say damn it, put it away, and have something else."

Renormalizing can have serious import if rheumatoid arthritis
strikes early in life, as it did with one young woman who, instead of
pushing to the limits of action, decided to redefine those limits. She
recalled her decision:

> At one point I was struck with fear. If I got interested in a guy I'd
> have to be on the go and I knew I couldn't go out one night and

then the next day. Maybe I set up enough blocks, so it didn't happen.

Increased frequency and duration of flare-ups will spiral re-normalization into lower and lower expectations. New coping mechanisms replace old mechanisms for tolerating uncertainty. For example, when constant use of a cane made covering-up impossible, one man adjusted with a substitute philosophy: "This cane opens many doors."

Eliciting Help

Part of the step downward, of renormalization, is the accepting of help. Arthritics in fact may have to elicit help—to be dressed, cooked or shopped for, helped in carrying out tasks at home and at work. If they live alone they may have to ask a neighbor for help with zippers and buttons. Once the need to ask extends beyond the immediate family, the act is weighed for importance. For example, one may consider asking a neighbor to unscrew the cork from a wine bottle but decide to forego the wine; however, when pain and stiffness make public transportation a forbidding prospect, one will ask to be driven to the clinic.

Eliciting help threatens the arthritic's psychological tolerance, for it reinforces his dread of dependency. Here is perhaps the most extreme illustration: one woman stood without moving for two hours, when her back froze while she was visiting a friend in a convalescent home. She would not ask for help but waited until she could walk home, one mincing step at a time. Throughout her interview she expressed her fear of "being a burden."

Hesitation in eliciting help also stems from the fear that others may not be responsive. Problems of justifying inaction surface again when others have stakes in action. One patient, who is supposed to wear braces on her hands at night and sometimes forgets to put them on, said: "It's too much of a strain to pull up the light comforter I use, let alone get out of bed and get the braces." Yet, no mention was made of eliciting help from her husband. This was the woman referred to earlier, who feels her healthy husband "really doesn't understand." Within their own families, arthritics have preferred tenders because of this matter of differential responsiveness. For example, one will only accept help from her son. His role was merged with his growing up. At onset of her disease thirteen years ago:

My son was then five years old, and he had to take care of me. I'd sit on the side of the bed at night and he'd put my legs up, he'd tuck

*me in. Many times he had to dress me from top to bottom. My older
daughter and sisters have tried to help me but I don't feel comfortable having them do for me.*

Eliciting help decreases the arthritic's potential for covering-up
and keeping-up. A case in point: the woman who took a leave of
absence from work because she could no longer perform to her own
satisfaction—she could not lift the heavy robes on her sales job and
could not stand having other workers do it for her since: "After all,
they're being paid the same thing as I." Deprived of her strategies
for normalizing, she could no longer view herself as self-sufficient
and capable as she wanted to be viewed by her co-workers. Lastly,
awkward or embarrassing situations may occur when eliciting help
and these only serve to highlight dependency. One man, for example, was forced to ask a stranger in a public toilet to zip his pants up;
his fingers are closed to the palms of his hands, and he had left his
trusty button-hook at home.

Since eliciting help is a tacit acknowledgment of the gain that the
physiological imperative is making on the activity imperative, an additional strain on psychological tolerance stems from the identity
problems which arthritics suffer when their eliciting of help results
in a role reversal. Thus, a young mother told of her distress at being
unable to pick up her baby. As he got older he learned to clasp his
legs around her. Now five years old, he must open milk cartons for
her. She is anguished at her reduced capabilities as a mother: "My
son wants to play games and I have to rest; I call him and he runs
away, knowing I can't run after him." Male arthritics who have lost
their dexterity must rely upon wives to carry heavy objects or open
garage doors. Women frequently complain of their diminished roles
as homemakers using language like:

*I liked being a housewife and keeping the house immaculate. The
house is my responsibility, and now my husband (sic children) have
to do much of the work.*

Role reversal may result in a permanent change in the household's
division of labor. Helping out has now become a new job. Then, tolerating the uncertainty has lessened and dependency need no longer
be a dread, for it is all too clearly a reality.

BALANCING THE OPTIONS

When tolerating the uncertainty, arthritics are ultimately engaged in
the precarious balancing of options—options somewhat limited because of their already reduced resources of mobility, skill, strength

and energy. Indeed, a balancing is involved in all of the pacing decisions (weighing the potential benefit of acupuncture against the
climb up two flights of stairs "that will just about kill me," or the potential withdrawal from church activity against the loss of social
interaction). The options are constantly presenting themselves, each
to be met with an ad hoc response: whether to keep up and suffer
the increased pain and fatigue; whether to cover up and risk inability
to justify inaction when needed; whether to elicit help and risk loss
of normalizing.

At the same time, another very worrisome balancing can be in
operation. Arthritics may be put on strict drug regimens: the drugs
hopefully provide control—to help the arthritic normalize. Patients
with long histories of frequent flare-ups often undergo sequential trials of potent antirheumatic drugs, all of which can have adverse side
effects. Some have difficulty in recalling the sequence of these trials;
frequently they were not told what was in their injections and did
not ask. For them, the balancing was weighted in favor of relief at
any cost: "When you're hurting like that you have to do something."
Even after an accumulation of drugs, and faced with total hip re-
placement due to osteoporosis, one arthritic attested she would have
taken the drugs even if she had known the results: "I'm glad to have
had those years of life." (Osteoporosis is a loss of bony substances
producing brittleness and softness of bones, likely to be particularly
severe during the course of cortico-steroid therapy.)

There is a varying degree of knowledge among arthritics as to
specificity of possible side effects. Usually the specific realization
only follows an actual occurrence; even then, direct causation is not
always fully comprehended. One patient who suffered from cataracts,
which is acknowledged to be a side effect of cortico-steroid therapy,
referred to her eye problems as "arthritis in the eyes." She was indeed also suffering from iritis, a recognized accompaniment of
rheumatoid arthritis, but she did not appear to have made a connection between the cataracts and her eight-year ingestion of cortico-
steroids. Some when warned of the potency of their drug purposely
do not ask for specifics: "If you know what to look for, your mind
overpowers you." They are avoiding the potential strain of
balancing.

Knowledge of the specific possible adverse effects of a drug
heightens the psychological tolerance by placing an additional responsibility upon the arthritic. ("I cut down on the Butazolidin when
I have a good week. Recently when I had a flare-up of neck pain I
had to increase it again."; "I know when I take more than sixteen aspirin a day my ears start to ring.") Pain increases vulnerability—an
arthritic may rationally resist starting on a drug with known side-

effects, but when the pain becomes intolerable such resolution is
tempered by the uncertainty of duration: "When the pain is this bad
you feel like you'll never come out of it." The psychological burden
is increased further by another uncertainty. What "works" (i.e. keeps
inflammation and pain controlled), for one day or one week, may not
work the next.

Balancing decisions are therefore constantly being reassessed.
One must decide what the options are, must decide between them
by calculating consequences, must face the consequences whatever
(uncertainty sometimes) they actually turn out to be; and one cannot
rest easily or for long on previous definitions and decisions about
options. Thus, about balancing there is at best only temporary certainty. This, too, the arthritic must learn to live with.

REFERENCES

1. The Arthritis Foundation. 1964. *Primer on the rheumatic diseases.*
    New York.

2. Bland, J. H. 1960. *Arthritis: medical treatment and home care.* New
    York: Macmillan.

3. Bunim, J., ed. 1957. Symposium on rheumatoid arthritis. *Journal
    of Chronic Diseases* 5:609–778.

4. Walike, B.; Marmor, L.; and Upshaw, M. J. 1967. Rheumatoid
    arthritis. *American Journal of Nursing* 67:1420–1426.

5. Davis, M. Z. 1970. Transition to a devalued status: the case of
    multiple sclerosis. Doctoral dissertation, University of California
    Medical Center, San Francisco.

Part 6

Trajectory and Technology:
Complex and Simple

Case History:
Technology and Pain

14

The case of Mrs. Noble is one in which relatively experimental medical technology was used to treat severe chronic pain—to no avail. The consequence was a surgical situation wherein the problematic aspects of pain management were maximized. As we discussed in Chapter 5, surgical situations where maximized problematic pain is likely to be involved include (1) experimental or pioneer surgeries and (2) surgeries to alleviate chronic pain. In Mrs. Noble's case, both these conditions obtained. The surgery performed was the implantation of a dorsal-column stimulator, in an attempt to relieve chronic back pain. The pain was due to rapidly spreading metastatic cancer—an additional feature of the evolving interaction drama.

Several factors maximized the problematic aspect of Mrs. Noble's pain management. First, the pain was intertwined with an unpredictable illness trajectory as well as with an approach to pain relief which was experimental and unpredictable. Because of the experimental nature of the pain-relieving surgery, the staff focused on the medical details of the surgical trajectory and paid little attention to understanding how the surgery related to the patient's illness, death, and pain trajectories. Also, since the surgery was a last, desperate attempt to control pain, the patient's anxiety was heightened, thereby posing pain-assessment problems for the staff. No less important is the fact that the surgery failed to give the anticipated relief. This further increased the patient's anxiety, resulting in a continued increase in interactional difficulties between patient and staff.

In addition, certain organizational difficulties were maximized because the patient happened to be housed on a general surgical unit where the nurses were less familiar with the surgery than nurses on a specialized neurology unit. In large medical research centers organized around medical specialties, the staffs on general medical or surgical units encounter tremendous difficulties in providing the same kind of care as that given in the highly specialized units. The medical specialists and house staff are less available to the nursing staff on a general medical or surgical unit than on a specialized unit. When the surgery is unfamiliar, the nurses feel that effective nurse–physician communication is crucial to proper medical and nursing management. The lack of institutional arrangements to facilitate the care of Mrs. Noble, then, resulted in immense interactional problems between her and the nursing staff, between the nursing staff and the physicians, and between the patient and the physicians.

We will discuss the case of Mrs. Noble first by giving a brief description of the dorsal-column-stimulator implant, then by a description of the case, interspersed with relevant theoretical comments.

THE DORSAL-COLUMN-STIMULATOR IMPLANT

The dorsal-column-stimulator implant designed to relieve chronic pain causes a tingling or buzzing sensation by discharging electrical pulses to the spinal cord, blocking pain messages to the brain.[1] This pain-relief approach involves extensive surgery of the spine and shoulders for the implantation, as well as considerable electronic gadgetry.

A laminectomy is performed to implant an electrode device over the dorsal column of the spinal cord at a level determined by the location of the pain. This is wired to a receiver implanted in the subcutaneous tissue just below the collar bone. Spinal-cord stimulation is provided by a transmitter and antenna device. The antenna rests on the skin over the receiver implant and is wired to the transmitter set. The patient controls the frequency and voltage of the electrical stimulation by dials on the transmitter set.[2]

Because many of these patients are dependent on narcotics prior to surgery and because of the extensive surgery itself, the postoperative pain is anticipated to be relatively high. Therefore, pain drugs are used rather liberally in the postoperative phase. Following a decrease in surgery-associated pains and discomforts, the electrical stimulation is started. As the electrical stimulation increasingly controls the pain, the patient is weaned from narcotics.

In addition to the possibility of postoperative complications such as infections, there are specific possible complications such as leaking of spinal fluid, malfunctioning of the unit, or the body's rejection of the implant.[3]

Intensive patient training is required for the proper use and maintenance of the transmitter. Patients are also instructed to avoid certain positions or movements which might compromise the surgery. The degree of pain relief achieved by this procedure varies greatly. Some patients get no relief; others have total relief. Between 70% and 85% of the patients seem to obtain some relief.[4]

TECHNOLOGY AND MRS. NOBLE

The head nurse and the nursing staff on a general surgical unit urged our researcher to interview Mrs. Noble. They described her as presenting an immense problem because she cried constantly in pain despite heavy doses of narcotics every two hours along with tranquilizers. A dorsal-column implant had been performed two weeks earlier, but thus far she had had no relief. Her care was further complicated by the unavailability of Dr. Osborn, the attending neurosurgeon, and the neurology house staff. The unavailability of the physicians was particularly important because the surgery was new to this nursing staff. They needed detailed information from experienced staff about the proper care of these surgical patients. The head nurse had gathered pertinent literature and had been attempting to arrange a nursing staff conference with experienced neurological nurses and physicians, but she had been unsuccessful in doing so.

From the medical chart and interviews with the patient and nursing staff, the researcher derived a brief medical and social history, plus the events up to the fourteenth postoperative day.

> Mrs. Noble, a 37-year-old housewife, married to a traveling salesman with two daughters in their late teens, was found by a local physician to have cancer of the colon. Prior to this illness she had been healthy—her hospitalization experiences being limited to childbirth. A colostomy was performed by a surgeon in her home town. Two months after the colos-

tomy she developed backaches. A laminectomy was performed along with the removal of cancerous nodes in the groin, followed by a series of radiation treatments. Neither the laminectomy nor radiation relieved the pains. She suffered a steady increase in sharp pains in both legs with some numbness along the lateral aspect of both legs.

Following the unsuccessful laminectomy she was at home. Because of the constant pain she could not maintain her management of the house; over the weeks and months the pain steadily increased, with minimal relief in spite of all varieties of pain drugs. By the time of the patient's admission to the medical research center, she was on 15 drops of Schlessinger's solution (morphine compound) every two hours along with tranquilizers.

While at home, Mrs. Noble constantly wept about pain. The family and the patient were desperate for pain relief. Finally the family physician recommended consultation for a dorsal-column stimulator at a medical research center located 70 miles from home. Thus, eight months after the initial colostomy surgery, with more surgery and radiation after that, and after suffering five months of intractable pain, she was admitted to the neurology unit.

Upon admission a variety of examinations and tests were made to determine if she was a good candidate for the surgery. These included a physical work-up, a neurological work-up, and a psychiatric interview to determine the patient's emotional stability. A trial electrical percutaneous stimulation stopped the patient's pain. Mrs. Noble looked forward to the surgery as the final solution to pain relief.

The medical work-up indicated that the staff's primary focus would be directed toward the pain surgery. There was little or no information about her cancer status except for the dates and kinds of surgery and therapy for the cancer. The psychiatric notes merely stated that there were no psychiatric contraindications for the surgery.

Mrs. Noble tolerated the dorsal-column-stimulator implantation well and was returned to the neurology unit, but two days later, because of a shortage of neurology beds, was transferred to a two-bed room on the general surgical unit. For the first week following the surgery the staff focused on her postoperative care. Narcotics were liberally used to control the surgical pains and discomforts. The patient wept from time to time about pain, but this crying was not considered unusual, considering the extensive surgery. Five days after the surgery, electrical stimulation was started, but the patient did not obtain relief. The lack of pain relief during this early postoperative phase was not considered unusual.

On the tenth postoperative day, under the assumption that the surgical pain was now minimal, the surgeon stopped all previous pain medications and substituted methadone. He also encouraged the patient to use the electrical stimulation and to become more physically active. This change in pain-drug orders occurred on Friday. The weekend, for both the patient and the nursing staff, was described as "dreadful." Methadone did not control the pain, and the electrical stimulation provided no relief. Neither the neurosurgeon nor the neurology house staff could be reached for a change in drug orders. Finally in desperation the nursing staff persuaded the unit house staff to restart the Schlessinger's solution. Meanwhile, the patient's weeping increased. Because the constant weeping upset her roommate, Mrs. Noble was transferred to a private room.

Over the ensuing week a variety of pain drugs were tried, along with tranquilizers. Increasingly the patient became a "clock watcher," demanding more frequent pain drugs, and accusing the nurses: "You don't give me the pain drugs on time." Or the nurses were cast as unsympathetic: "You don't have pain so you don't know how I feel." Day after day the nurses' notations read: "Patient in pain all day. Weeping most of the day."

During this period the head nurse cared for the patient for a few days, spending much time talking to her and trying all types of comfort approaches. A nursing staff conference was held, and a decision was made that pain drugs be given every two hours on schedule without making the patient wait. The patient was addicted to pain drugs prior to surgery, and since the success of the dorsal-column stimulator was still unknown, it was decided that persuading her to tolerate pain would only increase her anxiety and weeping. The head nurse felt the patient needed to weep and the nurses should not get upset about her weeping, and it was the nurses' responsibility to learn to cope with and tolerate her constant weeping.

The nurses varied in their individual tolerance to Mrs. Noble's weeping, but by and large it was tolerated. The patient cooperated in the general care. Her weeping was quiet, so that behind her closed door, it could not be heard in the hallway. As long as she received her pain drugs on schedule, every two hours, she did not argue with the nurses to increase the frequency. She waited, docile, for each two hours to pass.

From the medical history it is apparent that the rate of the cancer extension was rapid. Pain was intertwined with the cancer trajectory. Because of the uncertainty of the trajectory and the increasingly intractable pain, pain relief became the primary concern for both the patient and the medical staff. The connection between the cancer trajectory and its accompanying pain tended to be neglected by the neurosurgeon. He had been consulted about neurological pain, and the patient's hospitalization was primarily for pain-relieving surgery. Such narrowed perspective on pain and its management by the medical personnel, as Bonica[5] states, is due in part to a lack of systematic, organized teaching of medical students and physicians in regard to the proper management of chronic pain. Bonica adds that the trend toward specialization encourages tunnel vision in regard to pain. Also, we should note that when hospitals are organized along lines of medical specialization, then the absence of adequate institutional arrangements further encourages a narrowly focused approach to pain management.

Once surgery was decided upon for Mrs. Noble, the staff's primary concern became the management of the surgical course, hopefully without complication. Also, because of the experimental nature of this surgery, the nurses were particularly concerned with the complex medical details to ensure that the patient was kept on an anticipated course. As is usual with surgical patients, her pain was handled routinely with the expectation that it would be high for a few days and gradually taper off. In this case, exceptions were made because of Mrs. Noble's prior narcotic dependency and the extensive surgery.

Using the anticipated surgical timetable, the surgeon decreased the narcotics, anticipating that the dorsal stimulator would take over the pain relief. The patient's weeping increased when the stimulator did not bring about the expected response without adequate narcotic coverage. Pain-management problems occurred because of mistiming: the weaning from narcotics and the testing of the unpredictable stimulator occurred over the weekend when the physician and house staff were not available. The nursing staff had to cope with the patient's pain as well as her constant weeping, which upset the sentimental order of the ward.

Returning to the patient's medical history, we can see that in a very short period, and in rapid succession, she faced coming to terms with cancer, a colostomy, pain, and death. There was a possibility that the dorsal stimulator, the last desperate option for pain relief, might not work. She expressed her pain and general frustration by weeping. At first the nurses perceived her weeping as primarily a result of acute pain. As we will see, in the ensuing weeks the connection of this weeping with her chronic pain and spreading cancer became more apparent to the nurses.

> Weeping, with statements such as "I hurt so much," or "The pain is constant and won't go away," constituted Mrs. Noble's usual interactional pattern. In the midst of talking she would suddenly give way to tears. Communicating with her required considerable time because one had to allow her time to weep and time to control herself.

> During the researcher's first encounter with her, she maintained that the colostomy was not her problem, but rather pain. Because of the cutaneous trial stimulation prior to surgery, when she had pain relief, she had looked forward to the surgery as finally giving relief. Her constant weeping in pain at home was upsetting to the family, but she could not help herself. Both she and the family looked forward to the surgery. The neurosurgeon had informed her that pain relief was largely a matter of getting used to the stimulator, but thus far she had had no relief. If the stimulator didn't work then she had spent a great deal of money and suffered a painful surgery, all for naught. She wept for a period. The researcher commented that her weeping seemed related both to the possibility that the surgery might not provide the pain relief, and to the uncertainty of the future. She agreed, and wept again.

> When asked what the stimulator felt like, she answered that it was an odd tingling sensation which she didn't particularly like. When asked to describe the pain, and though supplied with numerous pain adjectives by the researcher, she could only weep and say it was a "terrible pain" in her back and along her legs.

> Mrs. Noble had few distractions other than television. Because of the great distance from home, she had few visitors other than her family. Her husband and family visited in the evenings and weekends, but the evening visits were not always regular, as the husband's work took him out of town.

> Nights were particularly terrible for her, for she slept only for short intervals. Her sleeplessness was partly related to fear that the nurses would not give the pain drugs if she were asleep. If the time intervals between the drugs were increased, it would take longer for the drugs to work.

> Mrs. Noble recounted her illness history and her unsuccessful juggling of pain drugs and tranquilizers to control the pain prior to the pain surgery and over the past week. She described at length the great shock and anxiety which accompanied discovery of the bowel cancer. The shock was particularly marked because, a year before her own colos-

tomy surgery, her mother had died of bowel cancer. The mother's cancer was discovered very late when she had metastases throughout her body. Her dying stretched out for several weeks and Mrs. Noble and her sister took turns sitting with her. The nurses kept her mother relatively pain-free with liberal use of narcotics.

To questions about the use of the stimulator to relieve pain, Mrs. Noble could give only vague answers and weep that "nothing stops the pain."

The researcher told the nursing staff about this conversation with Mrs. Noble. The nurses were unaware of the patient's experience with the mother who had died of cancer. They could see now why the patient was anxious. The nurses also stated that because of the increased numbers of new postoperative patients over the past week, they tended to relate to Mrs. Noble only when giving her the pain drug. Therefore, they didn't obtain social information about her.

They had great difficulty in assessing the degree of pain because the patient always wept and could only describe the pain as terrible. Also, she was on so much tranquilizer that assessment was further complicated. Furthermore, she was a chain smoker and they were fearful she might start a fire. Over the past week, in her grogginess, she had burned a hole in her mattress.

The researcher asked the nursing staff about the status of her cancer. Although the medical chart showed no indication of its rate or how long she had to live, considering its rapid progress she might well be closer to death than suspected. One nurse stated that she had been suspecting this because during the previous evening's chat with her husband, he indicated that Mrs. Noble didn't have long to live and he didn't see why the medical staff was doing all this "messing around." Give her all the painkillers she wants. What difference does it make if she is addicted? This was the first time that other nurses had heard about this conversation with the husband.

When the researcher commented that the medical notes were too sparse on the surgical status to make an evaluation, this opened up a barrage of criticism directed at the neurosurgeon. Not only did they feel he looked down on the nurses, but the times of his medical rounds were impossible. He made medical rounds before 7:00 AM, a time when the night staff was busy completing work for the shift, or when the night staff was reporting to the oncoming day staff. Although the nurses attempted to keep a sharp eye open to intercept him, they were often unsuccessful. Information from the patient about the patient–doctor communication was often suspect because the patient was groggy from sleep as well as from the pain drugs and tranquilizers.

As to teaching the patient to use the stimulator correctly: she was unwilling to "play" with the stimulator and the staff members themselves
did not have sufficient information to help the patient. The nurses re-
iterated the need for having more detailed information about this
technique. They told the researcher about another patient who had had
the same surgery and who did have relief from pain, but who developed
mechanical difficulties with the stimulator unit. The latter patient was in
terrible pain while the nurses had a difficult time locating the surgeon,
the surgeon being the only person who knew the intricate details of operating this electronic unit.

The nurses speculated about Mrs. Noble "needing" her pain—that perhaps she was afraid to go home, and that pain would keep her in the
hospital.

We have here a patient who could only express her pain and
anxiety by weeping. Not only had she a limited pain language, but
her weeping prevented effective negotiation with the staff. Moreover,
the weeping upset the nurses' composure. If the patient were given
sufficient time, she could eventually have managed to communicate,
but the ongoing ward work and the innumerable tasks connected
with keeping a large number of patients on their surgical courses
without complications prevented many extended patient–nurse interactions on this ward. Thus, the nurses interacted with Mrs. Noble
only during the act of giving pain drugs. Relevant psychosocial information was not gathered.

The patient, unable to negotiate effectively, could not rely upon
her husband because of his working hours and the great distance between home and the hospital. Compare this situation to a pediatric
unit where children also express their pain and frustration through
weeping, but have parents to interpret the crying to the hospital staff
and negotiate in the child's behalf.

For patients to negotiate effectively on the subject of pain relief,
they must have both interpersonal skill and knowledge of hospital
routine. It is noteworthy that during the period of Mrs. Noble's hospitalization, another patient with chronic back pain from a spinal
injury was admitted for evaluation for a dorsal-column implant. This
patient was not only knowledgeable about hospitals because of many
past hospitalizations, but was also exceptionally skilled in relating
to the hospital staff. Granted, her illness was less serious than Mrs.
Noble's, but still she was able to communicate and negotiate easily
with the very same physician. She found this neurologist willing

and cooperative in sharing information, and she described him as "brilliant."

In Mrs. Noble's case the nurses were faced with an increasing problem of assessing her pain because she could not articulate it herself, and of providing pain relief without endangering her. The staff's work routines ran counter to the physician's order concerning the time to give the drug, which posed additional difficulties. Also, unlike the husband, they were still thinking in terms of potential addiction rather than of comfort care for a dying patient.

Complicating the matter further, the nursing staff was dealing with a new surgical situation and a new technology without sufficient information and institutional arrangements to facilitate their care of this patient. (Indeed, the introduction of new procedures and technology by physicians without sufficient foresight of the organizational and nursing–physician interactional consequences was noted frequently during our research.)

The following week the pain-drug routine of Schlessinger's solution every two hours with two kinds of tranquilizers and phenobarbital was continued, with minimal relief. The patient was encouraged to use the stimulator, but was reluctant to do so. She was also encouraged to be more active. She continued to weep behind the closed door. At one point she had increased backaches. She was fearful of what this meant although it might be attributed simply to her increased activity. The nurses were beginning to doubt the stimulator would work, but they adopted the stance of "wait and see."

On the twenty-first postoperative day, Dr. Osborn checked the stimulator unit to determine if it was functioning properly and rechecked the patient's response to stimulation. He scolded her for not using the stimulator. She should get out of bed more and stop babying herself. As the patient related: "He bawled me out." "Do you want to lie around and be a junkie?" The patient was ordered to increase the stimulator use and start decreasing the narcotic. The doctor informed the nurses that he had read the patient the "riot act." In his testing he found the unit was functioning properly. Most important, he found the patient had a low toleration for the sensation of the electrical current; however, he did not inform the patient of this finding. He asked the nursing staff to start tapering off the narcotic while encouraging the patient to use the stimulator more often. The previous tranquilizers were discontinued and a new tranquilizer was ordered.

The head nurse and the assistant head nurse decided they would postpone the drug withdrawal to the following day instead of beginning during the evening shift. They reasoned that the evening shift had fewer staff members and more difficulty in contacting the house staff. So although the withdrawal would occur on the weekend, both the head nurse and her assistant would be on duty and the staff coverage would be fairly good should they run into problems. They also decided to discuss the withdrawal with Mrs. Noble and include her in this process.

Over the weekend when the nurses confronted the patient about reducing the narcotics, Mrs. Noble stated she knew nothing about this—she denied having had any conversation with the physician about this. The nurses were not sure if this were so or if the patient was confused, considering the large amounts of painkillers. However, they were inclined to believe that the physician had not made this information explicit to the patient.

Mrs. Noble expressed a desire to decrease the narcotics, but she was unwilling to do so until she had a more positive response from the increased electrical stimulation. She thought she might require a couple of additional days to get used to the higher current. Thus, the drugs continued as during the previous week.

Another complicating factor was that the changed tranquilizer had a depressing rather than a mood elevating effect. The patient had tried this same drug while at home and found the drug depressed her. The neurosurgeon could not be reached because he was out of town for a few days. Finally the neurology house staff was persuaded to change the tranquilizer, after which her depression decreased.

In most therapies there is a "wait-and-see" period to judge an outcome. This trial spans a more or less definitive time, depending upon the kind of therapy and staff familiarity with it. With new therapies, this trial period is likely to be longer. Mrs. Noble's physician, after a reasonable wait-and-see period, took active efforts to test the therapeutic effectiveness by checking factors which might be compromising the outcome. After checking the stimulator, he decided the patient was not using it properly, but he also discovered she could not tolerate the sensation of the electrical current. Yet, he was hoping his patient would become accustomed to the sensation.

As noted earlier, a common problem in procedures for pain relief is mistiming in the weaning of patients from drugs; patients are unwilling to give up a drug unless they have evidence that the new substitute procedure is working. In Mrs. Noble's case, although the nursing staff tried to avoid organizational pitfalls mitigating against successful weaning, they ran into difficulties because of the aforementioned factor (plus the substitute procedure being unpredict-

able!). In addition, both the staff and the doctor had different philosophies about how the weaning was to be accomplished. The nurses
believed it should be handled by an "open awareness,"[6] with both
she and they aware of how this was to be accomplished. The physician believed otherwise. During the ensuing week, the difference
in their views became more apparent.

Difficulties were also encountered because staff did not take into
account Mrs. Noble's past experiences with drugs—her pain biography—as illustrated by the side effects from the briefly substituted
tranquilizer.

> In the following days Mrs. Noble increased the electrical current, but
> she found little pain relief, so the pain drugs were delivered every two
> hours. She was unwilling to increase the time interval between the pain
> drugs without evidence of the stimulator's taking over. She continued to
> weep. In this period her husband went out of town on business.

> On the thirtieth postoperative day, a third attempt was made to wean the
> patient from the narcotics. The physician, without talking to the nurses,
> left an order to reduce the narcotic by three drops and to increase the
> time interval from two to three hours. The nurse in charge complained to
> the researcher that the doctor had not informed the patient about the
> weaning—"the bastard." The nurse assigned to care for Mrs. Noble in-
> formed her about increasing the time interval of the pain drug. The
> patient agreed that although it would be difficult she would try to co-
> operate, since she wanted to get off the hard drugs. The nurse did not
> inform the patient about reducing the drug dosage, however, reasoning
> that this was too much for the patient to bear, although she felt bad
> about deceiving the patient. Fortunately the patient tolerated the reduc-
> tion of drugs better than expected.

> The head nurse sighed in dismay. Mrs. Noble now had a seratoma (blis-
> ter) around the implant over her chest. The seratoma might absorb on its
> own or it might mean that her body was beginning to reject the implant.

> Mrs. Noble informed the researcher that she was sick and tired of the
> hospital. She had been playing with the transmitter but had found no dif-
> ference in pain. She could not judge whether her pain was less, or
> whether the pain drugs helped or not. Dr. Osborn had told her they don't
> know why she was not getting pain relief. Mrs. Noble wept as if her
> heart would break.

> Over the next two days, her weeping increased. The nurses thought the
> increased weeping was related to her discouragement over the stim-
> ulator, the development of the seratoma, and "jitters" associated with

narcotic reduction. The patient couldn't distinguish what was what, and neither could the nurses. They described the crying as a "weeping of despair."

The previous day the head nurse had confronted the neurology resident, complaining about the lack of follow-up by the neurology house staff. The resident agreed, but explained that he had difficulty keeping his head above water; the neurology service was very large and scattered throughout the whole hospital. Furthermore, he himself had difficulty in reaching the attending physicians and keeping up with the medical plans for each individual patient.

In spite of the patient's increased weepiness, she had been getting out of bed more often. The nurses encouraged the increased activity.

During the researcher's next encounter with Mrs. Noble, she wept for a prolonged period. She stated that the last several days had been extremely difficult. The many difficulties stemmed from her inability to tolerate the sensation of the stimulator, her growing conviction that the stimulator would not work, jitteriness from narcotic reduction, worry over the meaning of the seratoma, and the absence of her husband. Of particular concern was the fact that she could not get a straight answer from the doctor. Part of the problem in communicating was not only that he cut her off—and the untimely hours of his visits—but that with her increased weepiness she could not better manage the interaction. When asked if the nurses might intervene for her, she answered that the nurses had as much problem as she in contacting both the neurosurgeon and the house staff.

She had reached the point where she thought: "Nothing is going to help anymore." She didn't want any more "messing around" with needles or new surgery. "Everybody is helpless," she added. She thought the nurses didn't come to the room as often as before; she supposed they felt as helpless as she did.

When asked if a definitive answer from the physician about the stimulator, as well as answers about her cancer status, would help her situation, she responded that she couldn't stand the uncertainty much longer. She wanted to know the truth, no matter how dire the situation. She could not bear another week in the hospital and thought she would be better at home.

As the patient could not effectively relate to the physician because of her crying, the possibility was explored that her husband might handle the physician for her. Also explored was the role that her private physician, with whom she had good relations, might play.

After this discussion with the patient, the researcher discussed her with the head nurse, who had had a long chat with Mrs. Noble wherein she stated she thought she would never have relief from pain and wanted to go home. A change of environment might help. The researcher pointed out to the nurse that as matters now stood the nursing staff could not effectively negotiate with the patient. The possibility was explored that the husband or the private physician take a more active role in behalf of the patient. The head nurse stated that she was arranging to have an extensive conversation with the husband upon his return.

The researcher informed her also about the patient's comment that the nurses were avoiding her. The nurse answered that the nurses interacted less with the patient not to avoid her, but because they had a large influx of new surgical patients and also a very demanding, "acting out" patient who had the total ward in an uproar.

Over the ensuing days the head nurse spent some time talking to the husband, urging him to contact the surgeon. Then the husband had a long chat with the surgeon. He also spent much time talking to Mrs. Noble, after which she became less weepy. Her usual countenance—a worried, drawn face—became more relaxed. The husband stated that he had informed his wife that her cancer was spreading, and that they should make the best of what life they still had together, to live from day to day; that being upset and anxious would make the pain greater; and that dependence on narcotics should not worry her. Subsequently, the patient informed the head nurse that she would try to make the best of what life she had with her husband, and seemed less upset about the dorsal-column stimulator's not working.

On the thirty-fifth postoperative day she was discharged. She was doing more for herself and even packed her own bags to go home. The nurses all expressed amazement at Mrs. Noble's poise and behavior.

With the extended hospitalization, both the staff and the patient became increasingly aware that the desired pain relief was not forthcoming. The rate of their awareness varied; the patient learned experientially over time that she could not tolerate the electrical sensation, although the staff suspected this some weeks earlier. The failure of the last, desperate option left everyone helpless. The development of the new symptom (seratoma) posed further uncertainties. All of this increased the patient's weeping, posing further interactional difficulties for her and the staff.

In despair, the woman was faced with the task of being weaned from drugs, her one and only relief from pain. In the midst of this, she was faced with coming to terms with her disappointment over the stimulator and with continued pain. The absence of her husband during this trying period made those tasks even more difficult. The nurses could not help her because they also felt helpless; they were concerned with handling other, competing ward demands. This left only the husband to help her cope with unsuccessful pain relief efforts and an uncertain future, leading probably to an early death.

The case of Mrs. Noble illustrates above all that in spite of the head nurse's great sensitivity and her "one-to-one" interactional skills, the kinds of problems described here will continue on her ward and others like it unless there is a restructuring of ward organization. To improve pain management requires an understanding of the organizational context of pain management and a recognition of the limitations of a predominantly medical perspective. Implied in this statement is the fact that Dr. Osborn was perceived as a villain by the nurses precisely because he was totally unaware of the consequences of the new technology for the ward organization and its associated staff interactions. This lack of organizational sensitivity is, as remarked earlier, a common shortcoming of physicians.

New technologies are rapidly being introduced into the current medical scene. Often unpredictable, they pose new kinds of medical problems, and they sometimes fail. Consequently, it becomes increasingly important to develop organizational structures which will facilitate the dissemination of information and lend needed psychosocial support not only to patients, but also to staff members. Otherwise, medical and nursing care—and especially to chronically ill patients, whether or not in pain—will often be rendered ineffective.

REFERENCES

1. Melzack, R., and Wall, R. 1965. Pain mechanism: a new theory. *Science* 150:971–979.

2. Gaumer, W. 1974. Electrical stimulation in chronic pain. *American Journal of Nursing* 74:498–499.

3. Burton, C. 1974. Instrumentation for D.C.S. implantation. *Surgical Neurology* 2:39–40.

4. Fox, J. L. 1974. D.S.C. stimulation for relief of intractable pain, problems encountered in neurological pacemaker. *Surgical Neurology* 2:59–63.

5. Bonica, J. 1974. General clinical considerations. In *Recent advances in pain*, eds. J. John et al. Springfield, Ill.: Charles C Thomas, p. 74.

6. Glaser, B., and Strauss, A. 1965. *Awareness of dying*. Chicago: Aldine, pp. 274–285.

Birth Process and Pain

15

Unlike the pain discussed in previous chapters, the pain which accompanies normal (uncomplicated) childbirth has nothing to do with illness. The pain may even be welcomed because of its association with the joy of bringing a new life into the world. It is a "good pain"—or, at any rate, it is often a necessary and inevitable part of becoming a mother. (However, that does not necessarily make the pain any less painful!) Another difference from most other pain discussed in this book is that birth pain is well known to the general public. What is supposed to happen, what might happen, what has actually happened during birth is known to family, friends, even strangers, and of course to one's spouse and oneself. Furthermore, almost everyone has attitudes toward birth and how people are supposed to handle pain during the birth process. Those attitudes are culturally derived, varying around the globe and even within specific nations. They can also be linked with philosophical positions like the natural childbirth movement, the Lamaze method, or various perspectives associated with the increasingly powerful general movement toward the equalization of women's rights.

Interaction with and around a prospective mother in pain is so familiar that it hardly calls for special discussion. The rationale for focusing upon it at all is that certain complexities of interaction may occur. The conditions and consequences for those occurrences are especially interesting, in light of the usual simplicity of the birth-pain situation and how different even the complex instances are from most pain-in-illness situations.

GENERAL PROPERTIES OF BIRTH PAIN

Birth pain has various properties which are directly relevant to the usual pain situation. Most need little or no commentary:

1. Birth pain is expected, so that when it appears there is no problem in its diagnosis. (Only if another pain appeared and was mistakenly defined as birth pain would there be a misdiagnosis.) This is, of course, not true of many other types of pain, where there is a diagnostic hunt for its etiology.

2. While birth pain in general is expected, its specific details may vary a great deal for individual mothers or even for different deliveries by the same woman. When it occurs, how long, how often, and how much are all problematic. Even a past delivery or two may lead to expectations that are completely wrong for the current delivery.

3. Birth pain is finite, in the sense that relatively soon after the delivery, it is "finished." (We are referring to the contracting pains rather than any postepistiotomy or postdelivery pains, discomforts, and damage.)

4. The duration of the birth pain is variable; however, the range of variability is relatively small. The pain persists days at most, not months or years as with some other types of pain.

5. The amount and frequency of pain experienced are also variable, but here the range of variability can be very great, even for the same mother who may scarcely hurt during one delivery but be in excruciating and frequent pain during another.

6. Provided that drug and skill resources are available—and in developed nations today they are—then the relief of birth pain involves a relatively uncomplicated medical technology. Drugs are relatively nonexperimental, routine, and so are the usual surgical procedures (spinal blocks, epidurals, caudals).

7. The shared main task of staff members and mother consists of two items of business: to deliver a "good" baby and to conclude

that process with an unimpaired mother. Of course, different cultural or ethnic groups place differential emphases on those two goals, but certainly each takes precedence—as main tasks always do—over the relief of pain.

8. Pain relief is balanced against the main task. This balancing can be a delicate matter but is neither very prolonged (often minutes or hours, at most days not weeks) nor very complex (as compared with main other types of pain balancings).

9. The pain work, by mother and staff respectively, is relatively uncomplicated. Of what does it consist? The mother is supposed to endure her pain "within limits" while cooperating in the main task of producing both the healthy baby and an unimpaired mother. That means she must accept the staff's balancing of relief medication and main-task considerations. It also means that while enduring pain, she must also keep her pain expression appropriate. Cultural definitions of expression may, of course, vary widely, and what is thought admissible or appropriate in one cultural setting may be unacceptable in another; in the United States, those cultural standards may well vary between mother and staff members, or even among staff members. Another of the mother's pain tasks is that she must request pain relief "in time" (not too early, not too late) and in properly conventional ways. The responsibility for making those requests is certainly hers.

   As for the staff, they have pain tasks which match those of their charges. In brief, they bear the heavy responsibility of balancing wisely; otherwise they may relieve too fast or too much and so fail to produce a maximally healthy child. But within the boundaries of that balancing task, they must also be responsive to the needs for pain relief and to reasonable requests for that relief. To be otherwise is to be remiss, even callous. Also, they must endure whatever "appropriate" expressions of pain to which the delivering mothers may unintentionally expose them: moaning, groaning, crying, even screaming in medically difficult cases.

10. The organization of work and pain work needs little discussion here. Whether a midwife or an obstetrician delivers the child, or whether the delivery occurs "professionally" at home or in a hospital, the organization of work is basically a rather simple one. Typically in American hospitals, there are several mothers waiting to deliver, lying in different rooms or the same room. Unless they deliver unexpectedly, they will be taken to a de-

livery room to have the babies. Before the delivery itself, the nursing and medical staff are organized to adequately monitor the birth process (contractions, dilations, other bodily signs). Moving in and out of the rooms, their work includes listening to and judging requests for pain relief, as well as reducing the use of medication for relief by utilization of presence and other interactional tactics. In the delivery room itself, ordinarily or ideally, the staff will have the proper resources and skills to deliver the baby and protect the mother during and just after the delivery, and to give proper pain relief. Sometimes fathers are allowed to be part of the division of labor within the delivery room. Certainly they often are at work during the predelivery period lending support and presence—helping their wives to carry on with minimal loss of "control."

THE POTENTIAL COMPLEXITIES OF PAIN WORK

For even the usual or uncomplicated childbirth, the variability of pain (duration, frequency, amount) is so great that it is difficult to make generalizations about the associated experiences and interactions. Generalization is all the more precarious since there are great differences in women's capacities to endure their pain and to control their expression—complicated by different cultural or ideological "prescriptions." Likewise, those who assist in the childbirth may be differentially responsive to requests for pain relief, and differentially conservative or liberal in their balancing of relief versus birth-process considerations. They may also be more or less skilled in assessing pain or in utilizing relief measures such as epidural procedures.

It is quite possible, however, to itemize the kinds of "disturbed interaction" which occur under certain conditions. Some of these conditions pertain to medically complicated childbirths, but some may obtain even when the birth process is relatively run-of-the-mill and even when labor or delivery pain is relatively minimal. Keeping in mind the respective pain tasks of both staff and mothers, what then are those conditions which make for difficult interactions?

MEDICALLY DIFFICULT BIRTHS AND HIGH-RISK BIRTHS

When things are going medically well and the labor is not taking too long, then interactional tactics work relatively well to keep pain expression in check, or medication for relief can be given early and with relative safety. However, in difficult situations nurses have

been known to slap hysterical women (or physicians to give epidurals) to relieve pain sooner than anticipated. Nevertheless, *if* a
woman is able to keep good control over her expression of pain, then
a researcher's fieldnote about her is likely to read like this:

> *Her labor was prolonged and acknowledged by the staff to be very*
> *painful. After 11 hours of labor the staff was concerned about the*
> *slow progress and the fact that they could not give her anything un-*
> *til she had dilated more. . . . When I interviewed her 24 hours later,*
> *she told me the nurses had been very good about explaining ev-*
> *erything to her about breathing, not tightening up, waiting for the*
> *epidural, and that at the appointed time "the epidural worked fine."*

When labor is unexpectedly difficult or long and much pain
accompanies it, however, then the mother's control over her pain expression tends to weaken: she becomes increasingly tired or weary—
perhaps also anxious, frightened, even terrified or hysterical. So she
moves along a continuum of increasingly visible expression, from
stoic control evidenced only in bodily tension or slight movement,
through wincing, sobbing, moaning, crying loudly, yelling, hol-
lering, and screaming. While, of course, not everyone moves from
one end to the other of that continuum, control is certainly put under
severe strain, and a woman may "give in," going beyond where she
felt she wanted to—sometimes with consequent shame and guilt. Fathers may fail in agreed-upon assignments as effective control agents.
Not able really to help, they may abandon her room, fleeing in helplessness or despair. Staff members may similarly fail at helping the
woman to retain proper control, either because their interactional tactics prove insufficient or because the medication does not "hold"
her. They too may feel helpless.

Beyond this, the staff members may be balancing their main
tasks (healthy baby, unimpaired mother) against giving adequate or
any relief of the mother's evident pain. Thus they will withhold medication because "she is not far enough along in her dilating." In the
stern words of one nurse to a woman in labor:

> *You're just going to have to cope. You're the only one who can do*
> *it. I can't do it for you. They will give you what you need after you*
> *have dilated enough, but if it's too soon it will slow the labor and*
> *eventually it will just hurt again, so you'll just have to learn to*
> *cope.*

Even when medication is permitted, the amount is balanced
against medical considerations, such as its potential for slowing up

the contractions or delaying the delivery. In one instance, our field notes report that after many hours and some medication:

> When I left at 11:30 P.M., they were deciding whether to induce. . . . The next day she told me there had been two hours of pushing a certain instructed way, to get the lip of the cervix back into proper position, and finally the doctor pushed it back manually. Then two hours of pushing to get the baby's head to crown; still nothing, so into the delivery room (15 hours after hospital admission), where after much work, the resident called the chief, who . . . took the baby with forceps. In delivery, she had the full effect of the epidural, but the long period prior she described as terrible.

When births are anticipated as high-risk, the balancing becomes even more of a consideration and pain relief sinks to even lower priority. There is now far too much concern by the staff, frequently revealed to the mother, over potential damage to the infant—or her, or both—to allow for much relief of pain. We witnessed one high-risk birth complicated further by deliberations over "how much pain" because of the staff's estimation of the patient's social rank. First, the high-risk scene:

> When this woman came in she was not in labor. She had mild contractions, which the staff were ignoring, since they were secondary to her main problems which can only be multiple. She was hyperventilating and complaining of severe pain on the right side. They put her on oxygen immediately, and there began a tremendous commotion, with residents, nurses, and senior doctors running in and out of her room and conferring in the hall. The door was open and she would let out piercing screams when they touched her. They took a number of blood samples and a cardiogram. . . . At one point, there was an emergency request for a chest x-ray to be done in the room, which ran into a bureaucratic delay. The machine finally arrived after an angry exchange between the chief resident and the x-ray department. They gave her a shot of morphine, and she quieted down.

Then, the relevance of her "low social value:"[1]

> When things were quiet, I started to pick up some feelings about her from the resident who had been on during her last admission to this ward, a few months previously. He described her as an alcoholic, a pharmacist's assistant who prescribed drugs liberally for herself and her husband. . . . She had come in the last time in the same condition just described, reeking of alcohol. . . . I later heard the exact same description of that admission from the nurse who was presently

assigned to watch her, who described her as a "dingbat," and said "with that type of patient, it's hard to tell when she's acting."

During the night they had to induce labor, and she delivered—baby fine. She was still in serious condition; the anesthetist told me she couldn't have survived the bleeding from a Caesarean and they were lucky she had delivered vaginally. The student who had been with her all day and night said in the course of chatting with me, but not in reference to her: "An alcoholic will be watching for the next Demerol and will try to con a new nurse to give it earlier." This was generally the attitude toward this patient.

During the postdelivery period, the nurse quoted earlier made her remark about "it's hard to tell if she is acting," having had difficulty in assessing her postdelivery pain. And a couple of days later, another nurse reported the patient was asking her to sneak narcotics. Nevertheless, they were still watching her closely; there were still many tests—lung scans, x-ray, etc. The interactional and medical problems also continued, one nurse telling the interviewer that:

"We've taken away her cigarettes and her alcohol. She got very mad this morning and wouldn't sign [some paper] because we had put on the baby's birth certificate that the delivery had complications because mother is an alcoholic." Later in the day, the head nurse from postpartum came over to labor and delivery looking for the resident following the case. Nurse very upset: patient complaining of severe pain right side, hyperventilating, blood pressure up to 180.

In short: if the procedure is high-risk, then pain relief takes a back seat. If the situation is high-risk and the patient has "low social value," additional problems arise concerning correct assessment of pain and there will probably be less sympathy for pain and less pain relief.

IDEOLOGICAL VERSUS PROFESSIONAL CONSIDERATIONS

Even with medically uneventful births (let alone with difficult ones) the mother's cultural, personal, or ideological ideas about birth or birth pain may clash with those held by the staff members. Understandably, the latter's ideas may also be cultural or personal in derivation. We shall focus here, however, only on the personnel's conventional professional stances on giving appropriate pain relief, and pose those against the ideological stances of the delivering mothers.

First a word about the mothers' culturally derived perspectives. The range and mode of expressions of pain are, of course, affected by cultural training and definition. What is important for understanding the interaction between mothers and personnel, however, is how the personnel perceive a mother's expression of pain. If they see it only as idiosyncratic, they can blame or praise her accordingly. If they perceive it as culturally patterned, they may blame or admire her as a representative of her culture. When a woman is evidently in great pain but amazingly stoic, and if she happens to be a Chinese or Japanese American, then the staff is likely to explain her behavior by saying: "She is an Oriental." If her reactions are more disturbing to the staff or intrusive on their work, they may define her as "one of those too-expressive Italians or 'Latins.' " (In turn, the mothers and fathers may misread, because of their cultural backgrounds, the staff's professional behavior as cool, distant, impersonal, even callous).

Besides such culturally derived stances, there are, of course, personal ones. Nurses may be quite short-tempered about some women's lack of control over relatively little pain, or conversely quite empathetic with painful deliveries, because they themselves have had difficult childbirths. ("Now if they want to scream, I let them scream.") Some stances are not so much experiential as they are derived from familial or other public communication. For instance, one mother screamed more constantly and loudly, according to a staff resident,

> . . . than anything he had ever heard. He tried to calm her down, since he was sure she wasn't hurting that much, and she said: "Look, my mother screamed like this, my grandmother screamed like this, my sisters screamed like this, and I'm going to scream like this."

Both personnel and mothers may have perspectives that are ideological in character rather than personal or cultural. Usually the staff's are less apparent, at least to the mothers and sometimes even to their colleagues. For instance, a young nurse, recently graduated from nursing school, exemplified an up-do-date nursing philosophy combined perhaps with a contemporary "touch and feel" therapeutic ideology when she remarked that:

> I use my own form of hypnosis—speak to them in low soothing tones, telling them to breath deeply, it will be over soon. I am interested in what illness does to the self-image and would like to try more massage for pain therapy—massage for touching, contact. Very few

nurses touch a patient, unless they are actually doing something for
them. When you're hurting, or ill in any way, massage can make
you know that parts of your body are OK; they feel good. I've tried
to convince the nursing office of this, but they say people are not
ready for that. I've tried touching with patients in labor; some like
it, some don't.

Also, disagreements over what is more or less medically effective
may not simply represent discrepant judgments over efficiency but
quite literally differences among medical ideologies. (When recom-
mending a procedure, some surgeons tend to lean toward surgical
techniques and internists toward nonsurgical ones). Hence, various
physicians may manage the balancing processes somewhat differently
in timing, in amount and kind of medication, in delaying pain relief,
and so on.

More obvious and certainly more dramatic is the impact of a
mother's ideology upon the usual birth situation in hospitals. During
the early 1950s, some mothers converted to the natural childbirth
movement (well before physicians and nurses understood that movement, much less would bow to or agree with some of its tenets).
These mothers had great difficulty getting hospital staffs to agree to
birth without medication. Often they felt betrayed by their physicians who had agreed to nonmedication, but then would use it
during the delivery. Or their private physicians would agree but
house staffs would disregard or misunderstand the agreement. Today, methods like Lamaze are even taught within the hospital, and
on many obstetrical wards there is much more cooperation with the
explicit desires of mother (and father) to follow the Lamaze or other
methods. ("The anesthetist said one woman was on Lamaze and
screaming, so he offered some nitrous oxide but she said, 'No, this is
my second child, just let me scream;' and he was perfectly willing.").

Nevertheless, the persistent use of such methods on what is essentially foreign (medical) terrain may lead to interactional
difficulties, including those that pertain to pain management. For instance, a hint of what a determined Lamaze patient can, quite
unintentionally, do to an experienced nurse:

The nurse was getting irritated. After about three (more) hours, she
said the patient was "hanging on a cliff" and later mumbled "these
people who are so free with street drugs and then go in for La-
maze. . . . I'd rather they would take something (during de-
livery). . . . I feel helpless. *They're huffing and puffing. Why*
do they come here if they don't need help?"

That last query suggests the extent of the lay invasion of professional territory and the impact of that invasion on professional identity. On the other hand, some personnel develop tactics to handle these unconventional mothers and fathers. One resident explained his views to us:

> If a woman wants natural childbirth and she is only two centimeters away, I will encourage her to go on. It is not my place to inflict my feelings. But if she is a long way away: "Look you're only tiring yourself out." Usually she's ready to take something. The problem is with the husband, who feels he's failed. Then I tell him how great she is, but now she needs something.

In contrast, the extent of control over the birth process by an ideologically fortified team of mother and father is illustrated graphically by the following instance, which also illustrates that a given staff may be familiar with Lamaze ideology and methods but not necessarily with other natural childbirth alternatives.

> When this patient entered, it was announced she was on the Bradley method, a first for the ward. It was explained to me as a form of natural chilbirth, but that was all they knew. She was being watched by a nurse with ten years experience in labor and delivery, who commented at one point: "That woman is really a stoic. I think she's in a lot more pain than she says."

> She went through the delivery with no anesthetic, husband holding her hand and saying: "Be brave" or "I'm so proud of you." She would get extremely red with each contraction, eyes closed. The doctor had needle in hand, ready to give a local right before cutting, and the husband asked: "Do you have to do that?" The doctor explained and the husband said: "We heard that if the skin is blanched, she will not feel the episiotomy, that too many women are given locals and really don't need it." The doctor said: "It will hurt too much to be cut. I couldn't take it, if it were me. The local does not affect the baby." The husband was nervously insistent, so the physician said he would cut a little and see if she could take it. (Patient had said nothing, but was still very red, eyes closed, etc.) He cut a little, asked her if she felt it. She said: "Yes." Husband said: "OK," and she was given the local.

> The next day, I asked if she was disappointed that she needed the local, and she said: "No," since the doctor inspired confidence and told her it didn't affect the baby. But she didn't realize he was testing with a small cut. She thought what she felt was a needle and maybe she could have taken it. I asked how she felt when her hus-

> *band was insisting on no local. Didn't it make her mad? She said:*
> *"No, you can't handle it by yourself. It's impossible when you're in*
> *that much pain to say it will be over in 2½ hours. You have to*
> *have someone else saying it for you."*

In essence, the ideology supporting the Bradley method implies a far
greater degree of nonprofessional control over the birth process than
is usual in American hospitals. This particular mother said that every
time a nurse entered her room, she would tense up because: "I
wanted to do it my way. I knew none of them had heard of the
Bradley method, and I wanted to show them how well it worked."
The aim of the true missionary, in short, is not simply to exert nonprofessional control over her own delivery but to convince professionals to adopt permanently the new methods. A natural-childbirth
mother risks shame if she falters and asks for or accepts medication.
On the other hand, if she is only partly committed, she can succumb
more easily, and both she and the father can comfort themselves that
at least they got that far and that the philosophy did help.

> *She was glad she had the Lamaze training, even though she had not*
> *been able to go the whole way. . . . I asked if it was a disappoint-*
> *ment to have to ask for drugs, and she said: "I'm still disappointed."*
> *Her husband was indignant: "You shouldn't be." He was glad he*
> *had been at the delivery because he knew she had reached the point*
> *where she needed medication.*

This father's response to the entire experience of attempting to
follow through, as far as possible, on Lamaze methods in handling
both the labor and its pain, was: "I had no idea of how much responsibility I would have. But when she was frightened, she would
hold on to *me*, not to some strange nurse." So the experience had
brought the couple closer together. On the other hand, breaches can
open when following through on an ideological position:

> *She had thought she would have a natural childbirth, but ended up*
> *wanting more medication than they would give her. "I never ex-*
> *pected that pain could be so bad and hurt so long. I thought I was*
> *going to go into shock." Her husband kept saying: "I thought you*
> *wanted a natural." "I could have hit him. I wanted to throw them*
> *all out."*

This kind of conflict is probably more characteristic when the couple's commitment to natural childbirth is minimal or when one is
more committed than the other. Even when quite committed, the
parents may be very surprised during labor or delivery at the du-

ration or amount of pain, for which the Lamaze instructor or the book on natural childbirth left them unprepared.

The lengths to which staff tolerance and lay invasion of professional terrain can go are illustrated by the following scene which occurred in a delivery room. The mother-father team was committed to the Bradley method. When the mother was wheeled into the delivery room, a field-worker described the scene:

> She was clearly in a panic, yelling: "Help me, somebody help me. . . . How much longer?. . . . I have to push. . . ." She was close to hysteria. As she continued to yell and cry for help, the father gleefully said to me, "Looks like this is it." At one point, the nurse told him to help her breathe; he made a feeble attempt but clearly this was not your classic well-coached Bradley father. Then I heard the chief say sardonically: "He's busy with his camera." Throughout her delivery, the loudest I had witnessed so far, the father continued to snap pictures from every conceivable angle, apparently oblivious to the pain, and at one point leaning over her stomach to get a good shot of the afterbirth. The second the baby was out, she asked: "Is he all right?" and the father answered, snapping away and crying: "He's all right" but clearly they didn't know yet; the baby had been somewhat blue, they were still working on him. . . .

> I later heard the father in the waiting room telling his friends how many pictures he had taken. A friend asked: "Didn't you mind the blood?" and he said: "No, that kind of thing doesn't bother me. And it was such a beautiful shade of red I took a picture of the placenta."

Lest this man be judged as callous to his wife's pain and totally eccentric, it ought to be recognized that one of *his* main jobs— thoroughly agreed to by his wife—was to preserve a permanent memory of the great family event. As the patient said the day after, when queried by the fieldworker: "No, she was not annoyed. She was glad because in fact the staff, busily working away, had impeded her view of the mirror so that she couldn't see her child's entry into the world—a baby she wished to born the natural way rather than 'have someone take it out.' " Her husband could now present her with a vivid representation.

ORGANIZATIONAL CONSIDERATIONS

Besides the ideological and medical considerations, organizational factors also profoundly affect the interaction which accompanies the birth process. Since organizational structure varies widely from hospital to hospital, and doubtless from country to country, we shall emphasize only a few organizational conditions which are probably widespread throughout the United States (or wherever Western medicine is involved with birth pain).

To begin with, every hospital ward is organized on a 24-hour basis, hence is characterized by multiple (usually three) shifts of personnel. Communication among shifts may be less than efficient, with relevant consequences for the mother's pain relief. For instance, one woman had reached an agreement with her private physician that a particular drug, to which she was very allergic, would not be used to relieve pain during either her labor or delivery. Their agreement, however, was disregarded, lost in the shuffle of staff rotation, so that this mother suffered marked allergic reactions, including a "fantastic headache for a week after my delivery."

A mother who is in labor longer than the duration of one shift's work is even more likely to encounter personnel with different ideas about birth and pain. She is likely anyhow, in American hospitals, to meet up with divergent views, but one or two or more shifts of staff, and the variations will increase. Differences among staff views will be basically medical. A nurse from Norway is scandalized at the amount of medication used during labor in the United States; another nurse has definite ideas about coaching patients to breathe along with the contractions; while another either places no faith in that procedure or has never heard of it. Comparable differences exist among staff physicians, affecting labor, delivery, and pain, not to mention staff relationships, which in turn may affect future patients.

> The anesthetist gave her, on request for relief, an epidural. The nurse and resident doctor were annoyed because they felt she could have made it without anesthetic. . . . (When I asked the next day about this case) all they remembered was their annoyance at the anesthetist for giving an epidural when it wasn't needed.

As we have seen, the staff may also hold quite different cultural, personal, or ideological perspectives on birth and its accompanying pain. A kaleidoscope of ideological positions sometimes whirls around "the care" of the birthing woman, and the longer her labor, the more likely is she to be aware of those discrepant positions. If she has a firm one of her own, then some staff views will be more congenial and some will grate on her.

This general situation occurs in our hospitals because the ideologies are usually implicit. Sometimes, of course, they are explicit, as when the chief establishes a particular set of rules about pain relief and its associated medications; even then there will be at least implicit disagreement with him, and his rules run the hazard of being broken or sometimes at least qualified. It is indeed a rare occasion on obstetrical wards when the staff members sit down in explicit con- clave to discuss divergent views—certainly the views about pain management—and then agree together upon a set of procedures.

Consequently, under present organizational conditions, a sit- uation often occurs where, at a critical juncture during the birth process, a staff member whose ideas are congenial to the mother may be absent, or someone with a conflicting or even abhorrent position may be present.

A second organizational feature of obstetrical wards is this: al- though there are very slow periods and very busy periods, the number of staff members available remains the same. In slow periods (few mothers or early in the labor) there is much waiting; in busy periods the staff goes into action, and sometimes the action is hectic. Multiple deliveries may occur, or several mothers may be in difficult labor, or there may be more than one difficult medical case. Yet the ratio of staff to patients is usually not responsive to these variable conditions. Indeed, for one reason or another, there may be fewer staff members available exactly at the time when *more* are needed. (Once one of the authors found himself substituting for an assisting obstetrical resident who had been called elsewhere for an emergency, while the attending resident performed an episiotomy.) During night shifts, peak loads of laboring and delivering mothers may find them- selves in hard competition for relatively scarce personnel. (To quote one resident: "Once I had to do three deliveries without scrubbing in between.")

It is precisely at such peak periods when the nursing staff, at least, are happy to have the father as part of the ward's total division of labor. "He knows the patient better than we do, and he is better able to do things for her like rub her back"; or watch the monitoring machine, or help count with the breathing, or ask for pain medica- tion if he thinks it's time, or help the mother control the expression of her pain and her demands for medication.

Variations in staff skill are a third important feature of obstetrical wards which affects the carrying out of pain tasks. The personnel are likely to possess varied amounts of experience as well as to have profited differentially from their experience. In some hospitals, medi- cal students work regularly on obstetrical wards, and the monthly rotation of residents and interns brings to fairly low levels what one might term "the experienced–inexperienced ratio." Additionally, there can be a high turnover of the nursing staff. To underline the difficulties inherent in this situation, a patient may be as inex- perienced as the greenest intern, or she may have had a bit more experience than the nurse who is counting the contractions or even the resident who is delivering her sixth or seventh baby.

On the medical side, this inexperience may lead to error, or at least to staff disagreement, as in the following instance:

> She was relieved of her pain for a while, but two hours later the nurse was fretting that she wasn't getting any relief. This became a glaring example of the resident's job being impeded by the change in shifts. The first resident had felt she was 6 cm dilated, and had ordered her membrane broken and ordered the epidural; the second resident felt she was only 4 cm and grumbled: "She got the epidural too soon as far as I'm concerned." They measure a centimeter by the width of the finger, and all you have to do is look at the first resident's hand (male) and the second's (female) to see where there might be a discrepancy.

The degree of medical skill as it relates to inflicted pain is underlined by the comments of an experienced obstetrician about a test which requires the extracting of amniotic fluid: Too many unsuccessful tries can traumatize the patient (aside from damaging the placenta if the needle is not placed correctly). Besides, "fantasy-wise the worst thing you can do to a pregnant woman is stick a needle in and stab her belly. You are doing it because there is already suspicion of something wrong."

As with such inflicted-pain procedures, the patient can often know or guess the physician's skill or lack thereof. Mistiming or misjudgments about amounts of relieving medication also emphasize lack of skill, but hospital organization makes it difficult to accurately place blame. However, more sophisticated Lamaze parents may make accurate assessments—or at least believe they are accurate—of staff skills, and this may affect their reactions, both during the birth process and thereafter.

> They had been told in the Lamaze class that the last epidural injection inhibits the pushing, and he felt the anesthetist should have asked before injection. Forceps had been used, marking the baby's head; they knew of dangers, but "next time I will know better. I will tell them no injection and forceps unless absolutely necessary."

Staff members may also lack social skills and may not be able to interact successfully with the laboring or delivering mother to help her through the birth process. Sometimes drastic measures are called for when a mother is screaming or close to hysterics. More subtle means of helping the mother control pain expressions and to endure her pain include making encouraging noises, promising that it will soon be over, stroking arms, patting hands and heads, and generally encouraging the mother to hang on. These tactics are what we have previously termed "presence."

Some nurses and physicians are superb at such tactics; others use them scarcely recognizing them as tactics; other personnel consistently fail the mothers either because they lack such skills or because they are too intently focused on other tasks. In general, of course, there is even less organizational programming directed toward achieving consistency in such interactional skills than there is for the more straightforward medical procedures. Although failures of procedural and medical skill abound, at least staff are accountable for those; for interactional skills they are not. Specific staff members may be superb in their use of interactional skills, but for the ward as a whole, use of those skills is hit and miss. Accountability is, as usual, reserved for medical acts.

REFERENCES

1. Glaser, B., and Strauss, A. 1964. Social loss of dying patients. *American Journal of Nursing* 64:119–121.

Part 7

Juggling the Options

The Balancing Process

16

BALANCING AND CONTROLLING

We now turn to balancing—perhaps the most important process of all for understanding interactions that involve pain and pain tasks. Throughout this book—and indeed on almost every page—we have seen or sensed patients and hospital personnel making choices among various pain alternatives. Endure considerable pain in order to have a natural childbirth? Give relief with risk of addiction or wean the patient despite considerable pain? These choices among various options represent calculations and decisions concerning: What is to be done? When is it to be done? How is it to be done? Who is to do it? What considerations are to be taken into account in doing it? Balancing, the term coined to refer to those processes of choice, involves patients and personnel in innumerable contests over the control of their lines of action. Thus an analysis of balancing will inevitably plunge us into a consideration of genuinely political activity. And we have seen plenty of such politics!

When a person living at home needs to decide among options involving pain, then the only genuine issue of control is self-control. (One needs to bargain only with oneself.) Thomas Schelling terms this intrapersonal process "tacit bargaining."[1] As soon as other persons are involved, however, whether family or friends, then the balancing becomes directly or potentially a political matter.[2-4] Why? Because as soon as a decision impinges on others' lives, those others may feel they need to negotiate or contest that decision. They may even seek to control future decisions which pertain to their pain. Others' desires may not always coincide with the patient's. We are reminded here of two extreme instances. An elderly woman was told by her physician that to get relief from her pain she would need an operation, but that the operation would render her less mobile. Her husband and her several sons and daughters each had a different stake in balancing her present and future pain levels against her present and future mobility; none of their stakes were quite the same as hers! One would be unjust to characterize their balancings as "selfish"; unquestionably each person had a different life to live. Another example of conflicting desires: It is not unknown for football players to endure immense pain during an important game because they are urged on—or threatened by—exploitative coaches. Within hospital walls, this political activity called balancing is frequent and often quite visible. Sometimes battles are settled satisfactorily, but sometimes the explosions are tremendous and the "fallout" is highly detrimental to patient, to staff, or to both.

In the most general sense, the relationship between balancing and controlling can be understood by noting that hospitalized patients are temporarily required to cede to staff members considerable control over some (though not all) aspects of their lives, behaviors, and bodies. Mrs. Abel allowed the staff to manage her medical therapy but not her pain. The patients in burn units permit the staff to manage their therapy and even to inflict great pain during that management, but usually they retain the right to pace some of the therapeutic procedure. Insofar as everyone agrees on what is to be delegated—and when and to whom—there is little contest over balancing. When there *is* disagreement, whether or not it is clearly recognized, contests occur. That is why one burn patient, for instance, finally signed himself out of the hospital, refusing to undergo further debriding sessions. Putting more weight on avoiding the terrible inflicted pain than on the consequences of avoiding it, he refused the staff members the right to continue with their therapy. And that is why Wertenbaker refused to die in a hospital, reasoning that his main task—dying in his own manner, retaining his own style and his identity while dying—would be interfered with, and his essential rights infringed upon, in any hospital.[5]

What are seen as options and the choices among them are different for different people. The bases for those differential judgments may be personal, cultural, or social. They can also be positional, as when a patient, nurse, nurse's aide, resident, and private physician all weigh somewhat different considerations, or weigh the same ones differently. One additional condition which can profoundly affect the balancing pertains to what information is available. A patient, for instance, can only balance what he recognizes, so cannot weigh his potential addiction against pain relief if he does not know (as the staff does) that addiction is hanging in the balance.

The existence of those differential bases for balancing makes it very probable that there will be a fair amount of contest for control of pain management, despite the patient's delegation of control over body and behavior. How to get pain and related tasks done, in the face of differential balancing, is then a major problem for both the staff and the patients. Short of brute force or threat of coercion, this involves both parties in political processes such as negotiating, persuading, and eliciting or suppressing information. It is for this reason that although a psychologist might be interested in the intra-psychic mechanisms involved in an individual's juggling of the options, we have been interested rather in the interactional aspects of that juggling.

Since this book is replete with implicit and explicit discussions of balancing, we shall here focus on only two additional aspects: first, an outlining of the major features of balancing; second, an underscoring of the political aspects of balancing through a discussion of crises and fateful choices. A few examples will be presented, but readers can surely draw for further instances on data presented in preceding chapters, augmented by experiences of their own. The case-history chapters afford perhaps the richest, or at least the most dramatic, instances of such data, for balancing can become ever more problematic when the chronically ill patient remains hospitalized for a considerable time without much improvement in illness and pain trajectories. (Another case history focusing primarily on sequential balancing is presented in the next chapter.)

DIMENSIONS, MATRIX, AND CONTEXTS

The most basic questions about balancing are: What is balanced? Why? The answer to those questions, both in general and for particular interactions, can be approached by considering a grid (see diagram on p. 244). This grid consists of *dimensions* listed vertically and horizontally. The vertical ones pertain to various pain tasks. The

dimensions listed horizontally pertain to various matters that may be
affected by or affect the pain tasks: the illness trajectory, the maintenance of a life, the interaction itself, the personnel's work, the
sentimental order of the ward, and the identities of various interactants. If we think of these dimensions as "crosscutting," or
balancing each other (i.e., pain expression versus interactional disturbance), then the entire grid might usefully be referred to as a
balancing *matrix*.

To know what is being balanced in any given pain drama, or in
a scene from such a drama, we need to find out which dimensions
are being balanced by each interactant. Suppose that, for convenience, we call that particular calculus the balancing *context*. For
instance, a child is balancing crying against keeping outward poise
in the face of pain inflicted by a catheterization which he's agreed to,
while the physician is balancing the infliction of pain against needed
diagnostic information. If the child decides the pain is too much and
decides against further catheterization (i.e., the diagnostic test versus
enduring the pain), then the staff may utilize coercive measures since
their choice, unlike the child's, remains in favor of the diagnostic information versus the infliction of pain. If the press of work is not too
great, the physician may take the time (i.e., "work") to be more careful and gentle in the continued catheterization, thus minimizing the

A Balancing Matrix

Pain Tasks	Consequences For						
	Illness trajectory	Life and death	Carrying-on	Interaction	Ward work	Sentimental order	Personal identity
Diagnosing							
Preventing							
Minimizing							
Inflicting							
Relieving							
Enduring							
Expressing							

inflicted pain. Each of those contexts is different, and each can be diagrammed easily on the balancing matrix. This is done by putting a mark in the box (or boxes) where the vertical and horizontal dimensions cross. (Since the patient and the staff may not balance identical dimensions, use a different letter for each relevant interactant: "p" for patient, "n" for nurse, "d" for doctor.)

A very important condition for any given balancing context is the array of organizational properties bearing upon it. By this we have in mind such properties as the ward's ratio of staff to patients, the experience of the personnel, the pain ideologies of the staff, and so on through the large number of properties implicitly or explicitly discussed in preceding chapters. When an organizational property changes (the staff at night may be less experienced than the daytime staff, or there may be fewer personnel, or an inexperienced resident may take the place of an experienced one), this change may profoundly affect a balancing context. For example, recall what happens when an empathetic, psychologically oriented nurse attending a mother in labor goes off duty and her place is taken by a brusque, no-nonsense medically oriented nurse. To designate the most relevant organizational properties bearing on balancing, we suggest the term *organizational context*. Balancing never takes place in an organizational vacuum.

BALANCING, MISBALANCING, AND AWARENESS

Now let us see some implications of the scheme just sketched. To begin with, all participants will be balancing identically in a great proportion of pain dramas. Thus, all agree that a pain-inflicting procedure must be given (and endured) because life and death may be at issue, or that comfort care with its pain relief should now be operative because life-saving measures are senseless.

It is worth noting, however, that sometimes only one person, say the patient, is actually balancing. Thus, she may decide to endure the pain and not ask for relief, because she does not wish to interfere with a busy staff or because too many requests for medication will earn her a poor interactional reputation. Likewise, a physician may not let the patient know that she is about to run the risk of increasing pain because the physician must cut back on medication to achieve some medical goal. In such instances, there is a situation of "closed awareness," since only the person who is balancing options knows the balancing is being done.

Most of the difficulties discussed throughout this book, however, whether relatively inconsequential or of immense import for interaction and care, flow from *misbalancing* (i.e., differential balancing) by the various actors in the pain drama. There are various types of misbalances. First, two or more interactants may be balancing one or more different dimensions, rather than the same dimensions. Sometimes each may be aware of that differential balancing; sometimes only one may be aware. And sometimes none are aware. (In this book, we have related situations where the researcher was aware of differential balancing, but the interactants were not.) Second, the interactants may simply disagree on the priorities assigned to the same dimensions, as when a dying patient opts for morphine to relieve his pain knowing he is dying anyway, while the staff opts for a non-addicted patient and lesser relief of pain. Again, one or more of the interactants may not be aware of such disagreement between or among them.

Implicit in those distinctions and examples, of course, is that two staff members may agree or disagree, just as a given staff member may agree or disagree with the patient. And those two staff members may disagree with each other, while also disagreeing with the patient. Instead of disagreeing, however, they may be balancing different dimensions. Or the nurse may be agreeing with the patient, while the physician is differently balancing one or more items.

What makes this picture all the more complicated is the existence of different states of awareness that are possible concerning what the other interactants are balancing. The nurse may be aware both of the patient and physician's differential balances and agree with the patient, who may be aware only of their agreement, while the physician is aware only of a discrepancy between the patient's and his own balancing. (To make the matter still more complicated, sometimes an interactant is aware of the reasons for discrepant balancing among the implicated persons, but sometimes they are not so aware, or are wrong in their knowledge of "reasons.")

By now it should be apparent that all these various misbalancings resulting in contests over control can be illuminated by reference to the diagrammatic scheme outlined earlier.

CRISES AND FATEFUL BALANCING

A phenomenon which illustrates with dramatic if sometimes tragic clarity the relationship between control and balance—and the political nature of that relationship—is that of medical crisis. In its simpler versions, one sees this phenomenon in the emergency rooms of hospitals where a physician (with or without the patient's agreement or awareness) may have to balance, because of life-and-death considerations, quick medical action against the infliction of pain or the delay of pain relief. In general, when there is no agreement between patient and staff, and no time to persuade or to negotiate, the staff may deem it necessary either to use coercion for carrying out a critical task or to make the decision about the task (and do it) without the patient's (or even the family's) awareness.

On the subject of awareness: In one instance a patient was brought to the hospital terribly burned and also having a heart attack. The physicians had to decide quickly which critical medical task had priority, with pain relief and the awareness of the patient far in the background of this balancing context.

Crisis action tends to underscore the fact that control is in the hands of the attending staff, with the patient and family pretty much out of the decision-making process. An ironic instance of such professional control concerns a terminally ill patient, in despair over his suffering, who slashed his wrists. But a nurse quickly called the resident and together they saved him before they had a chance to wonder why they were acting so impulsively to save someone who was terminally ill and wished to die. *They* had reversed *his* balancing, a telling example of political power in the hospital!

Another phenomenon seen on occasion throughout this book is the dilemma involved in choosing between fateful or dire options. An acquaintance of ours, weary of intractable pain, chose voluntarily to undergo the severance of a nerve, knowing that he was trading relief for permanent blindness. Less drastic but still risky was the choice of a patient who continued using a hot water bottle because it yielded relief when nothing else seemed to, knowing it might contribute to the growth of her cancerous tumor. Indeed, many persons with cancer are engaged in precarious, if not fateful, decisions on a weekly or monthly basis, as they balance living longer against lessening their pain or against the side effects produced by chemotherapy. Some opt against the therapy despite sharp disagreements with family and with physicians too.

In making such decisions, patients, families, and staffs are sometimes forced to face clear and terrible options. Sometimes, the options are less certain but still awesomely risky: whether to undergo an operation for pain relief that may (but may not) result in deafness. The neurosurgeon argued for a procedure which might end in the patient's deafness, but the patient's sister, who was a nurse, persuaded her brother to try acupuncture instead. Happily it worked. In this instance, not only deafness but also death were at stake. Confronted with such a dire choice, the tendency understandably is to thrust the decision into the patient's or family's hands, with the physician only outlining the pros and cons, the possibilities and probabilities. But that is not inevitable, for in the following case history the physicians (and the husband) eventually whisked the patient

off to the operating room to save her from predicted awful pain, after
she had for some days resisted that plan but been unable to choose
between the options of swift or slow suicide.

Mrs. Abel's sad end is also most instructive because of what it
tells about political control in the hospital. Mrs. Abel controlled much
of her hospitalized life at the expense of a demoralized and "avoiding" staff. She also paid the ultimate price of being forced to face—
completely alone—the fateful choice of continuing with her pain or
chancing an operation that might relieve it but which she feared
might leave her "a vegetable." While she was balancing these options the nurses were, unknown to her, disapproving of the potential
operation; indeed some were aghast at its possibility. The physician
who had proposed it would not make the choice for her and disap-
peared from sight while she made the final decision. While she
doubtless would have died soon from her cancer, the operation did
actually kill her. Sad as that is, sadder still is the fact that no one
from the ward accompanied or saw her off to the operating room.
The final irony of her complex illness, pain, hospital, and social biography can then be read as follows: The staff allowed her control over
her own final balancing of options, but she was given virtually no
information about the dangerous operation and no support at all in
the balancing process.

Lest this chapter conclude on too grim a note, we quickly add
that not all dire choices end so unhappily, nor are they all made with
such lack of professional support. But the main point of our men-
tioning Mrs. Abel's dilemma—and the main point of this chapter—is
that a balancing of pain considerations against other considerations
is both endemic to "pain management" and is ultimately a most
politicized activity. In short, it is inadequate to conceive of pain
management as primarily involving a nurse or a physician in a one-
to-one relationship with a patient, outside of organizational and balancing contexts.

For the nurses and physicians, the stakes carried out within
these contexts are very high. As a further glance at the balancing matrix will show, and as data scattered throughout this book should
suggest, the stakes include not merely the maintaining of control
over conditions of work, but they involve many more subtle issues
pertaining to staff morale, professionalized identity, and personal
identity.

REBALANCING: BALANCING AS A PROCESS

Balancing always involves temporal considerations. Why? The choice
of one option over another usually is not an instantaneous decision;

the weighting of pros and cons about pain issues, the thinking, persuading, and negotiating may take many minutes, hours, even days. No matter how complicated such a decision, however, it is likely to be a relatively simple one when compared to those which are revised two or three times—or a dozen or two dozen times. Those revisions can be termed rebalancings. Even when acted upon, the initial decision is reconsidered and frequently altered.

The conditions which maximize the probability of rebalancing are quite varied. (1) Any change in the pain trajectory can bring about a different weighing of relief measures against a variety of other considerations. (2) Any change in the illness trajectory can bring about reconsiderations of available options.[6, 7] (3) Changes in organizational properties (ratio of staff to patient, a new resident) bring new contingencies to bear on an old decision, enhancing the probability of its reconsideration. Sometimes two or three conditions are changing simultaneously, or in quick sequence. In cases of chronic illness, when the patient is hospitalized for some days or weeks and when there is change—for better or worse—or instability of "condition," then the chances of rebalancing are very great. In addition, there are conditions that pertain to the patient's social trajectory, changes in what is happening to his family, his finances, his imagery of his own future, and his relationship to himself.

Cutting across all those considerations, as can be seen from the balancing matrix, is the added complication that the balancing process is not confined to the patient; many people may be involved. Reconsiderations of a previous decision may preoccupy exactly the same cast of characters (patient, spouse, physician, head nurse) or at least a slightly changed cast (a new physician, an additional consulting physician). Furthermore, where some persons may have seen eye to eye they may now disagree, or vice versa. New or changed contingencies may also effectively force some persons to reconsider faster than others, or the latter may either not notice that anything is different or not assess the situation as being different.

Finally, it is worth reminding ourselves that analytically one may think of the balancing process as cutting across other processes which also take place over time. Some of those other processes include the pain tasks: relieving, minimizing, expressing, enduring, even inflicting (as in rehabilitation therapy). It would be tedious for readers and authors both if, at this point in the book, we were to detail the linkages between balancing and those other processes. The main point is simple (although the specific connections can be complex); the pain processes may change over time. Thus more endurance is called for by the staff or is managed by the patient; less expression is permitted by the staff or the patient permits himself more expression. Those processes can also change because of altered or new contingencies.

Perhaps it will be confusing to assert, but assert we must, that rebalancing considerations may not only affect those pain processes but in turn may be affected by altered pain processes. (Thus, more overt expression may change the minds of staff members about how much relief is now necessary.) In short, those processes are mutually interactive with the balancing process itself. That makes the latter a very complicated process indeed. This is precisely why we regard it as the *primary process.* Unless we understand its complexity, we can never grasp the deeper complexities of pain management.

The next chapter, the case history of Mrs. Price, is largely about rebalancing—inevitable because of the full-blown complexities characteristic of uncertain trajectories and extended hospitalization.

REFERENCES

1. Schelling, T. 1960. *The strategy of conflict.* Cambridge, Mass.: Harvard University Press.

2. Luker, K. 1974. *Taking chances: abortion and the decision not to contracept.* Berkeley, Ca.: University of California Press. Esp. pp. 40–41, 78–111.

3. Mullen, P. 1974. Cutting back: life after a heart attack. Ph.D. dissertation, School of Public Health, University of California, Berkeley.

4. Reif, L. 1975. Cardiacs and normals: the social construct of reality. Ph.D. dissertation, Department of Social and Behavioral Science, University of California, San Francisco.

5. Wertenbaker, L. 1957. *Death of a man.* New York: Random House.

6. Kaehele, E. 1952. *Living with cancer.* New York: Doubleday.

7. Kesten, Y. 1968. *Diary of a heart patient.* New York: McGraw-Hill.

Case History: Cumulative Illness and Rebalancing

17

REBALANCING AND THE CUMULATIVE ILLNESS TRAJECTORY

The case of Mrs. Price is characteristic of a type of illness trajectory found more and more frequently in our hospitals. We call it a "cumulative illness trajectory" for reasons that will soon become apparent. Its chief features can be summarized chronologically. In order to keep a complex chronic illness under control, physicians utilize a variety of therapies, sequentially and in combination. These may or may not work for a while, but they inevitably add to the complications produced by the illness itself. To handle the complications and the new turns in the illness, additional tests, drugs, procedures, and therapies are utilized. Few of these are really experimental or untried, but their impact on the symptomology and illness of the specific patient may be relatively unpredictable. Over time, as in the case of Mrs. Price, the patient's physical condition can become more and more unbalanced, with increasingly varied medical interventions becoming necessary to manage the imbalances.

Pain may or may not be present during or at any point in such cumulative trajectories. Often, of course, it will be present, even constant. Sometimes, as with Mrs. Price, it will be an integral part of the cumulative trajectory, with *all* the pain tasks salient, necessary, and alas problematic.

Patients such as Mrs. Price are found in increasing numbers in our hospitals because of a corresponding increase in difficult-to-manage chronic illnesses, especially those in later stages when there is a deterioration of multiple bodily systems. Today elaborate technical resources permit multiple and sequential medical interventions which achieve or maintain physical balance, but that achieving and maintaining is difficult and precarious. Hence there is a constant—almost continuous—need to rebalance. As we shall see, the various actors in the drama may do that rebalancing differently, and the negative consequences for personal-identity care, work, and the ward's sentimental order are shattering.

We should add that the field researcher who followed the case of Mrs. Price observed both the specific hospital episode discussed here and the patient's previous one several months before. The researcher developed a genuine fondness and affection for Mrs. Price, who is intelligent, charming, and brave. Her agonizing dilemma could not but deeply touch the researcher, but then, so did the staff members' predicaments. There were frustration, anger, bafflement, personal desperation, and despair for virtually *all* involved during the evolution of this cumulative trajectory. The medical problems were very great; the organizational problems were perhaps just as difficult and fed back into and helped to increase the medical ones.

The case of Mrs. Price illustrates far more than the rebalancing process, of course, but we shall focus primarily on that process as it evolved over two months. (Mrs. Price actually was hospitalized for three months.) The story will be recounted sequentially, accompanied by occasional commentary.

THE CASE OF MRS. PRICE

Mrs. Price, the 45-year-old wife of a physician, was in for her fourth hospitalization. She had been diagnosed as having lupus erythematosus two years previously. Since then she had had three acute episodes requiring hospitalization, the last two occurring within the last year because of bleeding gastric ulcers which required surgical intervention. The ulcers were complications from steroid treatments to control the lupus. In both episodes there were flare-ups of lupus, so that hospitalization was extended two to four months. Also, the uncertainty of Mrs. Price's condition together with her low tolerance for pain resulted in narcotic dependency. There were conflicts between Mrs. Price and the staff over drug control. Weaning her from the drug proved difficult.

During this period of two years both the treatment and the disease had drastically altered the quality of her life. For example, Mrs. Price could not engage in her one great pleasure, gardening, because sunlight exacerbated the lupus. By her fourth hospitalization she had come to realize that her illness would eventually be fatal, that the treatment created other problems, and that the future was highly uncertain. At the time of her fourth admission she had a variety of disorders. As a result of her lupus she had (1) pericarditis, (2) pleuritis (both of which caused pain), (3) cerebritis, which caused some personality changes and a tendency toward tremors and convulsions, and (4) chronic obstructive lung disease from the lupus and her heavy smoking. Also, as a result of the steroid treatments she had (5) gastic ulcers and (6) cushingoid syndrome.

With each hospitalization she returned to the same nursing unit, a unit primarily for surgical patients where stays tended to be short. The nurses anticipated problems of pain management with Mrs. Price because she arrived on the unit with a previously formed reputation for being "manipulative" and "uncooperative."

> Mrs. Price was readmitted to the hospital because of continued chest pain. The lupus specialist, Dr. Nagel, suspected a pleuritic flare-up from the lupus and recommended hospitalization for reevaluation and readjustment of the steroid drugs. Mrs. Price informed the researcher that she couldn't tolerate the idea of hospitalization after the long siege of the past year and so delayed coming to the hospital, hoping the chest pain would decrease. With the increased pain and general worsening of her condition, and after several days of persuasion by her husband and her attending physician, she finally consented to hospitalization.

> The nursing staff members anticipated that this patient would become addicted and therefore decided to "set limits." They reasoned that in the past, since the numerous doctors on the case wrote conflicting drug orders, the nurses were caught in the middle. With only one doctor responsible for the pain drug order, they would avoid the patient "manipulating" the doctors for increased pain drugs. Dr. Power, the house staff member and assistant to Dr. Nagel, would be responsible for the patient's general care and the pain drug orders. Dr. Nagel would be out of town for two weeks for an important medical conference. A decision was reached that the patient be given 50 mg of Demerol and Talwin to

control the pain, and these two drugs would be alternated every three hours. All the nurses and house staff were alerted to this schedule.

The house staff was busy evaluating Mrs. Price's illness status during the ensuing three days. This involved innumerable blood studies, an electrocardiogram, and chest x-rays. Meanwhile, she was having increased chest pain.

On the third day she refused to have a chest x-ray done at the time scheduled because she was too uncomfortable, and she insisted that 50 mg of Demerol was not holding the pain. The physician who was handling the pain drugs and the nurses refused to alter the drug order. Mrs. Price phoned the psychiatrist, Dr. Perle, and Dr. Abel, the cardio-pulmonary specialist, asking each to alter the drug order. They decided to honor the decision that one person handle the pain drugs, reasoning that they could not risk another dangerous addiction problem.

Later in the afternoon the researcher found the patient dressed and packed, ready to go home. She recounted her inability to obtain pain relief, said she was tired of hospitalization and simply wanted to go home and take her chances. The nurse caring for her described her as a will-ful patient who couldn't get her way (an increase in pain drugs) and was using the threat of going home as a weapon. The nurse's attitude was that the decision, however, was up to her (going home), no matter how unwise. The husband visited the patient and confronted her with: "Alice, you can't go home in your condition. You know you can't manage at home. If you go home, I wash my hands of the whole affair." He left the room. The researcher spent some time with the patient, who talked about the quality of her life over the past year, the difficulty of living with uncertainty, and the pros and cons of remaining in the hospital. Later the psychiatrist persuaded her to stay.

During the next two days she was relatively free of pain, although the drug order was not altered. This was due in part to the distraction afforded by a sister visiting from out of town who spent most of the day with her. The necessary diagnostic tests were taken and showed increased chest involvement. Adjustments were made in the steroid drug. During this period of two days, the researcher's encounters with Mrs. Price were very pleasant. This behavior was typical of her when she was free of pain.

We have here a fairly straightforward balancing situation for the hospital staff members. They were concerned primarily with two issues. (1) The tests were absolutely necessary for determining the patient's illness status and the recommended course of treatment. (2) Pain relief must be such as to avoid addiction, which had occurred in the past. The staff members assessed her pain as not so

great as she insisted and said she was bluffing—her refusal to take
the tests was a bargaining tool for getting more of the pain drug.
Avoiding addiction was more important to the staff members, so
they maintained a united front against a "willful" and "manipulating" patient—one who was living up to her reputation. On her
side, the patient grappled with staying versus going home and taking her chances, but she was persuaded to stay by her husband and
the psychiatrist. Her enduring of the pain was rendered less difficult
by the sister's visit. As Mrs. Price's story unfolds, the balancing
problems become extremely complex as new symptoms continually
and cumulatively develop.

> On the sixth day, Fay, the nurse who had cared for Mrs. Price during
> previous hospitalizations, stated that the pain problem was currently
> worse than it was during the last hospitalization. The patient was be-
> coming more insistent that the 50 mg of Demerol was not holding the
> pain. She had been telephoning her husband and the psychiatrist to get
> an increase in pain drugs. Over the weekend she was able to persuade
> Dr. Abel to increase the Demerol by 25 mg for one dose. Fay described
> this doctor as being an "easier mark" than the other doctors for pain
> drugs. Fay feared the problem of addiction would "start all over again
> like the last time."

> On the previous day, Fay had been reassigned to care for Mrs. Price be-
> cause the patient did not trust the new nurse, preferring Fay. This
> created some tensions within the nursing staff since the other nurses'
> work was disrupted. Fay also expressed frustration that previous meth-
> ods of relieving the patient weren't working. An impromptu conference
> followed wherein other nurses expressed frustration about their inability
> to relieve Mrs. Price's pain. They were also concerned about her un-
> stable lupus status. Some nurses stated that they would prefer her
> having cancer to lupus—that cancer would be less uncertain. Fay was
> criticized by some nurses because she could not separate her personal
> from her professional involvement with Mrs. Price. Fay was chagrined.
> She thought maybe she shouldn't take care of Mrs. Price. The next day
> she decided not to be assigned to Mrs. Price, in part because she found
> it difficult to see Mrs. Price deteriorate, but also because she wished to
> avoid the criticism of other nurses.

> That evening Mrs. Price developed abdominal pain. In the following
> eight days not only did the abdominal symptoms increase, but new
> symptoms developed. The cause of the increasing abdominal pain
> could not be found easily; the early tests were all negative. A number of
> possibilities were posed: bowel obstruction, extension of the lupus, re-
> action to the steroids, or reactions to narcotics. During this period she
> had an episode of sudden, sharp chest pains. An electrocardiograph

was taken, but it showed no pathology. Then one night she could not be roused from sleep. The staff was concerned. Did this mean she was overmedicated with pain drugs and sedatives, or was it due to further brain involvement? An electroencephalogram was done the following day.

During the first few days after the appearance of abdominal pain, the staff took a firm stand that the pain drugs would be continued with no deviation regardless of the patient's objection. There were occasional flurries between the patient and the staff over drug control. Drug orders were changed; a tranquilizer was changed when it was discovered that the particular tranquilizer predisposed her to tremors and seizures. After an inability to rouse the patient, the phenobarbital (sedative) was stopped; it was restarted when the husband pointed out that the phenobarbital was necessary to prevent seizures and the patient was fearful of seizures, having had a convulsion in the past. Because of the abdominal pain, all drugs were administered by injection. Mrs. Price had little appetite.

On the eleventh day she became very nauseated. Continuous intravenous infusions were started because she was developing fluid and electrolyte imbalances. Some difficulty was encountered while attempting to get into a vein because her veins were poor from the numerous venipunctures done for blood tests during this and previous hospitalizations. After three attempts the patient refused any more attempts but was persuaded to cooperate further.

With her continued nausea the house staff decided that a gastric suction would relieve the discomfort. She objected because she had received this treatment in the past and could not tolerate the gagging and discomfort from the tube. Antinausea drugs were therefore added to her drug list.

She now began to balk about having any tests when her pains were at peak. Whenever possible the staff attempted to bring into alignment the uncomfortable tests and the pain drugs, but quite often this was difficult to arrange.

Dr. Ambrose, a gastrointestinal specialist, was next consulted. He suspected other possibilities, among them pancreatitis. The staff all realized that pancreatitis was extremely painful; however, Mrs. Price's pain drugs were not increased. Further tests were ordered: barium x-rays and a gastric analysis. The physician also recommended gastric suction. An intern attempted to put down the nasogastric tube but was unsuccessful because the patient had a hypersensitive gag reflex. Finally Dr. Ambrose convinced her of the test's necessity. Three hours after the tube was inserted, Mrs. Price pulled it out because it caused her much discomfort and did not relieve the abdominal pain. She reasoned that if the suction did not relieve the pain there was little sense in tolerating the gagging sensation.

To accommodate the possibility of painful pancreatitis, extra pain drugs were ordered whenever an uncomfortable test was done. "Give 25 mg Demerol now and revert back to the routine schedule."

With the appearance of numerous new symptoms the nurses began monitoring Mrs. Price's vital signs more closely. Thus, all stools were monitored. The nurses were disturbed by her continued deterioration.

During this period the sister's many visits partially helped her to endure her pain. In the researcher's encounters with the patient, she frequently talked about the problem of not knowing the cause of her pain and about the unexpected symptoms.

The psychiatrist continued to visit her daily but was not interacting to any great extent with the nurses. He was also much involved with the patient's husband who was often the victim of Mrs. Price's irritability, and he was looking more and more tired and haggard.

On the fourteenth day a definitive diagnosis was made: she had developed a huge gastric ulcer. Also, a chest x-ray showed broken ribs. Both were attributed to the steroids, yet they could not be stopped because the lupus would get out of control. Of course, everybody was terribly upset at this news. To some degree the nurses blamed the patient because she had not been very "cooperative" about taking the antacid routinely prescribed for patients on steroids in order to prevent gastric ulcers.

Her order for pain drugs now read: "Increase pain drugs. Addiction is not the priority now. Increased tension, irritability re. pain drugs increases gastric irritability." The order was changed so that she was to get from 50 mg to 75 mg every three hours.

The patient was both relieved and upset when told the cause of her pain; she realized that treatment would not be easy. To the researcher's comment that she tolerated pain relatively well for someone who supposedly had a low pain threshold she answered: "What else can I do? The only thing would be to jump out of the window, and I haven't quite considered that."

In some diseases, expected events may occur as the disease predictably evolves, but with such problematic illness trajectories as Mrs. Price's, unexpected events are frequent. Each day new symptoms developed, indicating that something was physically "out of balance." More and more tests were required. With each new symptom, new drugs and treatments were added or deleted in order to prevent, block, or neutralize the progression of the disease, or control the symptoms, or stem the general bodily deterioration.

When a painful symptom could not be readily diagnosed, the patient's anxiety and perception of pain increased, creating assessment and pain-relief problems for the staff. With the cumulative development of symptoms which required cumulative tests—some of which were uncomfortable—the patient began increasingly to resist the tests. Despite a definitive indication of pathology, the staff adopted the stand that addiction should be avoided. Nevertheless, as symptoms increased and tests became essential for diagnosis, Mrs. Price's pain drugs were temporally increased as a means of bargaining to gain her cooperation.

The continued uncertainty, the continued deterioration of the patient, and the growing frustration of the staff profoundly affected the ward's sentimental order. Also, Fay, the nurse closest to Mrs. Price, could not tolerate the continued deterioration of the patient or the criticisms of other nurses, so, as we mentioned earlier, she elected to be reassigned to other patients.

Once a basis for pain was discovered, addiction was not an issue in the staff's balancing. Relief of pain and lowering of tension were essential to preventing an increased gastric irritability.

> The definitive diagnosis of gastric ulcers and the broken ribs, particularly the ulcers, posed immense treatment problems. The medical choices were limited. Ulcers and broken ribs were the result of the steroids, yet the steroids were essential to control the lupus. In the patient's current physical state she was a poor surgical risk. Yet the size and the location of the ulcer, unless immediately treated, had dangerous consequences. Thus, there could be erosion of the ulcer into the peritoneal cavity or it might cause pancreatitis, both of which could be fatal, and at the least extremely painful. Indeed, this pain could be more painful than the ulcer pain.

> Numerous specialists were consulted. After debating pro and con, the decision was made to radiate the stomach to knock out the acid-producing cells and so prevent further extension of the ulcer. The radiation dosage would be low so that other organs, particularly the kidneys, would not be compromised. Concurrently, hyperalimentation treatment (special intravenous feeding through a tube placed in the subclavian vein, located in the neck) would be started in order to overcome the malnutrition. The physicians explained to the patient the limited choices, why the treatments were necessary, and that the radiation dosage would be extremely low. Hence the probability of compromising the kidneys should also be low.

Mrs. Price reluctantly agreed to the radiation treatment. She could not be convinced that her kidneys would not be affected by the radiation, a skepticism based on experiences of friends who had had radiation for cancer, and her awareness that lupus could also involve the kidneys. Explanations by her husband and other physicians that the radiation for cancer could not be compared to this situation and that there were no alternatives could not resolve her doubts. Her disbelief was also due in part to the fact that the radiology resident, unfamiliar with the patient's complex medical and social history, informed her that her kidneys might be affected by the treatment. Throughout the radiation treatment she wavered back and forth, wondering if agreeing to the radiation was a correct decision.

After the first radiation treatment, she informed her husband that she did not want anymore treatment because of possible damage to the kidneys. Her husband answered that this issue had been discussed many times, that there were no alternatives, and that the radiation dosage was very low. Mrs. Price continued to disagree. Finally her husband responded: "Stop being stubborn. We have to control the ulcers to stop the pain. If you want to commit suicide there are easier ways to do it. If we don't stop the ulcers you can have peritonitis or pancreatitis which are both very painful. There are lots of easier ways to commit suicide and I don't think you're ready for suicide." Mrs. Price agreed she was not ready for suicide. (It must be pointed out here that her husband was well regarded by the hospital staff and known as an extremely gentle and kind man.)

Aside from the doubts about the radiation, Mrs. Price dreaded the treatment because of the physical movement required to get on and off the stretcher and the radiation table, which increased the chest pains. The nursing staff made arrangements with the radiology staff to pace the pain drugs with the treatments in order to minimize her pain.

Just prior to the radiation treatments her sister returned home, which meant that Mrs. Price had fewer distractions which might help her endure the pain. By the twentieth day she was on 75 mg of Demerol every two hours instead of the previous every three hours.

On the twentieth day there was a change in house staff. The researcher informed the new resident of some of the psychosocial problems relevant to the case. He answered that at present he was more concerned with the difficult technical medical problems. Meanwhile the nursing staff informed the new house staff about the extreme uncooperativeness of this patient.

In the ensuing 12 days, her nausea increased and she had several days of diarrhea, all related to the radiation. She would frequently resist the treatment, either because she felt too ill or because she doubted the wisdom of the therapy. Some days she would be persuaded by the staff, but increasingly she resisted. Or she would agree that the treatment was essential in the morning, but change her mind in the afternoon. The staff was becoming increasingly annoyed with the resistance. Finally, in desperation they gave her intravenous tranquilizers just prior to the test to make her very sleepy and less resistant. The resident and the intern took the stand that they could not put up with the patient's constant refusal of treatment—that the patient must either cooperate with the therapy or go home. The hospital was a place for treatment and not a nursing home. The nurses supported this position.

Over the weeks innumerable specialists streamed in and out with no one person coordinating the patient's care. Dr. Osgood, the new resident, argued to the attending physicians that the complexity of this case required some agreement about who should be the major coordinator of care. Since the house staff was more aware of the day-to-day changes, and because the ulcers were the major problem, a decision was reached: the house staff and the gastrointestinal specialist would together be the major coordinators of care, and all new orders issued by the attending staff would be discussed first with the house staff. The nursing staff sighed in relief because at last the "mess" would be under control. However, the coordination continued to break down from time to time. When the patient could not get satisfaction from the house staff she would telephone attending physicians, crying pitifully. One physician in particular would telephone the nursing desk with orders based on his past experiences with the patient. This created much tension within the medical staff.

Blood studies indicated a low hemoglobin count as a result of the ulcers, as well as the lupus, so that blood transfusion was now done. Again hassles occurred between the patient and the house staff about both the timing of treatment and the inflicted pain. (It must be noted that both the resident and intern were very competent and usually related well with Mrs. Price; Mrs. Price trusted them.)

During the period when the radiation treatments were given, the nursing staff was very busy with several other critically ill patients. Also the staff was short because several members, including Fay, were on vacation. At the same time, with the hyperalimentation treatment given to Mrs. Price and the potential of many of her body systems going out of balance, the nursing staff had to engage in many treatment and monitoring tasks. The nurses were interacting more and more with her because of these tasks and when they were giving pain drugs. They were also becoming very weary of the daily hassles over the treatments.

On the twenty-seventh day the patient developed tremors of the hands and legs. Of course, she became very anxious since this was seen as a possible forerunner to convulsions, but because of her great anxiety the staff had difficulty making an assessment of her actual condition. The staff took the stance of "wait and see." The patient thought immediate action was called for. Again she phoned an attending physician who ordered drugs without consulting the house staff. The tremors did subside a few days later.

Because of continued nausea, all drugs were administered by injections, which required some 30 injections a day. The injection sites were becoming fibrous knots so that the drugs were not being properly absorbed. The nurses were very concerned not only about the poor drug absorption but also about the possibility of infections because of the high steroid dose.

On the thirtieth day the patient developed joint pains and swelling of her hands, elbows, feet and knees—all symptoms of lupus. The steroids were adjusted. Fortunately, in a few days the symptoms subsided.

With each new symptom Mrs. Price became increasingly discouraged. From time to time she would tell the researcher that she recognized she had a reputation for being uncooperative. She knew the staff was busy and all departments had their schedules, but: "There's only so much pain I can stand."

Early on the thirty-second day, the last day of the radiation treatments, she was exhausted from her cumulative pain and discomfort—chest pain, abdominal pain, nausea, and joint pains—and begged her husband to delay the treatment until another day. The husband acted according to medical protocol—he consulted the radiologist, asking if this was possible. The radiologist could predict no ill effects if the treatment were postponed. Although instructed to inform the house staff about all this, the radiologist forgot to do so. Hence, when the nurses called the radiation department saying that the patient was premedicated as arranged, they were informed that the treatment had been cancelled at the husband's request. The radiology technicians, of course, did not know the full or correct details. Consequently, the house staff and the nurses became very irritated, interpreting all this as meddling by the husband. The staff members—having had daily hassles about the treatment—complained that if she didn't have the treatment that day they would have to repeat the hassle tomorrow. The decision was made that Mrs. Price was to receive the radiation treatment. Intravenous tranquilizer was given to overcome her resistance to the procedure. Everybody sighed in relief when this last treatment was finally completed!

In chatting soon afterward with the researcher, the husband stated he was trying very hard not to interfere with the therapy. The psychiatrist's advice—that he "act the husband and not the doctor"—was very helpful. However, this was often difficult because his wife constantly confronted him with medical questions.

On the thirty-third day the patient developed burning during urination and began to run a low-grade fever. More tests were ordered. The test results were not definitive, and the symptoms subsided in a few days. In spite of the new symptoms, the patient was in a better frame of mind, if only from the relief of having completed the radiation treatments. She had less nausea and she complained less about pain. Food taken by mouth was now possible.

On the thirty-fifth day a staff conference (which included the psychiatrist, house staff, and nursing staff) was called. The conference was to decide the course of therapy and clarify the situation, so that the new house staff, due the following week, would avoid some of the "coordination" problems. The psychiatrist sketched the psychosocial background of the patient, and the resident responded that he wished he had known about this before. Decisions were reached. Now that the radiation series was completed, and the hyperalimentation treatment had controlled the ni-trogen imbalance (patient had gained 20 pounds), and because she was now taking food by mouth, they would discontinue the hyper-alimentation treatment. They agreed that there was a risk of infection with continued hyperalimentation. Medically, the patient now was fairly stable. They did not think they should try any more "heroics." It was now up to the patient to eat. They would do no more forced feeding. They were optimistic that the radiation would have its anticipated effects. An x-ray would be done within the week to check the effects of the radi-ation. Since the patient was now in a relatively stable medical state, the psychiatrist would be responsible for weaning her from the narcotic drug. There was considerable speculation about the possibility that the patient would try to starve herself. Physiotherapy would be started so the patient would begin to regain strength. Both the psychiatrist and the res-ident would inform the patient about the decisions. The house staff and the nurses agreed that the hospital was an "acute-care treatment cen-ter," a place of treatment and not a convalescent hospital.

In the days just described, while the staff was busy balancing and rebalancing complex medical considerations, the patient was jug-gling quite different sets of considerations—whether to endure the treatment, the wisdom of the treatment, whether the treatment and pains were really worth it all. From day to day and hour to hour she would swing back and forth, sometimes balancing the same items as the staff and sometimes not, and often weighing the same consider-ations differently.

With the appearance of new and cumulative symptoms, the pa-tient became more and more aware that she might die. A few nurses had recognized that she was struggling with this possibility. Fay cited Kubler-Ross's "emotional stages" in facing death, believing it was the anger stage which explained Mrs. Price's resistance and irritability. Mrs. Price herself recognized that her behavior disrupted the staff's work. Despite their mutual recognition of that problem, the patient would fight the staff constantly, driven by the overwhelming load of accumulated discomfort and pain, treatments and tests, and mounting anxiety with accompanying uncertainty. The daily fights over the radiation treatment began to wear down the nursing staff, especially as they had to balance Mrs. Price's demands against the competing demands of other patients. For the staff, the essential concern was to have the radiation treatment done. Hence, if the patient did not cooperate, they would use medication to blunt or break her resistance. The cumulative patient–staff tension reached such a peak that even when Mrs. Price had what seemed a legitimate reason to postpone the radiation treatment the staff would not accommodate her.

The most striking feature of the preceding series of events is the dominance of the entire staff's technical–biological orientation, which precluded genuine consideration of psychosocial factors when balancing. The problems of coordinating care were viewed as primarily medical, yet the psychosocial and interactional problems were major barriers in the medical care. The physicians and the psychiatrist reached a consensus. Now that the patient had attained a relatively stable medical condition, her pain management should be the psychiatrist's responsibility—a perfect example of the kind of separation which often exists between physical and psychosocial aspects of medical management.

The staff was hopeful that the radiation treatment would block the ulcer progression, but this was not to be the case. Here is the continued story:

> The staff took an optimistic stance, anticipating that the patient would be going home. She was placed on oral drugs, except for the pain drugs. The psychiatrist attempted to lower the dosage of the latter but met with little success. Everybody anxiously awaited the results of the stomach x-ray scheduled within a week.
>
> For a few days after the patient began to take food by mouth, she had diarrhea. The staff thought this might be a reaction to the sudden intake of food after three weeks of nothing taken by mouth. In spite of the diarrhea, the patient attempted to eat. Eating was not easy because sometimes the pacing of drugs and tranquilizers was such that she was too sleepy and groggy at the scheduled meal times.

For two days prior to the day the x-ray results were known, she was relatively pain free; that is, she complained less about pain even though the drugs were not delivered on schedule. The staff talked about the patient going home. Meanwhile, the patient was informing the researcher that she didn't think the ulcers were healing because her pain had not decreased.

On the forty-first day the x-rays showed no decrease in the ulcer's size. There was much troubled discussion among the staff. The patient was blamed for her uncooperativeness in taking the antacids and for her chain smoking which had increased the gastric secretions. The patient of course was upset. With great irony she remarked to the researcher: "I knew all along the radiation wouldn't work. All I probably got out of the radiation is kidney damage."

During the next days there was a great deal of discussion about the next course of treatment. A decision was reached that the only alternative was a subtotal or total gastric resection. There were of course surgical risks, and unpleasant consequences from having no stomach, but without intervention there would be the danger of peritonitis or pancreatitis and hemorrhage. The decision was to wait another week or so, at which time a gastoscopy test and an x-ray would be done for reevaluation. The general estimate was that with the surgery the patient might live for several more years. She was informed of the recommendation. The staff realized that her decision to accept surgery would be a difficult one.

For the next three weeks, she agonized over whether or not to have surgery. Her husband was of the opinion that it was the only alternative. The psychiatrist thought the patient, if discharged home, would "drive the husband crazy," and that she would not consent to a nursing home. So surgery, they reasoned, should be done.

Because of the danger of addiction, Mrs. Price's tranquilizers were increased instead of the narcotics. Also, the narcotics had made her groggy, which meant she often fell asleep with a lighted cigarette. Because of a shortage of staff on the night shift, a sitter was hired to watch the patient so she would not burn herself. Mrs. Price told the researcher that she shouldn't smoke, that it aggravated her chronic obstructive lung disease and pleuritis. But she had given up so much in the past year, and had so few pleasures, that she was going to continue to smoke. She didn't have long to live, so what difference did it make?

In the ensuing days there were more confrontations between patient and staff about increasing her drugs. The staff's and husband's explanations that she would become dangerously addicted only infuriated her. "What difference does it make?" she would angrily answer. (It must be pointed out here that Mrs. Price never lost her polite social manners: she would thank staff members for small favors and was polite in making requests. Her husband, however, was often the victim of her frustrations. He told the researcher that Dr. Perle, the psychiatrist, was extremely helpful in helping him cope with his wife's anger.)

The patient increasingly talked to the researcher about the frustrations of living with uncertainty, and her wish that she could die. She said the same things to her husband and the psychiatrist. All three wondered how seriously she wanted to die. Although the psychiatrist and the researcher encouraged the patient to talk about wanting to die, she could not pursue this line of talk beyond a certain point.

The psychiatrist, husband, and researcher were having more and more discussions among themselves about her sad dilemma and how to help her. She did not burden the nurses with her dismal thoughts. The researcher spent more and more time with her and less with the staff. The staff had difficulty in talking about as well as interacting with Mrs. Price.

On the fiftieth day a great qualitative change in the patient's mood was noted. She was very subdued and talked at length about what her illness was doing to her husband and herself and of her ambivalence about dying. She commented: "I wish I could tolerate pain better." Both her husband and the psychiatrist were very pleased that for the first time she could talk openly of her anxieties about dying. When the researcher asked the nurses if they noted any mood change in Mrs. Price, they said "no."

It is worth noting here that during the early days of the hospitalization, when the patient would resist treatments, the nurses would have troubled discussions about the ethics of euthanasia. At one point, having difficulty in persuading the patient to take the gastric suction, one nurse had commented: "I know it's the right of the patient to take or not take treatment. And the patient has the right to make the decision to live or not live. But where is it the patient's and staff's responsibility?" The nurse became very teary. This type of troubled discussion was a frequent occurrence throughout the patient's hospitalization.

On the fifty-fourth day a gastroscopy showed continued acid secretions. For 24 hours following the gastroscopy the Demerol was increased from 75 to 100 mg but was later reduced to 75 mg.

For the next four days the patient wavered back and forth on whether to have the gastric surgery; it was becoming more evident that the surgery was required. Mrs. Price frequently stated that she had been saved from death two times, and she didn't know if she wanted to be saved again. She would take her chances with no surgery, and so hemorrhage and die. She was weary of all the uncertainty. In the past year the lupus remissions had been very short. In periods when she did not have pain she would talk less of wanting to die; in periods of increased pain would talk more about wanting to die. At times she would ask the researcher to chat about "something nice, to get my mind off myself."

Now she was eating less, in part because meal times did not coincide with the pacing of the drugs. The tranquilizers were altered so she would be less sleepy. The staff members were becoming concerned with her continued weight loss. They wondered if she was trying to starve to death. Her eating and not eating alternated, depending upon her nausea, pain, and mood. The intern wrote an order to start the hyperalimentation treatment again, but it was cancelled. This was due in part to the staff's earlier decision that they would not force feed her, and in part to the infection risks; also the husband threatened that if she didn't eat they would start the hyperalimentation. She decided to eat rather than suffer the discomforts and general nuisance associated with the treatment. Because she had difficulty being alert enough to eat, or had pain at the scheduled meal times, she was ordering foods like sandwiches which allowed greater temporal flexibility than hot foods. This meant she was eating at odd hours: 10 P.M. or 2 A.M., for example.

She was talking more about wanting to commit suicide. Often the discussion was wistful and flavored with fantasy. The psychiatrist consulted a suicide expert, who stated that the probability of this patient's seriously considering suicide was low. Still, the staff could not dismiss this possibility. As a precaution, her clothes were taken home and money and drugs were removed from her purse, because she was talking about taking a taxi and jumping off the bridge. The psychiatrist requested that the nursing staff make closer observations and record them. Fay was now back from vacation and was assigned more frequently to Mrs. Price. With the exception of Fay, the observations made of Mrs. Price were quite sparse. Fay spent much time talking to the researcher about her frustrations in managing Mrs. Price. Other nurses did not want to talk about Mrs. Price. For example, during coffee break Fay began a discussion with the researcher about Mrs. Price; the nurses requested that we discuss Mrs. Price elsewhere. They were on a coffee break and wanted some peace.

On the sixty-seventh day the x-rays showed an increase in the size of the ulcers. There was total agreement among the physicians, including the psychiatrist, that a gastrectomy was required and this should occur while the lupus was stable. Two days earlier, the lupus specialist had discussed with Mrs. Price the possibility of trying new drugs to reduce the steroids. Mrs. Price was positive about this possibility.

For the next seven days she agonized over the decision to have a gastrectomy. The surgeons, husband, and psychiatrist tried to answer as best they could any questions she might have. Mrs. Price consulted other attending physicians. They all agreed that a gastrectomy was essential. Her husband was looking tired and haggard. A relative visited in this period and persuaded her that surgery would be the only solution. She finally signed the consent slip for surgery. But, having signed, she wavered until the very last minute. She was transferred to a gastrointestinal surgical unit.

Our account of the hospital episode will stop here. The surgery was successful, and the patient was weaned from the hard drugs, but not without considerable interactional difficulties between staff and patient. Indeed, the surgical-pain trajectory orientation of the staff maximized the interactional difficulties. On the one hundred-twelfth day, she was discharged home.

The medical staff had optimistically anticipated the radiation treatment would block the ulcers, but when this was not the case the patient and the staff were faced with a crucial and agonizing decision. The decision made after the radiation treatments—that nobody would force feed her or try any more heroics—was rebalanced and altered.

Temporally the situation was exceedingly delicate, because the surgery had to be performed at a time when the lupus was relatively stable. If it were not stable, steroids would have to be increased and this would compromise the surgical outcome. Extended waiting and the patient's inability to eat would increase the nitrogen imbalance and also compromise the surgical outcome. Yet, she must be allowed time to weigh and accept the decision about surgery. Surgical intervention required considering all the possible risks, and there was a question whether the surgery should be a subtotal or total gastrectomy. The surgeons and physicians were busy balancing and weighing all the medical considerations. The decision about surgery was related to their making an educated guess about how long she might live. Having estimated that she had several more years, they decided that narcotic addiction should be avoided. After making this decision, the tranquilizers were increased to control pain, which in turn increased grogginess, which in turn both interfered with eating and increased the danger of causing a fire because of the patient's chain smoking.

Meanwhile, Mrs. Price weighed and balanced living against not living. From day to day and hour to hour, she wavered back and forth, rebalancing one way and another—all of which altered her willingness to eat or not eat, or to confront or not confront the staff with requests for increased pain medication. The amount of pain suf-

fered at any given time altered her thoughts about dying or not
dying, and in turn her thoughts about dying altered her threshold for
pain.

Her husband and the psychiatrist were trying to help her make a
difficult decision. This required assessing how she felt about dying—
not an easy task. They estimated she would opt for surgery as in the
past. They leaned heavily toward surgery. In the end, she gave in to
all these pressures. The psychiatrist's comment about Mrs. Price was:
"She's the most difficult patient I've ever had. She's a 'tough' lady,
she'll fight you all the way, but her 'toughness' gives her staying
power. She's gone through some tight situations and has always
come up fighting."

TECHNOLOGY, ORGANIZATION, AND
"THE CUMULATIVE MESS"

The case of Mrs. Price illustrates vividly and dramatically the constant rebalancing of multiple considerations that accompany
cumulative illness trajectories. We have followed a course of illness
which not only moved progressively downhill, but in which everyone became angry, frustrated, and desperate. They become so not
merely because of the worsening illness, but because of complications setting in from the interplay of the disease and the various
technologies utilized. "Coordination of care" went to pieces, periodically being patched together again only to disintegrate once more.
Morale plunged. Personnel, including the various medical consultants, moved in and out of involvement; many eventually withdrew
psychologically and indeed even in terms of giving conscientious patient care. Fears of narcotic addiction were prevalent, and the sense
or senselessness of the risk of addiction was debated by people with
very different moral and medical philosophies. Ethical issues were
raised, fought over, and left unresolved.

Many factors contributed to what the staff, in the case of Mrs.
Price, called a "mess." (Indeed, it was a "cumulative mess.") They
include: the availability of a host of alternative technologies—sometimes experimental—tests, drugs, machines, procedures; technicians
and specialists skilled in those technologies; the possibility of utilizing those technologies with their potential side effects; and the
numbers of personnel streaming in and out of the picture. It was all
very much like a classical Greek tragedy, with everyone caught in a
fateful drama. Sad to say this kind of dilemma is not now unusual. It
occurs repeatedly, without the staffs ever seeming to solve the issues,
including those which pertain to the accompanying pain tasks and

interactions. Part of the difficulty no doubt rests on the problematic features of the chronic illnesses themselves. Another part of the difficulty rests firmly—if invisibly—with the organizational inadequacies of medical and nursing care, a care which is based, as we keep repeating in this book, on a disease-oriented, acute-care perspective. The problems associated with this kind of pain management will simply not be solved without organizational reform.

Part 8

Politics, Pain,
Patient Care, and Ideology

The Necessity for Organizational Reform

18

THE PARADOX OF PAIN MANAGEMENT AND THE ACUTE-CARE MODEL

We hope the foregoing chapters have made concrete and visible the paradox posed in the opening pages of this book. Hospital wards and their personnel are organized to manage the pain of their clients, and though often they manage it well, more often than not they manage it badly. In those cases where the evolving situation becomes increasingly desperate, the fault lies not simply with the ineffectiveness of medical technology but with a failure in the organization of work.

The heart of our paradox is a "trained incapacity" (to borrow Thorstein Veblen's pregnant term). The organization of the ward and its work are so well geared to acute medical care that the personnel as working units are unorganized or disorganized when it comes to the social or psychological aspects of acute care. Further, the ward's organization is astonishingly inadequate to deal with the nonacute (medical or nonmedical) aspects of chronicity. (The chapter devoted to arthritics at home suggests how few medical services are organized to care for the effects of arthritic pain on arthritic sufferers' life styles.)

To say all this is not to deny the interdependence of pain tasks
and straightforward or vital medical tasks. The major issue, however,
is that those relations are not at all timeless; they are embedded in
historical moment and movement. We have not developed a univer-
sal theory in the sense that it pertains to pain management under
any and every condition, at all times—past, present, and future—and
in all places. Details of our theory can vary radically depending on
conditions. Change the organizational settings in which the medical
and pain tasks are embedded, and their relationships will alter correspondingly. We believe that this theory of pain management will not
be invalidated by such changes, but will be strengthened because it
will be systematically qualified. Our primary concern and hope is
that contemporary hospitals and other care settings will change in accordance with a more realistic view of their clients. These clients are
mainly the chronically ill who need treatment and interaction different from, or at least supplementary to, those guided by a disease-
oriented, acute-care imagery, however implicit that imagery may be.

We despair of making effective suggestions for improving the
care of patients in pain unless hospitals begin to reorganize in terms
of nonacute models of thought, action, and organization. To quote
one of the authors from a policy paper on chronic illness:

> The complex character and increasing prevalence of chronic illness
> requires a major reassessment of the traditional manner in which
> illness and its care have been conceptualized. Only in the course
> of such a reassessment can we hope to achieve the organizational
> and policy changes needed to make chronic-illness care effective.
> . . . Reconceptualization and reorganization of care for chronic
> illness must focus on the overall need to solve the patient's prob-
> lems. This requires a reorientation of medical work, or hospital
> organization. . . .[1]

To change that organization and the acute-illness assumptions sustaining it will be quite a task. Although a 180-degree turn may not
be necessary, a change does require some radical additions to and al-
terations in the settings, their organization, their personnel, the
personnel's training, and the work performed there.

The likelihood of quick or radical change is unlikely. Aside from
the political resistance one can expect, deriving from institutional in-
ertia and vested interests, even those who seem to be most desirous
of humanistic change unwittingly manage to adopt most of the acute-
care model. For instance, the death-and-dying movement, for all its
surge and vigor, has focused primarily on changing the individual
practitioners, the patients, and their attitudes (although the movement is moving toward pressuring for more humanistic legislation)

and leaves the physicians virtually untouched and "unrecon-
structed." More important, it does not understand that hospital
organization has to be altered before very much improvement of "living while dying" can be managed. The emphasis now is more on self
and other understanding—on psychology—not on organizational
relevancies.[2-5]

Nevertheless, it is possible to list some trends likely to bring
about substantial changes in the organization of hospitals (and in
other health-care institutions) which will also benefit patients in
pain, whether acute or chronic. These include: the sheer increase in
the numbers of the chronically ill and their growing visibility; the increasing attention to the elderly; the rising public concern with
certain "bioethical" issues (side products of an improved but "out of
hand" medical technology); the death-and-dying movement as it
spreads among laymen; the immense concern of taxpayers and their
legislative representatives with the rising costs of medical care; and
the increasing strength of various consumer movements.

CONDITIONS FOR REORGANIZING CARE

What suggestions can be made for getting some changes in organizational conditions which might help to improve the care of patients in
pain?

Education

One obvious step is to change or at least supplement the education
of the principal personnel in hospitals. Obviously that is not going to
be easy. Though medical education may be far from static, the current trends do not particularly emphasize either a chronic-illness
orientation or even a focus on the social or psychological aspects of
acute care. Although it is the physician who officially runs and often
sets up a ward, he or she is assumed to know how to do that job
without any formal training whatsoever. This century's discoveries in
social and behavioral science and in organizational and administrative theory have scarcely been recognized, much less assimilated.
Given the doctrine of current medical education plus the continued
competition among largely disease-oriented specialties for a place in
the crowded medical curriculum, the practicing physician is likely to
remain innocent of the relevance of organizational or behavioral science literature.

Schools of nursing, and in-service programs in hospitals, are
much more aware of that nonmedical tradition. But there are two
problems that we see. One is that although the nursing profession

has been extraordinarily sensitive to writings about and the practice of interpersonal relations and group therapies, nurses are exposed to very little that would make them think organizationally either about the settings in which they work or about the work itself. The second problem, of course, is that even when they do have an experiential or pragmatically administrative sense of organization, they are not really in command. In the long run, even if and when nurses think more systematically about organization, the radical reorganization of wards still will have to run the gauntlet of physicians who are generally far less trained in the organizational facts of life. Also, insofar as the physicians' power and prestige manage to keep the other para-medical personnel thinking in relatively nonorganizational and nonsocial terms, their training is unlikely to emphasize those aspects of patient care. Perhaps the one exception to this prediction is the so-cial workers, whose professional base is in professional schools away from the medical centers.

In any event, curricula in the medical and nursing schools ought to place significant emphasis on the social and psychological (if not organizational) aspects of pain management. Otherwise an unfortu-nate discrepancy will continue between professionalized technical behavior focusing on medical aspects and what is essentially lay be-havior focusing on the social and psychological aspects. That change is the very least we might desire. In schools of nursing, the change would not be enormously difficult to accomplish, although putting one-to-one clinical nursing (of the patient in pain) into an organiza-tional–interactional framework would be much more difficult, we believe, because very few nursing educators have thought in those terms. As one of the authors once wrote about terminal care: "In short: the educational reform that we advocate goes beyond merely humanizing the curriculum a little more in order to make . . . care a bit more human."[6]

Accountability

Although physicians and nurses may exhibit considerable technical knowledge and skill and much conscientiousness and compassion when handling the pain of patients, their behavior with regard to the psychological and social aspects of the pain is actually outside the province of professional standards. In terms of work, staff members are not required to report to each other (or to their superiors) what has transpired between patients and themselves. They are account-able—that is, responsible—for only the technical aspects of their work.[7]

Of course, a certain amount of information is communicated because the patient is interesting or difficult, or perhaps for reasons
that are quite fortuitous. When what we have termed "mutual biographies" develop between certain patients and the personnel, there is
likely to be a fair amount of communication among the staff, informally or even formally at staff conferences, about the less technical
aspects of the case. (We have seen that happen with each of the case
histories.) For the most part, however, what is reported to the physician by the nurses, what is reported by the nurses or the physicians to the head nurse, and what is written on the charts about the
nonmedical or nonprocedural aspects of pain and the behavior of the
suffering patient, is accidental and fragmented. It is not ordinarily
requisite.

Our research has demonstrated how different the patterning of
events, as they pertain to pain, can be on different types of wards.
We would hazard that everywhere, on similar wards, one would find
similar patterns. Even if we were wrong—if organizational or other
conditions were so considerably different as to modify those patterns
—nevertheless, some patterns would exist and could be detected.
Our research correspondingly implies that insofar as those patterns
represent inadequate handling of *any* aspect of pain (medical, social,
psychological, organizational), that the organization of care needs to
be thought about and pertinent features of it be made explicit. People must be made accountable in new ways. This may mean hiring
new people to be responsible for new tasks.

With regard to pain management, this kind of corrective reform
would clearly be rather radical. It would require that staffs really look
hard at their problematic cases—usually repeated cases with the same
types of problems—and ask tough questions about what so often
goes wrong and why. And then the organization of work must
change correspondingly. Also, as is evident from our discussions of
the burn unit and the routine-surgery wards, even when things don't
seem to go wrong, staffs ought to listen very hard to the implicit
messages given by their patients and answer some of those messages
with explicit accountability.

There is also considerable need for a rational scrutiny of what
happens regarding pain when new technologies are introduced to old
wards, as well as when new types of wards are formed. Each of those
innovations brings about new social and organizational issues relevant to pain management. Ordinarily, of course, the staff is sensi-
tively alert only to medical or technical features.

In addition, all wards need to develop mechanisms for insuring a
wider awareness of degrees of agreement and disagreement about

what is to be done to, for, and around patients in pain. Rarely do the personnel agree entirely about these matters and sometimes they disagree sharply, yet many times they are not even aware of their agreement or disagreement. As our monograph vividly illustrates, consensus and dissent are patterned. Each ward needs mechanisms for discovering its patterned agreements and disagreements—among the staff and between staff and patient—and for mitigating their destructive impact on the care of patients, and on occasion even on the sentimental order of the ward itself.

One last point pertaining to accountability: Since many patients in pain are repeatedly hospitalized or move between hospital and clinic, features of chronic illness need also to be considered in terms not purely medical or even financial. Similarly the connections between home and hospital or clinic, as far as the less strictly medical features of chronic or repeatable pain are concerned, are currently virtually nonexistent. (Again, the arthritic patient illustrates our point, but so do cancer patients.) This last issue moves us into the realm of supraward and extrahospital planning and responsibility, but the virtual lack of organization for those aspects of care only underlines how little of it exists on the far simpler terrain of the ward.

In developing new, accountable actions pertaining to pain, staff members will have to decide among themselves what needs to be added, changed, and destroyed. These issues are divorced neither from questions of power and authority nor from political processes running the gamut from open negotiation to scarcely visible guile to downright conspiracy. As we have remarked so often, there simply is no realistic way of dealing with pain management without coming to terms with political management as well.

In the game of organizational politics, the patients can be expected to gain more power. Of course, it has been evident that in many situations they win particular battles but lose the wars to the hospital personnel. But fortified by Lamaze or Bradley ideologies, mothers and their husbands increasingly take control over management of the pain of childbirth. Increasing numbers of young nurses and physicians on obstetrical wards are themselves touched by the social movements represented by Lamaze and Bradley methods. On pediatric wards, analogous philosophies (personal, cultural, ideological) of childrearing also increasingly influence the staff's command of pain management. New attitudes toward death and dying must certainly have their impact upon what will transpire in hospitals. Perhaps even surgical wards will be affected by movements originating outside of "medicine." It is just possible! Whenever lay beliefs assert themselves in a collective manner—and especially when the

staff members are participants in the movements associated with
those benefits—then changes in what is currently deemed
accountable in hospitals are likely to take place. Those changes will
be visible in altered divisions of labor, new types of work, even in
new items written on the charts. They may also be visible in the disappearance of old items like certain common, stereotypical characterizations of patients in pain.

Suggestions for improving accountability   There are no easy recipes
for improving accountability, in the sense of that term as we have
defined it. After all, each work situation will vary in such features as
its organization, resources available, staff relationships involved,
kind of illnesses, and readiness of the personnel to change in the direction of improved accountability. If the authors were to be called to
a specific ward or work situation and asked to act as consultants,
they would certainly use their organizational-work-interactional perspective, but they would always use it in relation to the specific
features of the locale. They would look at and ask questions about
patterns pertaining to the matters discussed in this book. What are
the predominant illness biographies of the patients? The pain biographies? The medical-organizational biographies? What are the
predominant pain tasks, both of patients and of personnel? What are
the predominant patterns of normal work for the various kinds of
personnel? What are the main features of organizational structure?
The analysis of how to improve accountability then would proceed in
terms of the current matching and mismatching of pain work with
the various items just touched upon in these questions.

Having made that analysis, what advice would be give? What
priorities would be emphasized? Which things would be instituted
or changed first? One cannot possibly answer those questions without knowing the specifics of the situation. What is generally plain
enough, however, is that some changes would be relatively easy
while others would be tremendously difficult to institute and to
maintain. On the burn unit, for instance, adding one or two staff
members skilled in interviewing and counseling would not particularly upset the more medical aspects of patient care or the ward's
work and sentimental order. But every reader can easily imagine the
difficulties of instituting changed accountability on given wards if
greatly increased costs were at issue, or direct challenges by nurses
or social workers to the physicians' general authority.

Without calling in consultants, what steps can the personnel
themselves take to improve accountability in pain interactions and
tasks? There are two suggestions we can make that would lead to

fairly specific steps. The suggestions are based on the fact that most hospital wards have patients who are problematic in their illness or pain trajectories as compared with those considered routine and non-problematic. Each type of patient offers different opportunities for honing in on the critical problem of accountability.

Routine, nonproblematic patients.   Routine, nonproblematic situations might well be an opportune starting point for staff self-examination, because what staff members take for granted as nonproblematic and routine may be very problematic indeed for their patients. Also, the relatively unambiguous and predictable nature of routine illness conditions provides a situation for the personnel to come to agreement about the *what* and the *how*, the *when* and the *who* of pain management. Routine situations differ from highly problematic ones, where the effectiveness or ineffectiveness of staff interventions are difficult to evaluate. The many contingencies and balance problems are here less prominent. More important, improved accountability occurs when the staff knows they can cope with a given problem. Too often the staff focuses on pain only when the patient becomes a "problem pain patient,"—a point at which personnel are confounded and ineffective because patients were not managed well in previous, manageable situations and negative patient reputations have developed with subsequent distrust between patient and staff.

True, part of the problem may be related to nurses' disagreements with physicians, but nurses must recognize that the disagreements may be due to differing pain philosophies, as well as to differing work priorities. It is also true that in the politics of pain management, nurses are in a less powerful position than physicians. This means that nurses cannot effectively negotiate with physicians until they themselves come to an agreement that pain management needs improvement; they must have worked out the what, who, how, and when of pain care within the nursing staff. They can then present a united front.

A crucial starting point is the sharing of personal pain philosophies. As pointed out in previous chapters, many of the pain interactions between patient and staff are based on and confused by the staff's unshared pain philosophies. Pain philosophies involve such questions as: On what basis is tolerance to pain assessed? What kinds of pain are more legitimate than others (organic, psychosomatic)? What information should patients receive about pain and discomforts that they can anticipate during their hospitalization? Who should give this information? How much control should a patient have in managing pain? How important is medical versus comfort care or the various psychological approaches to pain management? At what point should the patient have less pain or endure more pain? When is addiction a problem? These kinds of questions are important because they relate directly to the way nurses assess, minimize, prevent, and relieve pain; how they make judgments about pain expression and endurance. They also pertain directly to the division of labor in handling the patient's pain.

We noted in our interviews with patients that they described the differences in nurses' management of their pain in terms of some imagined personality defect (sadistic, mean, unkind), when in reality the nurses' actions were based on differences in their pain philosophies. Then, too, nurses criticized each other in terms of personality defects, unaware that different pain philosophies existed among them. Discussions about differing philosophies would enable the staff members to utilize the vast literature and research on pain. As Bonica[8] states, there is much written about pain, but little has been applied in clinical practice.

General discussions of pain philosophies, however, will not be productive. These usually end up with people voicing such platitudes as "reassuring the patient is important" or "relieving patient anxiety is important." To learn about the differing philosophies and at the same time to establish organizational accountability calls for utilizing concrete situations on the ward. Preferably, these would be the most common, routine, run-of-the-mill cases on the ward. Areas which might be aired and clarified might include: What kinds of psychosocial information from the patient would be helpful in making a more accurate pain assessment? What kinds of information might be given to the patient about available relief measures and their limitations? What is the patient's responsibility in pain assessment, prevention, relief, and minimization? What are the mutual responsibilities of staff and patient in pain management? What is the physicians, LVN's, aide's, and RN's respective responsibility regarding pain tasks and how is it to be communicated among them? Through their discussions and debates, hopefully, the staff members will identify what they are accountable for and what they must report to each other. In effective pain management, patients' cooperation is gained through giving them explicit information and cues. Because of the usual lack of explicitness, patients are at loss as to how to behave. An additional point: The vast variety of comfort measures for minimizing pain—often volunteered according to the staff's personal philosophies or individual inclinations—must be made accountable.

Since patients are an important resource for improving accountability, interviews with them are essential to discover how they feel their pain is being managed. A patient feedback system would be useful for discovering areas of pain management which require attention, for evaluating nursing effectiveness, and also for improving the general care of patients.

Staff members might be anxious about the increased demands on them as a result of improved pain care. For example, nurses might anticipate spending more time with the patient—time they cannot spare. But our interviews with patients indicate that it is not the amount of time spent with the patients, but *how* the personnel interact with them that mostly needs change.[9] Also, the interviews indicate clearly that a few well-phrased statements can effectively communicate pain-task information from staff to patient. In all the clinical units we observed, there were some nurses who were very effective in managing pain. Hence, it would be well to discover what they do and say to achieve such success.

Furthermore, since pain work is part of the ongoing work, the members of each work shift need to examine how their other work might interfere with pain work and figure out what kinds of work readjustments might be required. Staff might also explore how pain tasks might be incorporated into other work. For example, during the induction process into the hospital, patients should automatically be interviewed about their pain. In most hospitals an admission interview is required; in fact, most have a special interview form. Observations of patient–staff interactions and examination of charts reveal that pain information is very sparse, even when patients are hospitalized specifically for pain relief. Perhaps other work takes precedence, or the staff needs assistance in interviewing skills.

In concluding this discussion of routine, nonproblematic situations, it is important to add that improving accountability also requires clarifying the physicians' responsibilities, so a dialogue involving them is absolutely necessary. The traditional physician–nurse relationship characterized by differential status may be a barrier to this dialogue, but accountability cannot be effectively accomplished without dialogue. Hopefully, physicians might even learn to initiate it.

New relationships must be established—however difficult the task—with the personnel on other services with whom patients have contact. Some services (x-ray, physical rehabilitation) receive and then send back the patients; others send personnel to the bedside (medical technicians) to do procedures. In either case, as we know, the care of patients in pain can be much affected. So these personnel and those services need to be brought into the circle of improved accountability for pain interactions. Again, the staff on a given unit

ought to analyze the standard, routine patterns of contact between
their patients and "outside" personnel; it is with those specific personnel and their departments that persuasion and negotiation should
be employed. Otherwise energy is simply scattered without focus
and with little likelihood of improved conditions for the patients.
Those outside departments ought also to think through their own
patterns of work with patients in pain and build that understanding
into departmental accountability. The personnel of some departments, like physical rehabilitation, are quite clearly aware of the
problem of pain; others, like x-ray, tend to be so focused on their
main tasks that pain hardly enters their consciousness unless a patient complains.

Problematic patients.   Each ward has its share of nonroutine, problematic patients. In addition to building organizational accountability
for the routine pain cases, the staff must also be prepared to cope
with its problematic ones. As discussed throughout this book, most
hospitalized patients today have chronic disorders. Thus, explicit efforts must be made to determine each patient's multiple biographies
(illness, pain, hospital, and social) and to predict how they might
affect pain during hospitalization. This means that the staff members
need much help in improving or acquiring interviewing skills.[10, 11]
Learning how to interview competently is essential. Also, many patients must be allowed greater participation in the decisions, both
about their general care and their pain management, because of their
own experiential knowledge. This change will require a new orientation and novel patient–staff interactions. It is hoped that the
message throughout this book—that pain, illness, hospital, and social
biographies are intertwined—will help that new awareness to evolve.
    Questions which might be raised during interviews with a pa-
tient are: How long has pain been a problem? What was done about
pain relief? Has he had problems legitimating his pain? In previous
hospitalizations what kinds of problems did he encounter? What
kinds of medications did he take at home? How effective were they?
Does he have routines at home to alleviate pain which might be
helpful now during hospitalization? How does he think he tolerates
pain? What are the usual ways in which he expresses pain? The
reader can obviously come up with many more questions. The next
step is to institutionalize such interviews.
    When wards consistently have certain types of problem patients,
efforts must be made to resolve the standard problems. Staff's discussions might include airing ideologies about these patients and
their pains, focusing on the social, illness, hospital, and pain biog-

raphies relative to the pain problem, and identifying aspects of pain work (assessing, enduring, expressing, legitimating) which are creating difficulties for the patient or the staff. For some of this, appropriate consultation may be required because anger, irritation, and frustration may be high enough to prevent clarifying or convincing discussion.

One warning, however, about calling upon consultants: there is a tendency to request help from the liaison psychiatrist, either with the problematic patient or with the general situation itself. Well-trained and insightful psychiatrists certainly can be of aid, but sometimes they are not. The primary reason is that they are too focused upon the psychiatric aspects of the situation and not nearly enough upon what has gone wrong because of organizational failure. (Certainly there are very emotionally disturbed patients who pose pain-management problems, but the intrapsychic emphasis tends to prevent or minimize organizational accountability.) With their particular training and practice, psychiatrists are not always prepared to understand the ward and its work. To be maximally useful in improving accountability, the psychiatrists will need both more training in understanding organizations and more time spent on the hospital floors.

Nursing staff especially must be alert to the "snowballing effect" of the problem patient. Anyone who is the "pain patient of the day" can easily become the pain patient of the week or month unless an organized way for coping with his type has evolved. Currently when someone becomes the "patient of the week," the probability is high that nothing will stop the downward spiral of interaction around him. Explicit approaches must, therefore, be built into ward organization to handle this type of situation. When the patient is still the pain patient of the *day*, staff discussions must occur, more information should be gathered about the patient, talks with the family should be instituted, staff reactions should be examined, and so on.

Every ward has its pain patient of the week or month. Usually the staff members discharge these patients with a sigh of relief, hoping that another will not soon be thrust upon them. Yet the likelihood of a repetition is always present. A direct and analytic focus on these patients would be a useful tool to improve care rather than ignoring the problem, feeling angry and guilty, and allowing it to occur again. Indeed, in our research the problem patients were especially useful for discovering where health personnel differed in their pain ideologies, as well as the difficulties faced by both patient and staff along with the organizational hitches in pain management. Problem patients exaggerated the organizational shortcomings which were not apparent in ordinary, routine illness conditions. Likewise, a discussion of the series of problematic events might assist staff members in discovering where in the vicious cycle specific intervention might have stopped the downward spiraling, and what kinds of resources might have been required—and *will* again be required! These discussions should help identify the areas for needed in-service training, the organizational shortcomings, and the new kinds of institutional arrangements which will be required to cope with problematic patients. Presumably these changes will also improve the care not only of routine pain patients but also of patients in general.

We say "will" because it is our observation that each ward repeatedly encounters the same types of problem patients. To coin a phrase upon which we shall elaborate in the next chapter, the ward generates its own *organizational failures*. These repeated failures should raise basic organizational issues: How should we change our work and work patterns? How should we break our stereotypical conceptions of these patients? Are we using the wrong technology to handle this patient's pain even if, on the face of it, it should be effective? Need we add to the resources available to our ward, or perhaps change them around and/or use them differently? In what other major ways need we change the organization of this ward to reduce the probability of making these patients into problems for us and themselves?

In short, an *equation: repeated organizational failure equals repeated organizational patterns;* therefore, the necessity for *fundamental organizational changes.* Presumably, the changes would also improve the care of routine pain patients and of patients in general.

PAIN MANAGEMENT AND CLINICAL PRACTICE: FAITH OR SCIENCE?

In the preface, with seeming rashness, we remarked that without attention to organizational contexts one can never know for certain "why a given approach or procedure [for pain management] does or does not work except on faith, believing it's for purely pharmacological, physiological, or clinical reasons." That assertion should not appear so outlandish if one considers the following. When, for instance, the pharmaceutical company representatives visit the physician and offer literature, or explain the actual effects of drug usage under laboratory conditions, the physician inevitably thinks and often says: "Well, let's see how it works under clinical conditions. The lab's one thing and my experience is another." It is not merely that the physician mistrusts laboratory research; rather, he or she is in-

sisting that under the specific conditions of practice and with
particular kinds of patients, too many nonlaboratory, uncontrollable
variables are at play. Clinical research, of course, attempts to specify
some of those variables.

Now introduce the drug into a hospital setting. The staff will not
trust it either until they have had a trial period, using it under a variety of clinical conditions. Once the usage becomes routine, they
will tend to account for departures from expected results by blaming
either "drug error" or the patient's psychology, or perhaps they will
seek a clinical reason (the patient's unusual weight or unusual tolerance of the drug). When the drug is an experimental or newly
introduced one, then everyone tends to be alert to effects which have
departed from those reported in the literature, and since these drugs
are often used with medically difficult cases, unexpected departures
are accounted for physiologically, pharmacologically, clinically, and
sometimes psychologically.

They are never—or almost never—accounted for by reference to
organizational variables. Yet we have seen on almost every page of
this book that medication is not just ordered and given; it is given
by a variety of agents, under a variety of interactional conditions
(some of them very complex), and the medication effects whatever
results are ascribed to it in a situation influenced by attending physicians, house physicians, nurses, aides, social workers, family, and
of course other patients. When the patient interacts with himself, the
staff thinks in terms of his "psychology." If the situation is defined
as warranting help, the consulting psychiatrist is called. When the
uncontrolled variables are organizational in nature, no one calls
anybody.

There is need, in short, for clinical research that *would* take organizational variables into account. As social researchers, we lack the
competence to do those studies. But they should be done. Otherwise,
to make another rash assertion, the clinical use of pain medication
(any medication) and other pain therapies will continue to be merely
experiential, pragmatic, and however useful in specific instances, ultimately a set of hit-and-miss techniques.

TWO IMPORTANT ISSUES: COSTS AND
DEHUMANIZATION OF CARE

Costs

In these last pages we shall briefly address two important and related
issues to which our findings are relevant. The first is the rising cost

of health care, a justified concern in all industrialized countries today. "The costs of health care continue to rise more than most other
costs, and more of the increase is due to rising prices without improvements in the quality or quantity of services or increases in the
number of people cared for."[12] Philip Lee, whom we have just
quoted, suggests several possible means of cost control:

1. Control of prices (i.e., charges for services).
2. Deductibles and copayments (requiring individual beneficiaries
    to share the costs at the time services are rendered).
3. Incentive reimbursement schemes, to stimulate payers and pay-
    ees to find ways of curtailing costs.
4. Limitation of services provided.
5. Control of the availability of health-care resources (e.g., hospital
    beds, physicians).
6. Global budget for the entire program and special budgets for the
    various components.[12]

   In that list of possible ways to control costs, there is no direct
reference to the operations of the health facilities themselves. Aside
from the fairly obvious issue of maximizing operational efficiency, in
the usual administrative sense of that term, our book raises other
questions about possible monetary savings through the kinds of organizational changes suggested. It is doubtless true that those
changes sometimes may require additional funds for training or personnel, but they should also help to cut costs, perhaps in a startling
manner. We cannot support that assertion with quantitative data,
since our consideration of costs is very much an afterthought, a question addressed only subsequent to the issue of accountability.
Nevertheless, we believe it is worthwhile to outline, in admittedly
somewhat speculative and qualitative terms, what our findings on
pain interactions suggest about hidden costs. We shall organize our
discussion around several topics, notably: length of hospitalization;
drugs, tests, and procedures; addiction; manpower; impact on work;
impact on sentimental order; costs to the family.
   The costs of *extended hospitalization* are among those which cause
the total costs of health care to skyrocket. What can we say, or at
least speculate, about savings that might have accrued if the hospitalization could be shortened by more organizationally sensitive
and sensible handling of those ward-wracking problem patients in
pain? When we addressed that question to Mrs. Price, the lupus patient who was hospitalized for over three months, we decided that if
her vicious downward spiral had been broken early she might, at

most, have remained in the hospital for only eight weeks. Then think about Mrs. Abel who remained in the hospital for about two months (disregarding the two additional months when she became a research patient) because the physician's conscience bothered him. We estimate that her stay could have been cut in half, to about one month. We estimate on the conservative side. If the respective staffs had been able to avoid the rapidly evolving cycle of mutual aversion and avoidance or just plain interactional difficulty, then both the pain and medical problems could have been handled much more speedily and efficiently.

What about the excess costs of *drugs and tests*, given problematic patients like Mrs. Abel, Mrs. Price, and Mrs. Noble? And what about the costs of *addiction*, since patients such as these tend to become addicted to narcotics. While it is difficult to estimate after the fact what proportion of painkillers and other drugs like sedatives, mood elevators, and tranquilizers might have been dispensed with earlier if the drastic trajectories of these patients could have been corrected, it is clear that a considerable reduction in medication could have been effected—perhaps as much as 30 to 50 percent. (In the instance of Mrs. Price, not only would she have been on less medication while she was hospitalized but also she would have been on less if she had been able to return home for a time between necessary hospitalizations.) As we have seen, when these problematic patients begin to complain about increasing pain, they are eventually given increasing amounts of painkillers and related medication, or given it at shorter intervals. They also are likely to receive more expensive medications, like narcotics or experimental drugs. Also, more than likely, they are subjected to tests and therapies in excess of what is standard, since there may be need to counter side effects deriving from the various painkillers, sedatives, and tranquilizers.

An additional important consideration in estimating the financial costs of medications and tests is this: As the patient enters into a very difficult or highly problematic trajectory (composed of both medical and interactional elements), there tends to appear a "rippling effect"—a spreading series of circles of impact, including impact on the use of medications and therapies. Interactional difficulties feed into the patient's symptomatology and tolerance for pain; both are then handled by medications and sometimes additional tests, which in turn may, and probably will, have symptomatic side effects as well as create additional interactional difficulties between staff and patient, which then have to be handled by more medication and tests.

It is understandable why addiction frequently accompanies these extended hospitalizations with downward problematic trajectories.

Addiction, of course, is of great concern to patients and staff members alike, and both attempt to avoid it as well as to shake loose from it when it occurs. To the direct costs of the narcotic drugs one must add the costs not only of those additional measures needed to counteract the side effects of the narcotics but also of the extra days or weeks of hospitalization needed to effect the weaning from narcotics. Mrs. Noble, for example, remained an extra two weeks so that weaning could be accomplished.

In general, battles over drugs and additional tests result in much psychological wear and tear on all parties. The psychological costs for individuals are certainly considerable, and of course there is also much disruption of ward work and of the ward's sentimental order. We shall touch on those "costs" next.

What about the hidden costs of excess *manpower*—hours of "work" which need not have been expended on the care of a problematic patient? It is possible to make some qualitatively based estimates. We have in mind the following types of expenditures of time and energy that might have been saved for the patients described in our case histories.

Mrs. Price was visited approximately 50 times by a psychiatrist who stayed 30 to 50 minutes each visit. Most visits were because of her continual problematic status—problematic to the staff, herself, and her husband. In addition, the psychiatrist spent many hours consulting with the staff members, explaining the patient to them and counseling them on their own reactions. Also, we should count the many hours the staff spent in discussing this case—where "discussing" stands for many verbs: arguing about and attributing her motives; analyzing and interpreting her behavior; planning new and reviewing failed courses of action; and so on. Some discussion took place in team conferences and staff meetings, but much occurred in the corridors and at the nursing station. A fair amount of time went into nurses' attempts to reach the house staff and the attending physicians, as well as in telephone conversations with them at all hours of the day. Also, the patient's chart became filled with written commentary far in excess of that ordinarily called for by a nonproblematic patient. Finally, it is probable that some of the physicians called upon as consultants, and some of their visits, were a consequence not simply of Mrs. Price's medical difficulties but of the staff's total reaction to the larger context or "gestalt" of the case.

It ought to be quite clear that each problematic patient has a considerable impact on the ward's *organization of work*—what we have termed the work order. A problematic patient, especially one with a drastically worsening cycle of interaction with the staff, uses up a re-

markable amount of time, attention, and energy. Such a patient is
always in strenuous competition with other patients. The problematic
patient may not know this, especially if the staff pulls back and
avoids her room, but as long as they are talking about her, debating
about her, or planning what to do about her, to that extent they are
spending less time and energy thinking about or working with other
patients. Not only patient competition, however, is involved, but
also a general skewing of the ward's work order. Adaptations have to
be made. The ward's schedule must accommodate consultants' visits
and also the patient's visits to those other departments where she is
given extra tests, and so on. This skewing is especially obvious to
the personnel when they feel overworked or overwrought. Of course
when there are two problem patients simultaneously on the ward,
then. . . .!

   Sentimental order is also profoundly affected. "A disruption of the
ward's organization of work is paralleled by a shattering of its characteristic 'sentimental order'—the intangible but very real patterning
of mood and sentiment that characteristically exists on each ward."[13]
The monetary costs of that disturbance of sentimental order—let
alone the costs of disturbed personal identity—must be considerable.
We did not attempt to measure those costs in quantifiable terms, but
it would be possible to do so if one designed a study specifically for
that purpose. Quantification aside, clearly the negative impact of a
problematic patient on sentimental order and staff morale is profound. And surely not only is patient care affected but so are the
monetary costs of running the ward's enterprise.

   Costs to *the family* are also considerable. Here we can easily imagine that, aside from unnecessarily lengthy hospitalization, the costs
pertain to additional in-hospital drugs and consultation visits; also
the extra trips to the hospital and time taken off from work. The extra
"psychological costs" must sometimes be frightful (remember Mrs.
Price's husband).

   The areas where heightened costs appear (extended hospitalization, drugs, additional manpower, sentimental order) should not
be regarded as separate. Rather they are intertwined. It is only an ar-
tifact of an analytic perspective that allows one to speak of them
sequentially rather than simultaneously. It is really all just "one big
ball of wax." Speak of one area, and all the others are implicated.
When the costs in one area rise, the others also are likely to rise. As
mentioned apropos of drugs and tests, those increases are likely to
proceed by virtually geometric progression when the vicious interactional cycle spirals further downward. The only way to avoid the
costs is to avoid the vicious cycle itself. How are hospital staffs to do
that except by instituting and sustaining organizational changes?

Dehumanization of Care

Dehumanization is a term used by both laypeople and health professionals when they criticize certain failures in health care. Criticism tends to emphasize one or more of four themes: the impact of strict professionalism; the impact of modern technology; the increasing size of health facilities; and the economic and social inequities in American life.[14-16] In conjunction with such themes, we believe two other conditions underlie this increasingly insistent critique. One is the major point emphasized throughout this book that *medical* ideology shapes medical facilities, training, and care. Care appears to be or is actually dehumanized because it is perceived and carried out according to that ideology. The psychological and social (the more human) aspects of care are slighted or neglected. We have insisted that an argument made merely to gain additional attention for those human aspects is unlikely to have much impact on either health care or the health facilities.

A second point pertains to "the implications of illnesses that cannot, on the whole, be cured but only 'managed' and that, in any event, must be lived with."[17]

> *One set of implications certainly pertains to how our facilities need to be reorganized to take into account the illness-health-care-social (and pain) biographies that precede, accompany, and persist beyond visits to the facilities. We must understand that organizational restructuring is necessary not merely for humanitarian or humanistic reasons, but quite literally to keep some people alive and certainly to give them better medical and nursing care.*

As for monetary costs: "Such care would be cheaper in the long run, keeping more chronically ill persons away from more facilities for more time. . . ."

In short, we believe that the cries about increased dehumanization and increased costs of care reflect twin problems. Neither can be understood without understanding: (1) the institutional crisis brought about by the disproportionate percentage today of chronic as opposed to acute illness, and (2) health care, health education, and health facilities which are organized according to an essentially acute-care ideology. Hence the paradox that modern medicine is both progressive and retrogressive, breathlessly improving and yet in its organization of care more than a little antiquated. In assessing the situation thus, it is not at all our intention to assign blame (nowhere in this book have we done that). To allow this paradoxical situation to continue *would,* in the most general sense, be very blamable.

REFERENCES

1. Gerson, E., and Strauss, A. 1975. Time for living: problems in chronic illness care. *Social Policy* 6:12–18.

2. Feifel, H. 1959. *The meaning of death*. New York: McGraw-Hill.

3. Fulton, R. 1965. *Death and identity*. New York: Wiley.

4. Kastenbaum, R., and Aisenberg, R. 1972. The psychology of death. New York: Springer.

5. Weisman, A. 1972. *On dying and denying*. New York: Behavior Publishers.

6. Glaser, B., and Strauss, A. 1968. *Time for dying*. Chicago: Aldine.

7. Strauss, A; Glaser, B.; and Quint, J. 1964. The non-accountability of terminal care. *Hospitals* 38:73.

8. Bonica, J. 1974. General clinical considerations. In *Recent advances in pain*, eds. J. John et al. Springfield, Ill.: Charles C Thomas, p. 274.

9. Copp, L. A. 1974. The spectrum of suffering. *American Journal of Nursing* 74:491–495.

10. McCafferty, M. 1972. *Nursing management of patients in pain*. Philadelphia: J. B. Lippincott, pp. 11–66.

11. Strauss, A. 1975. *Chronic illness and the quality of life*. St. Louis: C. V. Mosby, pp. 139–141.

12. Lee, P. 1975. Epilogue. In *Humanizing health care*, eds. J. Howard and A. Strauss. New York: Wiley, p. 312.

13. Glaser and Strauss, op. cit., *Time for dying*, p. 14.

14. Freidson, E. 1967. Review essay: health factories, the new industrial sociology. *Social Problems* 14:493–500.

15. Mechanic, D. 1967. Human problems and organization of health care. *Annals Academy of Political and Social Science* 399:1–11.

16. Howard, J. 1975. Humanization and dehumanization of health care. In *Humanizing health care*, eds. J. Howard and A. Strauss. New York: Wiley, pp. 57–102.

17. Strauss, A. 1975. A sociologist's perspective. In *Humanizing health care*, eds. J. Howard and A. Strauss. New York: Wiley, pp. 277–284.

Social Worlds, Ideologies, Organizations, and Work

19

In the preface and in Chapter 1, we asserted that hospitals and the activities of the people who work in them are organized in terms of a most pervasive disease and acute-care-oriented ideology which is dominant throughout the Western world. We will now raise some implied questions about the relationships among organizations, the social worlds in which they are embedded, their work, servicing agents, clients, and above all the ideologies held by their dominant members as well as by their clients. Our intent in the following pages is, then, to address more general issues by taking cues from the specific medical context documented in this book.

The concept of social world seems applicable to "the world of (Western) medicine." While the concept of social world is, of course, commonly used in everyday discourse, it has scarcely been examined or discussed technically. We shall not do that extensively here, either, except to follow two analytic discussions in the sociological literature. One is by Tomatsu Shibutani, who some years ago in pointing to worlds like those of drama, opera, and medicine, remarked that each social world is "a universe of regularized mutual response," an "arena in which there is a kind of organization," and a "culture area" whose boundaries are "set neither by territory nor formal membership but by the limits of effective communication."[1] Shibutani was essentially emphasizing the existence of networks characteristic of modern mass societies, and of participants linked through "channels of communication"—mainly particular types of media and language—into something apparently intangible yet very real. Such links have been recently described by sociologists of science, who have looked closely at various loosely knit networks of scientists, scattered internationally, who have worked collectively to develop new scientific areas.[2, 3]

Anselm Strauss has commented further on certain characteristics of social worlds.

> In each social world, at least one primary activity (along with related clusters of activity) is strikingly evident: climbing mountains, researching, collecting. There are sites where activities occur: hence space and a shaped landscape are relevant. Technology is always involved—inherited or innovative modes of carrying out the worldly activities. Most worlds evolve quite complex technologies. In social worlds . . . organization inevitably evolves to further one aspect or another of the world's activities. . . .

> Two other major processual features seem inevitable and immensely consequential. First, the intersection of social worlds. They intersect under a variety of conditions: where services are needed, technology is borrowed . . . where alliances are deemed useful, where other worlds impinge—as when worldly action is questioned as harmful or illegitimate or inappropriate for certain times and places. . . . Another important process is the segmenting of social worlds. Most seem to dissolve, when scrutinized, into a congeries of subworlds . . . their activities result in a neverending segmenting.[4]

It does not seem amiss to refer to the "world of medicine" (along with its subworlds—the various medical specialties). It has its characteristic activities, technologies, organizational forms, sites, and language. And, in Shibutani's terms, membership in that world or those subworlds is not in accordance with formal membership nor territory, but "by the limits of effective communication" and "shared perspectives." As we and others[5, 6] have noted, scientific medicine established itself in Europe and elsewhere, including the United States, during the years just before and after the turn of the century. The reform movements which led to modern medicine (or just plain medicine—as if there were no rivals) were rooted in a disease-oriented perspective, diseases which were predominantly acute (communicable and parasitic) in nature. This perspective exists, we would maintain, as a pervasive ideology within the extensive world of medicine, which means it exists as a predominantly taken-for-granted imagery, model, or set of assumptions. Even though attacked sometimes by outsiders to this world, and sometimes in part by insiders, certainly most health practitioners do not recognize themselves as "ideology bearers."[7-9] Even those who would amend the acute-care model (for instance, some psychiatrists, social workers, psychiatrically oriented nurses, and medical sociologists),[10] tend like most reformers to accept the basic philosophy but wish to expand it to make it less biological and more psychological or social. This ideology is so pervasive that many outsiders to the medical world have accepted most of it; if there is radical disagreement with it, that certainly is rooted in people who are either complete outsiders to the world of medicine or at least more marginal to it than the health practitioners.

As clients (patients), laypersons may resist the implications of this ideology without always knowing that they are resisting. When fortified with explicit ideologies of their own, they are much more likely to define the dominant medical one not merely as somewhat dehumanizing but as downright wrong or perverse, even when they are forced to deal with the medical institutions where necessary work is done. Such clients are representatives of other worlds as they intersect with that of medicine. (If conflicts become violent enough, the medical world is affected by legislation or malpractice suits won in accordance with legislation not advocated by the medical world.)

What we are saying is that organizations are often embedded in social worlds (hospitals in the medical world, universities in the academic world, museums in the art world). As such, they can be understood neither apart from those worlds nor apart from the ideologies which are dominant in those worlds. There is, of course, no one single ideology in each of those worlds—indeed each is likely to have one or more important ideologies—but certainly a single ideology or a very few ideologies may deeply affect the operations of given organizations.[10] When reform movements with their own specific ideologies sweep these worlds resulting in changes in extant organizations or the founding of new reform-based ones, those movements are still likely to retain major elements of the same prevailing ideology as unexamined assumptions. Furthermore, co-option is often probable because the more established organizations are also likely to have a great deal of power in the way of resources—financial, political, legal, organizational, psychological, and from alliances forged with other powerful or influential worlds which in-

tersect them. (That is why even though advocates of community
medicine, or of ethnic-controlled medical centers, made some reform
headway in the 1960s, they were relatively open to co-option by the
main medical establishment.)

Let us return to the medical scene in order to emphasize another
aspect of the relationship between ideology and organization. Patients, as we have seen, are a part of the hospital's division of labor;
their cooperation and their proper activity are needed to get the work
done. (Perhaps it is easier to see them as part of the work force because they are physically inside a hospital, as are students in a
university, rather than external to an organization as are most clients
or customers.)[11] Although the work gets done, it is complicated by
innumerable contests for control between patients and staff members.
Part of that conflict certainly stems from the way personnel organize
their work in accordance with their unexamined assumptions about
acute care. Also, patients who don't behave in accordance with judgments based on the assumptions are regarded as difficult and are
likely to be labelled uncooperative. They are regarded not only as
getting in the way of work, or as making more work, but also as
causing some work to fail.

Subunits (wards) each have a kind of organizational shape[12]
which can accommodate only certain kinds of patients and behaviors.
When a patient does not fit, he is pressured to conform, is shipped
to another ward with organizational properties better able to handle
him, or is sent home if the hospital seems completely unable to deal
with him. In such situations the organization and the patient are
mismatched principally because the former is unwittingly organized
in accordance with acute-care assumptions for too narrow a range of
client. In short, the organization produces—in patterned ways—its
own misfits.

Hospitals also seem to produce certain kinds of work failures
precisely because they are organized in accordance with an unstated
ideology. Some failures are obvious to everybody (not, however, the
reasons for these failures), if only because the staff members feel so
frustrated or helpless in their work with a patient (who is usually
quite complaining or furious about their work with him). Other failures are, quite literally, not perceived by the staff. This is partly
because the patient does not complain, accepting in silence what
both he and they would consider a failure or an error. Or the staff
may simply not define certain tasks as part of their work, so they do
not see what they are failing to do. For instance, the burn unit personnel didn't comprehend the patients' anxieties about their future
social biographies or even the part those anxieties might play in enhancing their current pains. All three case histories presented in this

book illustrate major failures produced, at least in part, by the personnel's inability—an inability produced by adherence to medical ideology—to perceive certain tasks as necessary in order to achieve central goals. In a genuine sense, these are patterned failures, manufactured by the organization itself. The hospital careers of Mrs. Abel, Mrs. Noble, and Mrs. Price did not need to take the forms they did, nor did their corresponding illnesses and pain trajectories.

Health practitioners can rarely perceive the social organizational bases for failure precisely because the ideology prevalent throughout the medical world defines reality in nonorganizational terms. Failures are seen in predominantly individualistic (or at most in "team" or "group") modes: incompetence; inadequate skill; poor judgment; fortuitous conditions like fatigue, haste, headaches; or inadequate resources, like drugs, machinery, or other technology, or requisite knowledge. Success at caring or curing is attributed to social organization, but in general neither the patterns of failure nor the organizational bases for those patterns are perceived.

In the past, hospitals were primarily organized for servicing patients with acute diseases (communicable and parasitic), whereas today the clients are predominantly in the acute phase of chronic illness. Nevertheless, the work organization is deeply affected by acute-disease conceptions, and this results in servicing many patients in inappropriate ways.

What are the further implications of this for the student of organizations? The general answer is that organizations ought to be scrutinized for the prevailing ideology or ideologies which profoundly affect the goals of its members, the means chosen to attain the goals, and the general articulation of activities within the overall structure of an organization. Many errors, mistakes, and indeed the failures which characteristically occur can be traced to the operationalization of ideology by the structuring of the organization and the work of its members. Cues to those structured failures are given, our examples tell us, by the complaints of the clients (and the staff about the clients) as well as by the conflicts between them, where each is likely to characterize the other as negligent, incompetent, uncooperative, and/or inconsiderate. Insofar as the ideologies are unexamined and taken for granted, the actors will not be aware of the source of their characterizations, complaints, and conflicts.

An additional point bears on the contests over controlling conditions of work. In most of the relevant literature,[13, 14] those contests are conceived of in terms of such employee–employer stakes as wages, hours, levels of performance, amount of work, and fringe benefits which may be both formally and informally contracted for (the right to have a radio playing while working).[15] Ideological con-

siderations, however, may also enter; for instance, young people who
are part of the counter culture may fight to wear beards or alternative
styles of clothing on the job. On the hospital wards we have seen
ideological considerations enter, sometimes as major elements, into
what interactants, including the patients, consider important features
of their work situation. In the most general sense, when a patient
wishes the work done in one way but the staff wishes it done in another, then the staff's medical ideology shapes the debate over the
conditions of work. If we view the client not simply as someone external to the organization or the servicing groups, but as a special
kind of coworker, then important ideological dimensions are added
to the general question: What kinds of relationships exist between
clients and helpers?

Berenice Fisher has suggested several possible responses by the
servicing agent's group when clients react negatively (rejecting, complaining, criticizing) to the agent's attempt to be of help.[16] First, the
servicing group may alter its ideology and claim. Second, it may attempt to change the reactions of the clients. Third, it may change the
makeup of its clientele. Fourth, it may alter its own structure to effect
better their original claim. Applying this scheme to American physicians and their assisting personnel, what do we see?

1. Our data reflect that the first option—to alter the basic ideology
   and claim—is actually pretty much rejected. (We shall discuss
   this point later.)

2. Attempts to change the reactions of complaining or rejecting clientele do not seem a prominent current strategy of the health
   practitioners. If anything, they appear to be somewhat on the
   defensive about such issues as impersonality and the high costs
   of medical and nursing care.

3. Changing clientele to reduce the numbers of critics has
   doubtless been a strategy for particular practitioners or medical facilities. The health practitioner professionals and nonprofessionals have, if anything, enlarged their clientele in recent
   years to ethnic and other groups who are likely to be, or at least
   feel, critical of many standard practices.

4. It is the fourth option—altering some of the structure of the servicing groups in order to affect the original claim (i.e., to
   promote health, conquer disease, block further illness, manage
   symptoms)—which seems the major strategy used by health
   practitioners in the world of Western medicine. Let us see why
   this might be both the preferred strategy and the most general
   reaction of the practitioners.

Potential outcomes of interaction are shrouded in a kind of ambiguity if one views the hospital both as an organization structured by the dominant ideology of the social world in which it is embedded and as an arena where ideology bearers interact during the course of their work. By ambiguity we mean several things. The prevailing ideology can be fortified by the experiences of angry and frustrated personnel who must deal with deviant clients. That seems the most likely and usual outcome. Some personnel, however, can be partly swayed by the complaints, accusations, and arguments of clients; in the face of the most articulate, ideological arguments, they can begin to doubt at least portions of received medical practice. (Fisher suggests several ways of altering the basic ideology and claim, but we can adapt her list to changing the structure of helping. Her list includes changing scale, scope, time schedule, location, and technique.[17] It is the last three which medical facilities have principally adopted—adjusting schedules more to clients' convenience, for instance, or building neighborhood clinics—but mainly the fights both with laypersons and among practitioners have taken place over modifying techniques to suit ethnic populations, children, geriatric clients, and the like.)

Since personnel can also be members of other social worlds, they may seek to introduce elements of ideology and practice from those worlds: for instance, group therapy concepts, EST techniques, co-counseling, Zen meditation, and—with special reference to pain—acupuncture. Health practitioners even make deliberate forays into other worlds to "try them out" in the hopes that offbeat techniques and philosophies, when combined with standard medical ones, can lead to better care for patients who currently are not well served. Here are two recent notices taken from the bulletin board of the Medical School of the University of California at San Francisco:

The Bay Area Family Health Fund
presents
"A Course in Homeopathy: Scientific Natural Medicine"

and

The University of California Continuing Education, and
in cooperation with
The Institute for the Study of Human Knowledge
"Ways of Healing: Ancient and Modern"
A Weekend Symposium

Including lectures on:
>   Meditation and Self-Regulatory Therapies
>   The Tibetan Art of Healing
>   Chinese Medicine and Acupuncture Theory
>   Curanderism: Latin American Folk Medicine

Here, servicing agents rather than clients introduce operationalized elements of those other-world ideologies.

The ambiguous outcome of this is not likely to be a radicalizing of in-world institutions but an adaptation and co-opting of other perspectives in the service of the prevailing in-world ideology or ideologies. A really radical ideology bearer is likely to drop out of medicine, for instance, washing his hands of it. Clients, however, tend rather to live with medical institutions for reasons noted earlier, but they often fight hard in specific contexts, or they accept some recommendations or commands and reject others—complying for instance with some regimens, some of the time, in some but usually not all respects.[18] They give up on medical institutions altogether, choosing alternate forms of health healing. Most often perhaps, in the United States, they juggle two or more kinds of healers sequentially or simultaneously, including one that is "regular medical" and one(s) that is not.

The reasons for those choices are not simply that "the doctors don't help my pain," but that ideological considerations are being juggled. Much as Chinese-Americans may patronize an herbalist for one set of symptoms, follow Chinese dietary rules for another, and go to a regular physician for yet another,[19] so may other Americans go to a surgeon for a seemingly necessary operation, follow an ideologically based dietary regimen for arthritic pain, and perhaps try acupuncture because "that old Chinese philosophy" might have some value after all. Put one of those patients into the hospital for one chronic illness or another, and he can be expected to contest the hospital's diet and doubtless some of its procedures, not out of pure temperamental obdurateness but for ideological reasons rooted in worlds other than that of medicine.

In short, much of the balancing and controlling that takes place within the organizational arena can be usefully conceived of as part of the intersecting processes among different social worlds. The representatives of those worlds are not usually aware of being actors in that larger drama. The health practitioners generally are not aware of it, since they are, after all, captives of their own construction of reality.[20]

A final note: Careful analytic distinctions should be made among three phenomena pertaining to social worlds and subworlds. First, in this book, guided by our data, we have often emphasized a single dominant ideology which pervades the world of medicine and its institutions. Second, there are quite obviously, however, many subworlds within the medical world (mainly the various medical specialties and those linked with different kinds of practitioners—physicians, nurses, medical social workers, etc.) These tend to have their own perspectives and ideologies.[21, 22] Within each subworld there are also likely to be contesting positions. Consequently, even though an organization is embedded in one world, it can be organized in accordance with more than one ideology, or its various parts may be differentially affected by various ideologies. The representatives are quite aware of many of their battles, but if the ideological positions are ambiguous, or buried in the history of a specialty or specialization, then the contestants may be unaware of the reasons for their disagreement. (Readers will have noticed examples of both heightened awareness and little awareness of such subworld ideology.) Third, there is the phenomenon of intersecting social worlds, hence the contest between representatives of different social worlds.[23] If one adds subworld membership, then there can be an intersecting of subworlds. (Thus Bradley mothers can interact with anesthesiologists or medical residents or with old-time nurses or nurses trained in new-style nursing philosophies.) For a full picture of organizational functioning, the researcher needs to touch on *all three* phenomena, though he or she may choose to emphasize, in accordance with data and interests, one or more of them.* In any case, what needs to be integral to the study are the *political* processes —such as negotiating, balancing, controlling—which are inherent in the intersecting of social worlds and their ideologies on organizational terrain.

REFERENCES

1. Shibutani, T. 1962. Reference groups in social control. In *Human behavior and social processes,* ed. A. Rose. Boston: Houghton Mifflin, pp. 128–147.

2. Mulkay, M. 1974. Conceptual displacement and migration in science. *Research in the Social and Historical Dimensions of Science and Technology* 4:205–234.

---

*In a terminology suggested by Barney Glaser, these political processes are "basic *social* processes," and they cannot, as we note, be properly understood without linking them to a larger context of ongoing "basic *structural* processes." The latter, as suggested here, include the intersecting of worlds and the interacting of ideologies.

3.   Mulkay, M; Gilbert, G.; and Woolgar, S. 1975. Problem areas
     and research networks in science. *Sociology* 9:187–203.

4.   Strauss, A. 1975. Social worlds. Paper given at meeting of the
     Society for the Study of Symbolic Interaction, August 1975.

5.   Woodsworth, J. R. 1973. Some influences on the reform of
     schools of law and medicine: 1890–1930. *Sociological Quarterly*
     14:496–516.

6.   Markowitz, G., and Rosner, D. 1973. Doctors in crisis: a study
     of the use of medical education reform to establish modern pro-
     fessional elitism in medicine. *American Quarterly* 84:109.

7.   Lauer, R. 1974. A medium for mental health. In *Religious move-
     ments in contemporary America*, eds. I. Zaretsky and M. Leone.
     Princeton, N.J.: Princeton University Press, pp. 338–354.

8.   Schatzman, L., and Strauss, A. 1966. A sociology of psychiatry.
     Social Problems 14:3–16.

9.   Strauss, A. et al. 1964. *Psychiatric ideologies and institutions.* New
     York: Free Press of Glencoe. Esp. pp. 8–10, 359–368.

10. Ibid., p. 3.

11. Simon, H. 1948. *Administrative behavior.* New York: Macmillan.

12. Strauss et al., op. cit., *Psychiatric ideologies and institutions,* pp.
     298–301, 356–359.

13. Becker, H.; Greer, B.; and Hughes, E. 1968. *Making the grade.*
     New York: Wiley.

14. Dalton, M. 1959. *Men who manage.* New York: Wiley.

15. Morgan, D. 1975. Autonomy and negotiation in an industrial
     setting. *Sociology of Work and Occupations* 2:203–226.

16. Fisher, B. 1969. Claims and credibility: a discussion of oc-
     cupational identity and the agent-client relationship. *Social
     Problems* 16:423–433.

17. Fisher, B. 1972. The reconstruction of failure: ideologies of edu-
     cational failure in their relation to social mobility and social
     control. *Social Problems* 19:322–332.

18. Strauss, A., and Glaser, B. 1975. *Chronic illness and the quality of
     life.* St. Louis: C. V. Mosby.

19. Louie, T. 1975. The pragmatic contest: a Chinese-American ex-
     ample of defining and managing illness. Ph.D. dissertation,
     School of Nursing, University of California, San Francisco.

20. Berger, P., and Luckmann, T. 1966. *The social construction of re-
     ality.* New York: Doubleday.

21.   Bucher, R., and Strauss, A. 1961. Professions in process. *American Journal of Sociology* 66:325–344.

22.   Schatzman, L., and Lonner, T. 1975. The psychiatric paraprofessional in community mental health: the new social manager. Unpublished paper, Department of Social and Behavioral Science, University of California, San Francisco.

23.   Kling, R., and Gerson, E. The social organization of the systems world. Unpublished paper, Information and Computer Sciences, University of California, Irvine.

Appendix:
The Method

The research reported on in this book evolved from previous research on terminal care in hospitals, carried out during the early 1960s by Anselm Strauss, Barney Glaser, and Jeanne Quint Beneliol. That work stimulated the study of hospitalized patients in pain—whether dying or not. In *Awareness of Dying*[1] and *Time for Dying*[2] we included an analysis of the problems confronted both by dying patients who suffered from pain and by the staff responsible for their medical and nursing care. Later, we did exploratory interviews and about four months of field work in a large hospital, observing and interviewing nonterminal patients in pain and the personnel who worked with and around them. We also did an analysis of a long case history of a woman (Mrs. Abel) who had suffered much pain and eventually died from cancer.[3]

Thus, the research on pain management reported here was not undertaken *de novo;* rather the earlier work yielded the beginnings of a substantive theory (or at least a theoretical perspective) about pain management, some of the concepts developed here, and a number of hypotheses about activities such as assessing, legitimating, and relieving pain. (All of this emerged from analysis of our data, rather than from the literature on pain or on others' re-

ported research.) We conceived the main task of our new research to
be the verifying or qualifying of hypotheses and the developing of
new hypotheses, as well as the evolution of a conceptually designed
and integrated theory bearing on pain management.[4] The researchers' motivations for pursuing this research were then primarily
theoretical in thrust, including the aim of extending a previous line
of theorizing. A secondary aim, quite important to us, was the practical application of this research, for effective theory should have
both immediate and long-range applicability.

THE FIELDWORK

Our two years of fieldwork encompassed observing and interviewing
in 2 clinics, approximately 20 wards, and 9 hospitals (San Francisco
Bay Area) including a university medical center, a small-town hospital, a county hospital, 4 sizeable community hospitals, a large
extended-care facility, and a university-linked private hospital. Two
field researchers gathered data "on and off" during one year, and a
third gathered data for two years. They studied different locales.

The researchers were generally able to work with a fair amount
of speed for two reasons. First, the problems of accessibility to wards
and to the people there were minimal, and our interest in pain was
shared by many and seemed to threaten nobody. Second, two fieldworkers were skilled nurses so they were familiar with hospitals,
although they did not always study the kinds of wards on which
they had previously worked. The research team as a whole, however,
had a great deal of combined work-and-research experience with
most of the wards that were used as locales for studying pain interactions. We should add that all five researchers who comprised the
project team shared in the analysis of data.

The amount of time spent at each locale varied, depending on
such conditions as the difficulty in gathering data on the particular
terrain and the importance of the data for generating and qualifying
the theory. Fieldwork for the more extensive case histories and case
studies took much time. The particular phase of the research also
affected the amount of time spent at locales, as well as the type of
fieldwork done there. In closing phases, for instance, we did a fair
amount of "pinpointing" collection of data.[5] Pinpointing techniques
consist essentially of highly directed interviews and observations,
which can be very efficient precisely because the study is drawing to
a close with relatively few "holes" remaining. An example is the interviewing of the chief of an x-ray unit about his views of its work in

relation to pain infliction and pain minimization—which work we had already observed—but we did not have evidence on how the chief's views might differ from those who actually worked with or "on" patients. The last locales on which data were collected were the geriatric wards. The several days of observation and interviewing there were highly directed, partly because the researchers already had much experience on such wards from previous research (though with no focus on pain management) and partly because what they were pinpointing was so well anticipated on theoretical grounds.

A word now about the fieldwork and interviewing techniques, but only a word for there was nothing very different about them. They involved the usual range of techniques described in *Field Research* by Leonard Schatzman,[6] in *Psychiatric Ideologies and Institutions* by Anselm Strauss et al.,[7] and in similar publications on fieldwork and interviewing in field settings. We did no interviewing that involved asking exactly identical questions of a number of people, even when interviewing patients with similar disorders. In fact, as in most field studies, we did very few "formal" interviews; rather we relied on interviews and conversations *in situo* which varied widely in style and type. Even the prearranged interviews followed no particular format, but the interviewer followed through on areas deemed relevant or on leads offered by the interviewee.

The most persistent and often intensive interviewing and fieldwork observations were done while collecting data and checking hypotheses pertaining to the extensive case histories. Fieldwork for these case studies involved concerted efforts to follow closely the evolving sequence of events and to get the perspectives on these events held by the various participants. Also, it was when doing this particular fieldwork that Shizuko Fagerhaugh, a nurse as well as a sociologist, deliberately allowed herself to be drawn into advisory and even mediating relationships with personnel and patients. This involvement yielded some of the project's richest data.

THEORETICAL SAMPLING

Following the advice we laid out for ourselves in the *Discovery of Grounded Theory*,[4] we planned to collect data on a large number of wards and in five or six hospitals, being guided by our emerging theory and in accordance with theoretical sampling. Interested readers can find the logic for that kind of sampling discussed in *Discovery of Grounded Theory*. We quote here two sentences which are especially relevant: "Theoretical sampling is the process of data collection whereby the analyst jointly collects, codes, and analyzes his data and decides what data to collect next and where to find them, in order to develop his theory as it develops. This process of data collection is controlled by the emerging theory. . . ."[8]

Operationally, what did this mean for the researchers on our project? We shall give a few examples of the steps. Guided by our emerging theory, we chose several different types of hospital wards on which to observe interaction around patients in pain. Initially the fieldworkers were asked to collect data on three different wards. The first two represented locales where inflicted pain should be much in evidence; we wished to get information quickly on that type of pain since we had little from previous exploratory research.

> An intensive care unit for severe burns. Theoretical rationale: weeks of infliction of severe pain by the staff, on top of ongoing burn pain, with patients called upon to endure that infliction in the service of proper healing.

> A cardiac care unit. Theoretical rationale: regimen pain, post-operatively, balanced against the great necessity to do the regimen (deep breathing). We also wished to look at the management of anginal pain as an indicator of physiological condition, and in terms of its relief because it is potentially "dangerous."

> An obstetrics ward. Theoretical rationale: expected pain—relatively short in duration, finite—and with diverse cultural, personal, and ideological conceptions concerning pain expression, pain endurance, and the phenomenon of birth; with pain relief balanced against the requirements of a "good birth."

The fieldworkers were then sent to three additional types of wards, in order that we might observe more pain trajectories and follow through on some major theoretical dimensions including legitimating, assessing, and inflicting.

> Physical rehabilitation. Rationale: inflicted regimen pain, calling for endurance and control of expression by the patient, and co-operation between the patient and the inflicter-therapist; their respective pain tasks persisting for many weeks or months and with some frequency.

> Neurology and neurosurgery. Rationale: the issue of legitimating might be salient there, because of ambiguous etiologies for the pains.

> Routine surgery. Straightforward, expectable surgical and pain trajectories and routine organization to handle those trajectories.

This would contrast with:

> Medical ward. Multiple chronic-illness trajectories and pain trajectories.

On all these wards we made "internal comparisons" along the
theoretical dimensions. That is, we continued our theory-directed
sampling: for instance, high-pain regimens versus low-pain regimens; experienced inflicters of regimen pain versus new inflicters;
delivering mothers who had the fathers supporting their efforts to
endure pain versus those who had no such supporting or controlling
agents. Meanwhile, we were also looking at an activity that spanned
separate wards and which would maximize variables as they related
to pain infliction. We followed a number of personnel who drew
blood from patients. We observed some who were very experienced,
some who were not; some who were able to work in a leisurely fashion, some who were not; some who met "first-time" patients, others
who met patients very experienced at this particular procedure; some
who encountered patients with much ongoing pain and some who
did not; some who had recently had experiences with accusations of
incompetence and some who had not.

This kind of sampling led us to look eventually at other locales
including x-ray (mass production work, stream of "stranger" patients, with potential pain infliction atop of ongoing pain of various
degrees); emergency (pain relieving has lesser priority than managing the emergency); kidney transplant unit (pain relief perhaps has
low priority versus long-term life/death considerations); cancer ward
(pain relief and expression in the context of dying and comfort care).

The essence of this methodology consists of a multitude of theoretically directed choices; in this study, choices included locales
where the researchers expected to gather data on theoretically relevant events. In the course of gathering that data, specific hypotheses
were verified or qualified or discarded, and new ones formulated.
The latter were checked by more directed sampling, either on the
same ward or on a new one. (For instance, pain relief for routine surgery should not present radically different features in a small town
hospital, except when affected by such variables as, say, the more
closely linked mutual biographies of nurse or physician and patient
because many people from small towns are more likely to know or
know about each other.)

Lest the reader think that everything is strictly planned, we hasten to add that while sites and even the people interviewed are
chosen with some care, a great deal is observed that is, happily,
unanticipated. While the unexpected event can pertain to the
verification of hypotheses, its more exciting function (and this is not
possible in many kinds of research) is to suggest formulations not
previously conceived. In our research, which began after considerable exploratory fieldwork, the happy accidents tended to relate the

unexpected to what was already conceptualized. As an example: the case of Mrs. Noble taught us, rather early in the study, to think about unfamiliar technology as a condition which might affect such matters as the patient's ability to get the staff to accept her pain as truly legitimate, and thus influence the staff's handling of pain-relief tasks. Later this kind of conceptualization about new or unfamiliar technology affected both our choice of new locales to study, and analysis both of old and new data. Thus, delivery pain was reconceptualized in terms of the relatively simple technology (medication) involved in its relief. Later, while analyzing data pertaining to Mrs. Price, we realized that although the staff was familiar with the drugs given to her, it never knew quite what their impact would be, alone or in the many combinations given, on this patient who was very ill from lupus. In analyzing her case history, all this gave unexpected analytic thrust to a consideration of sequential balancing (rebalancing) in such an uncertain illness trajectory and furthered our analysis of balancing as a basic process in the politics of pain management.

THEORY DEVELOPMENT AS A PROCESS

This kind of theory generation and verification is based on a conception of theory development as a *process:* that is, the theory evolves over time, and there is a vital, essential, and repeated interplay between gathering and analyzing data, which is directed in accordance with the evolving theory itself. We cannot hope even to outline this research project's multitude of actual steps, including the precise sequencing of choices of theoretical samplings of which the preceding are only a few. It may be useful, however, to know something of how the data were actually handled after collection, as well as about central conceptualizations which developed during the course of the research.

As the data were collected, they generally were not allowed to pile up waiting for later analysis but were analyzed quickly. This allowed the speedy discovery and elaboration of categories, the detailing of their relationships, and a comparative analysis of data already at hand—to be followed quickly by queries about possible theoretical sampling for the next rounds of data gathering. For example, initial data pertaining to the category of "inflicted pain" were coded for properties, tactics of the infliction, and for persons inflicted upon. Some of the theoretical samplings to maximize variations and enable comparative analysis have already been mentioned; but we might note the other variations we sought, such as those conditions which maximized the already discovered categories of "accusations of negligence and incompetence."

Our style of analytic coding involves careful examination of any given item in a specific fieldnote, then the typing up of the coding. As these analyses accumulate, the total conceptualization becomes increasingly dense and the relationships increasingly numerous and elaborated, but also increasingly precise. Hypotheses of course are qualified, discarded, or related to others. New data gathered primarily via directed theoretical sampling, plus many happy accidents, are coded; generated theory also directs the analyst back to his old data for recoding.

From time to time analytic memos are written. These tend primarily to be directed toward clarification of core categories: in this study the various pain tasks and processes like balancing, legitimating, and assessing. These core categories and their elaboration have integrative functions[8] both in directing the research (especially through theoretical sampling and comparative analysis) and in the final writing of the theory in manuscript form. Realistically speaking, the final integration is not accomplished until the completion of the manuscript, since that forces additional coding of old data in the light of the theorist's sense that something pertinent might have been missed despite all previous analyses. The writing may, of course, also force new pinpointed data collection in order to fill in unexpected holes in the previous data.

Because this particular research had its origins in several years of previously related work, most of the core categories were discovered then. To render that complex and not always verbalizable process more concrete, here are some examples of the sources for core categories. Balancing as an important process, for instance, was first clearly apprehended in the form of a memo titled "the balancing of priorities." We had observed a patient with cancer whose mouth was extremely sore and rendered more painful whenever she ate or drank. We noted that she would balance taking nourishment against otherwise increasing her pain. Several weeks later, when Mrs. Abel's case began to evolve, we began to see many events in terms of differential considerations being balanced by the different actors.

We had for a long time used another core category represented. by the term legitimation because of the frequently expressed doubts by staff about patients' pains and their use of placebos to test their doubts. But Mrs. Abel brought home the great difficulties that could be experienced by patients in convincing the staff of the degree or even the existence of their pains. We had a tendency to overestimate, at the time, the amount of legitimating activity that one might find in hospitals, only later thinking about and checking on the more precise conditions that made for legitmating behavior. Our detailed focus on assessment, especially in relation to legitimation issues, also derives from Mrs. Abel's case, although its link with relief as a pain task goes back to the terminal-care research.

A relative latecomer to the cluster of core categories was that of inflicted pain. Of course we had witnessed that phenomenon for years, but we had never particularly focused on it. During a teaching session describing features of pain interaction, one of the students described a scene she had recently observed. A urologist was catheterizing a series of young children. He achieved acquiescence by giving promises which he did not keep ("it won't hurt very much," "just a little while more"). With the telling of this incident, the connection between staff jobs and the infliction of pain moved into central focus for us, and among the first elaborations of the concept were "inflicted pain atop of ongoing pain" and "accusations of negligence." The latter term later changed, because of additional data, into accusations of incompetence or negligence.

It should be clear from the brief descriptions just given that the so-called "emergence of categories" involves a complex interplay between "what's going on out there" and "what's going on inside" the researcher's head. Rather than explore that complicated relationship, we prefer to touch on three other points that may lead to a clearer understanding of the way our theory developed. First, the sources of ideas can be diverse—including even hearsay accounts. Ideas at that stage, of course, have a completely different logical status than after the research has taken further steps. Second, even if those first ideas turn out to be good, they may not be the central concepts which will eventually guide, inform, and integrate the research. Their effectiveness in those regards must also be discovered, through a complex and continual interplay between data collecting and data analyzing. Third, the interplay of analysis and data collection (via theoretical sampling and comparative analysis in our study) leads also to conceptual clarity, elaboration, and overall conceptual density. We should add that it is not only new data that is instrumental to those ends; but the review of old data is necessary too. (An example is the reobservation of pain ar.d comfort care during the last stages of dying in comparison with pain and comfort care on the geriatric wards, as well as with the pain of nondying patients.)

Two major considerations also altered the original conceptualization derived from the study of terminal care. By 1972, the year this research project actually began, we had come to appreciate the larger meaning of chronic illness, both for the general population and medical institutions, and we had made a number of inquiries pertaining to the "problems of living" faced by people with chronic illnesses.[9] Consequently, we now realized that many if not most hospital patients in pain were chronically ill, and that this would undoubtedly affect certain of the pain interactions we would be observing. This conception became an important part of our data collection and analysis. (For example, one of the first conceptualizations involved the realization that chronically ill patients may have had pain trajectories prior to those associated with current hospitalizations.)

In contrast, the focus on the unstated ideology of health professionals did not become prominent in our thinking until the third and last year of the research. It was when we began to review and write up the cases of Mrs. Noble and Mrs. Price, and the chapter on chronic surgery, that we began to think more intensively about the context within which the pain of such patients is handled—such considerations as how the care is organized, how the ward is organized, how the perceived relevancies are balanced, and what the assessments of the staff appear to be. Hence, in the first draft of the manuscript we emphasized, as part of the larger conceptual framework, the unstated ideology's influence in shaping hospital organization and its work. Some chapters, however, were written before we realized the profound organizational and behavioral implications of the ideology. Perhaps for that reason this aspect of the total conceptualization is less integrated into the structure of each chapter than are others (including the one pertaining to chronic illness). Nevertheless, this broader integrative conceptualization is not merely laid atop the analysis, because its origins lie in our puzzlement over phenomena we witnessed. We followed with an investigation of some historical sources of this dominant medical ideology and a close scrutiny of our data to see how the ideology was operationally translated into hospital and ward structure and into the work of the staff.

Perhaps we should note also that underlying both the initial and later theorizing were certain assumptions that rested on how pain interactions might fruitfully be viewed. We mean specifically that we are sociologists with trained capacities to think in terms of the sociology of work and professions. We assumed hospitals were workplaces and the staff there was at work. (Such assumptions had previously proved useful in our research on terminal care.) By preference, we are also "interactionists," which means we held further assumptions about the necessity of getting the participants' viewpoints in order to analyze interactions taking place among all the people involved in the developing dramas we observed. Also, we held certain views about the necessity for linking social structure, interaction, and process.[10, 11] The researcher is not necessarily aware of all the assumptions deriving from such perspectives—certainly not at every stage of his or her inquiry—but he or she is more or less cognizant of the perspectives and what these signify for the enterprise. The specific steps in developing the core and minor categories, relationships, and hypotheses are quite something else. We mention this only to emphasize that we certainly entered the field with a particular "sociological eye"[12] or what used to be termed "an apperceptive mass." In this particular substantive area, however, where little or no sociological research had been done, we necessarily relied very little on extant studies or theories for our concepts and hypotheses. (We did utilize such studies as Zborowski's *Patients in Pain* as sources of stimulating data.) Realistically, too, the early conceptualizations lay so deep in our previous research as to keep us almost totally immersed in our own theorizing.

THEORY, CASE STUDIES, AND CASE HISTORIES

In writing our analysis, we decided against presenting it as previously (in *Awareness of Dying* and *Time for Dying*), in the form of a discursive theory. Rather, we opted for a style of presentation that would maximize reader interest in three directions: (1) substantive theory about pain interactions, (2) "concrete detail" pertaining to organizational (ward and hospital) action, and (3) the drama of actual events. For that reason, the analytic chapters are written on three levels of abstraction. Some are organized around discursive presentation of *theory* (inflicting pain, relieving pain, etc.) Some consist of *case histories* of particular patients in pain and the interaction around them, "over time." In *Anguish*, we wrote about the case history of Mrs. Abel that:

> The focus of a case history is a full story of some temporal span or interlude in social life–a biography, an occupational career, . . . an illness . . . and so forth. . . . The research goal . . . is to get the fullest possible story for its own sake. In contrast the case study is focused on analytic abstractions and constructions for purposes of description, or verification and/or generation of theory. There is no attempt at obtaining the fullest possible story for its own sake. Fullness of description refers only to what data are needed for the constructions designated by the abstract purposes of the researcher. . . . In sum, the case history gives prominence to the story –and to the "story line"–whereas in the case study the story is subordinated to abstract purpose.

We also stated that:

> *This task of doing a case history is at one end of the continuum of abstraction in sociological work. At the other end is the generation of theory by multiple case studies and comparative analysis. (Between the two are the studies which involve descriptions and verifications, the former being closer to case histories.)* The fullest understandings of social phenomena come, we believe, from dense case histories on one end of the continuum and from densely generated grounded theories on the other end. . . .[13]

Our presentation here has utilized both ends of that continuum, but it has also included specific case studies or interaction on specific types of wards.

We wish also to emphasize that the presentation of the particular case histories and case studies was directed by the final evolution of our theory of pain interaction. It is true that relatively early we decided, on theoretical grounds, that the burn unit, say, should be presented and that the case of Mrs. Noble should be written, but the final analyses of these cases could not be properly accomplished until further conceptual closure had occurred on matters such as inflicting or legitimating pain. Other cases could have been selected for presentation—we had such a wealth of data—so why these? Mainly because they combined dramatic interest and analytic clarity *and* illustrated a range of variation of the phenomena under our scrutiny. It seems to us that each case brings out central aspects of the total theory—an important aim.

For readers who have special interest in method, it is vital to us that they recognize these cases were studied initially for the precise reason that theoretical sampling directed us toward them. We did not stumble on the case studies of the specific wards. However, when we did stumble across interesting case histories, we pursued their evolving stories carefully and diligently, with an eye to their theoretical relevance, having quickly recognized that relevance. We think of this selection by theoretical sampling, combined with systematic presentation in intimate relationship to a substantive theory, as somewhat novel.

We note now an especially important series of points. It should be evident that the case histories and studies provide numerous events to be coded in the process of developing a theory. It may not be so evident that each case—as a total unit or story—also may function to generate, qualify, and validate theory. The case history also contributes to an understanding of important features of the hospital ward on which various dramas take place; besides, its major features as a case lead to new theoretical considerations or qualify or validate old ones. In turn, the case studies of particular wards lead to more astute interpretations of case histories but also to more specific coding of their constituent events. Of course, case studies yield essential data for supracase analyses, as in all sociological research where such analyses are sought through case studies. In this research, all those modes of operation were utilized. Effective theory can, of course, be built without much or any concentration on building elaborate case studies or case histories. However, we believe that the use of one or both can lead, depending on the specific research situation, to additionally rich data and thus perhaps to additionally dense and integrated theory. The cases need not be presented as such but may be included if the researchers decide that they can render the presentation more effective because of either their evidential or their "illumination" value.

CREDIBILITY ISSUES

The last paragraph raises issues of credibility. This is a large and complicated topic, hence we shall confine our remarks to only a few relevant issues. The key to validity and hence to credibility in "grounded theory" lies in theory viewed as process—the continual interplay over time of data collection and analysis, principally through comparative analysis and theoretical sampling. Theory developed in this way keeps the inquiry grounded in data, and yet it does not allow the researcher to settle either for theory which is conceptually thin or for a theory which, though it may be brilliant and even grounded, is not especially well integrated. Theoretical sampling and comparative analysis not only force integration and conceptual density but also keep those features of the theory grounded in the data. Readers should sense that grounding of the theory through its density and integration.

Then too, the comparative analysis and theoretical sampling lead the researcher to "theoretical saturation."[14] Eventually she finds herself discovering nothing particularly new, since most of the seemingly important issues, hypotheses, and categories have been pinned down and interrelated. Of course she may feel saturated, but what about her readers? In addressing that question, we shall take the liberty of quoting from one reader of the two earlier monographs on terminal care, for he puts his finger upon what the researcher must additionally count on in persuading others of the credibility of her presented theory:

The usage of the constant comparative method *throughout [these books] is literally constant and overwhelmingly effective. . . . The well-organized manner in which the reader is confronted with an extremely persuasive array of cross-hospital and cross-ward analyses . . . analyses of patients' social and health characteristics, and analyses over time, is an example of the methodology of qualitative social research as an unquestionably effective research tool. . . . One cannot help but be impressed . . . by the frequent and informative references to the different types of dying trajectories . . . and their associated settings (e.g., institutional dying, dying at home, dying at the hospital), the relationship between particular wards and expected or acceptable dying trajectories . . . the admission process to several different kinds of wards, and even the macrosocial organization of hospitals. [The authors'] reformulation and application of the comparative method is unequivocally the cornerstone of their strategy for qualitative research. Their success in conveying credibility is, I think, directly related to their ability to satisfy the reader's curiosity as to the upper and lower limits of the theory's explanatory capacity. . . . Though I have only alluded to a very small number of specific case histories (or cases in which aspects of an individual's case history are examined) . . . [they] have perfected the technique of blending an element of critical "realism" in the form of case histories with a more general theoretical framework in yielding quite interesting and persuasive documentation of their empirical generalizations. In my estimation, if they had excluded one or the other, they would have been open to criticism either for presenting a theoretical argument pitched at too great a level of generality or for engaging in a highly impressionistic summary of a succession of theoretically unrelated events.*

In the present volume, the theory is presented with a more extensive use of case histories and studies. Concerning this particular theory's credibility, what can we claim for it? We could ask readers: Do not these case histories and their accompanying commentaries read like "reality"? Do not the case studies equally "feel right" as constructed and presented? Do they not all hang together as a total unit, especially when combined with the more abstract analytic chapters?

One need not, however, rely completely on those arguments since other points can be made. To begin with, the case studies were selected through theoretical sampling, and additional data was also collected also by theoretical sampling; they were finally constructed by selecting from among the multitude of witnessed events and interviews in accordance with an evolving theory. On the other hand, the case histories were discovered in the course of fieldwork, but recognized as theoretically important because of the same evolving theory. The data for the ensuing narratives were carefully collected both in accordance with usual fieldwork standards and with our sense of what should be pinpointed because of theoretical considerations. Again, the decisions of what to select from among the large number of field notes, and how to shape this mass into a readable narrative, were guided by further theoretical considerations. These latter involved not just the initial interplay of data analysis and collection, but an interplay between final theory and final "understanding" of the case history. That understanding shaped the selection of items, the organization of the account, and of course the embedded theoretical commentary.

Credibility also rests on how—in a kind of "critical realism"— the data and its analysis strike the reader as hanging together. In this particular book, it is a question of how three types of analysis (case studies, case histories, and the more abstract theoretical discussions) hang together.

As researchers should, we invite replication with similar data. As every theorist should, we hope that this theory will quickly be qualified by the introduction of additional variables. And as practical people, the authors trust that their theory will prove useful to practitioners. Applicability to the real world is after all one of the genuine payoffs for a good theory, if not one of its best tests.

If in the course of time the conditions which we studied become changed because participants better understand previous conditions and act on that understanding, then we would be very pleased, provided the handling of pain were rendered either more humane or efficient. Good theory might conceivably lead to such change. ("[The] very discovery of a stable social sequence must inevitably . . . act to some degree as a new and unique element in the stream of empirical events that make up social and behavioral interaction.")[15] Researchers then would necessarily share the responsibility and the challenge of rewriting—that is qualifying the original theory—taking the new conditions into account as well as the disappearance of some older ones.

If the conditions change under the impact of unforeseen contingencies, then both the ways and the degree to which the theory remains valid will depend, it seems to us, very much upon which old conditions remain and in which specific combinations with the new. That is—is it not?—one of the principle advantages of having an effective theory spelled out in such a form, whether propositional or discursive. Thus, both complex and varied explanations can be made; they will eventually be modified when new conditions occur or are discovered.

REFERENCES

1. Glaser, B., and Strauss, A. 1965. *Awareness of dying*. Chicago: Aldine.

2. Glaser, B., and Strauss, A. 1968. *Time for dying*. Chicago: Aldine.

3. Strauss, A., and Glaser, B. 1970. *Anguish*. Mill Valley, Ca.: Sociology Press.

4. Glaser, B., and Strauss, A. 1967. *Discovery of grounded theory*. Chicago: Aldine.

5. Ibid., p. 173.

6. Schatzman, L., and Strauss, A. 1973. *Field research: strategies for a natural sociology*. Englewood Cliffs, N.J.: Prentice-Hall.

7. Strauss, A. et al. 1964. *Psychiatric ideologies and institutions*. New York: Free Press of Glencoe, pp. 3–37.

8. Glaser and Strauss, op. cit., *Discovery of grounded theory*, p. 68.

9. Strauss, A. 1975. *Chronic illness and quality of life*. St. Louis: C. V. Mosby.

10. Glaser, B., and Strauss, A. 1971. *Status passage*. London: Routledge and Kegan Paul.

11. Glaser and Strauss, op. cit., *Time for dying*.

12. Hughes, E. C. 1971. *The sociological eye*. Chicago: Aldine-Atherton.

13. Strauss and Glaser, op. cit., *Anguish*, pp. 183–186.

14. Glaser and Strauss, op. cit., *Discovery of grounded theory*, pp. 61–62, 111–113.

15. Friedrichs, R. 1970. *A sociology of sociology*. New York: Free Press of Glencoe, p. 180.

Index

Accountability
  for inflicted pain, 98–99
  in pain management, 69–70,
    81, 276, 285
    suggestions for improving,
      279–285
Acute-care model, 273–275
Addiction to drugs, 124–125
Anticipation of ineffective pain
  relief, staff, 39–40
Anxiety, pain and, 109, 111
Arthritic pain, 75
Arthritis, rheumatoid; see
  Rheumatoid arthritis
Assessing pain; see Pain
  assessment
Asthma, 73
Autoeuthanasia, 165–166

Back pain
  discrepant perspectives in,
    117–119
  endurance of, 118–119
  etiology of, 117
  intractable, 22
  relief procedures in, 118
  signs or visibility of, 118
  social background of patient
    with, 23–24
  treatment of, disagreements
    over, 118
Balancing matrix in pain, 244
Balancing process in pain
  dimensions in, 243–245
  misbalancing, 245–246
  rebalancing, 248–250
  relationship to controlling
    pain, 242
  staff involvement in, 248
Behavior, effect of pain on
  patient's, 129–130
Birth
  difficult, pain, 225–227
  organizational considerations
    in, 233–237
Birth pain
  general properties of, 223–225

ideological versus
  professional considerations,
    228–233
Birth process and pain; see Birth
  pain
Burn pain
  children, 110
  controlling, 103-104
  enduring, 106
  expression of, 103–104
    management of, 104–105
  features of, 102–103
  gradients of, expressions of,
    108–109
  learning by comparison, 106
  patient group support in,
    106–108
  trajectory of, 102–103, 106
Burn patients, social trajectories
  of, 24
Burn unit
  characteristics of, 102
  theoretical rationale for study
    of pain on, 307

Cancer
  lung, 75
  ovarian, 73
Cancer patient; see also
  Terminal patient
  case history of, 28–55
  chaplain and, 49–50, 53
  comfort care of, 46
  drug stockpiling by, 43
  estrogen therapy for; 51
  narcotics and, 42, 44, 45, 48
  pain talk of, 45–46, 48
  psychiatrist and, 47–48
  social worker and, 48, 52–53
Cancer wards, ongoing pain in,
  20
Cardiac care unit, theoretical
  rationale for study of pain on,
  307
Care
  conditions for reorganizing,
    275–285

costs of, 286–290
dehumanization of, 291
Chaplain, cancer patient and,
  49–50, 53
Childbirth; see also Birth and
  Birth pain
  Bradley method, 232–233
  Lamaze method, staff and,
    230–231
Chronic disease, pain infliction
  and, 97–98
Chronic illness, pain and, 71–81
Chronic pain; see Pain, chronic
Clock watching, 124–125
Comfort, dying and painless,
  156–166
Comfort care, 46
Communication failures, 75
Consultants in pain
  management, when to call,
  284
Control
  on patient, 33
  patient having, 38–39
Cooperation
  pain work and, 21–22
  staff and patient, 86–87
Cost of care, 286–290
Credibility issues in researching
  pain, 315–318
Crises and balancing pain,
  246–248
"Crocks," 125–127
Crying, pain legitimating by, 38

Death
  expectations, differential,
    157–158
  letting the patient die,
    161–166
  pain and, 33, 42
  painless comfort in, 156–157
  patient balancing life against,
    37
  patient's awareness of, 34,
    169–170
    pain relief and, 158–160

sedation tactics in, 163–165
terminal patient and thoughts
  of, 52
"Death work," 77
Dehumanization of care, 291
Diabetes, 73
Diagnostic procedures,
  legitimating painful, to
  patient, 89–92
Disability, severe, patient
  reaction to, 25–26
Doctor; see Physician and Staff
Doctor's orders, contrary to
  normal procedures, 34
Doctor-nurse conflict, in dealing
  with pain, 31, 33
Dorsal-column stimulator
  case history of patient
    having, 209–221
  implantation of, 207, 208–209
Drug(s); see also Medication
  cost of, 288
  overdose of, deliberate,
    149–150
  pacing use of, 107
  patient's "demand schedule,"
    31
  patients snowed by, 160–161
  patient-staff disagreement
    over timing of, 30
  reliance on, in surgical pain,
    65–66
  stockpiling by cancer patient,
    43
  for surgical pain, 62
  usage in rheumatoid arthritis,
    203
Drug addiction, 36, 107, 124–125
  avoiding, 254
  staff causing, 151–152
Drug dependency, 65
Dying trajectory, 35

Education, medical, 4–6
  disease-oriented, 6
Elderly, care of; see Geriatric
  ward
Endurance of pain, 21
  as part of implicit contract, 91
Estrogen therapy, for cancer
  patient, 51
Expression of pain; see Pain
  expression
Extended-care facilities,
  organization of, 184–186

Faith in pain management,
  285–286

Family
  dealing with patient's pain,
    41–42
  pain and, 26
Fieldwork in pain management,
  305–306
Force, used in pain
  management, 8

Geriatric ward(s)
  biographies on, 188–189
  burden of care on, 190–191
  illness trajectory in, 182
  organization of, 184–186
  pain on, 181–191
    inattention to, 188
  pain trajectory in, 182–183
  pain work on, 186–188
  priority on, 189–190
  social contract on, 184
  social isolation on, 189–190
  social trajectory in, 183–184

Hospital(s)
  acute-care, 59
  organization of
    changes in, 275
    work in, 293–301
  organizational derivation in,
    3–7
  organizational setting of, 9–12
  rhythmic features of, 11
  rules of, 11–12; see also Staff
    rules
  space arrangement in, 10
  work failures produced by,
    cause of, 296–297
  work rhythms of, 11
Hospitalization
  extended, 78–79
  length of, 287–288
Hypertension, 23
Hypnosis, self-, to control pain,
  107

ICUs; see Intensive care unit(s)
Ideologies, work and, 293–301
Illness trajectory
  changes in, rebalancing
    caused by, 249
  cumulative, 251–252
    considerations that
      accompany, 268–269
    rebalancing and, 251–268
  death and, 156
  geriatric wards and, 182–184
Inflicted pain
  accountability for, 98–99

accusations of incompetence
  or negligence elicited by,
  94–97
chronic disease and, 97–98
control of, 98–99
experienced patient and, 96
legitimation, grounds for, 86
nature of, 85
necessary, cooperation in, 99
necessity of, 87
organization properties of,
  88–89
patient properties in, 88
properties of, 87–88
staff properties in, 88
staff tactics to control, 93–94
staff work causing, 88
tabooed bodily area or
  activity and, 93–94
variable conditions in, 87–89,
  93–94
work activities causing,
  control of, 89–92
work properties of, 88
Intensive care unit(s)
  organizational features of, 19
  staff work in, 19
Interactional context of pain
  management, 9
Interactional downward spiral,
  consequence of, 39
Intractable pain
  ideological considerations,
    167–171
  organizational considerations,
    167–171
  relief of, modes of, 171–177
  wards, 172–173

Legitimating pain, 24
Limits, setting for patient, 41
Lung cancer, 75
Lupus erythematosus, case
  history of, 252–267

Malingerers, 127–128
Manipulators, 128–129
Medical education, 4–6
  disease-oriented, 6
Medical ward, rationale for
  study of pain on, 307
Medication; see also Drugs
  amount of, to effect relief,
    149–153
  frequency of, 211
    pain relief and, 153–155
    tension and, 153–155
  routines of, 32–33

schedule for, 34
Medication nurse, 43
Method for research, 304–318
Model, acute-care, 273–275

Narcotics
    cancer patient use of, 42, 44,
        45, 48
    for surgical pain, 62
Negligence, 44, 75
Negotiation in inflicted pain, 99
Negotiators, 128–129
Neurology, rationale for study
    of pain in, 307
Neurosurgery, rationale for
    study of pain in, 307
Nurse; see also Staff
    medication, 43
    mother surrogate role of, 47
    as relief messenger, 40, 41
    vocational, 53
Nurse-doctor conflict, in
    dealing with pain, 31, 33

Obstetrics ward, theoretical
    rationale for study of pain on,
    307
Organizational context of pain
    management, 9
Organizational failures, 285
Organizational patterns, 285
Organizational politics,
    patient's role in, 278–279
Osteoporosis, 203
Ovaries, cancer of, 73
Overdosing, deliberate, 149–150

Pain
    alerting patient to possible,
        90
    anticipated, 89
    anxiety and, 109, 111
    arthritic, 75; see also
        Rheumatoid arthritis
    assessing; see Pain
        assessment
    back; see Back pain
    balancing options, 241–250;
        see also Balancing process
        in pain
    behavioral signs of, 129–130
    burn, 102–103; see also Burn
        pain
    children and, 110
    chronic
        assessment of, 117
        dorsal-column stimulator
        used to control, 208–209

inattentiveness to, 181–191
    surgery for, 80–81
chronic illness and, 71–81
comparisons of, made by
    patient, 90–91
control of, distraction used
    in, 123
convincing others of, 120
credibility of
    conditions and calculus,
        140–142
    tactics and countertactics
        in, 142–144
death related to, 42
denial of, 120
diagnosing meaning of, 20
endurance of, 21, 108
    on burn care unit, 101
    low-back, 118–119
family dealing with patient's,
    41–42
finite, ideal surgical model of,
    123–124
inattention to, on geriatric
    wards, 188
incisional, 62
inflicted; see Inflicted pain
intensity and duration of,
    patient tactics to control,
    90–91
intractable; see Intractable
    pain
legitimate, 31; see also Pain
    legitimation
minimizing, 20
    necessary, 90
    variations of, 20
nonlegitimate, 47
ongoing, 20
options in, 247; see also
    Balancing process in pain
organizational-work-
    interactional perspective,
    18–27
origin of, 19–20
patient's claim to, 50
patient's distinction between
    necessary and unnecessary,
    95
patient's means of
    controlling, 107
patient's response to, 8
patients who "use," 127–128
preventing, 20
previous experience of,
    relationship to present
    pain, 30
psychological, 24, 33

real, 24, 33
relief of; see Pain relief
signs or visibility of, 118
staff response to, 8
surgical; see Surgical pain
tractable; see Tractable pain
treatment-inflicted,
    controlling, 103–104
unnecessary, causes of, 95
Pain assessment, 24, 31, 115–116
    chronic, 117
    differential of, 31
    informational base for, 119
    interactional aspects of, 120
    patient legitimation, 116
    patient responsibility in, 122
    patient's credibility in,
        140–144
    physical versus patient input,
        138–140
    psychogenic, 127
    researching, 304
    staff and, 116
    staff personal experience with
        pain and, 122
    status-forcing, 120–121
    testing tactics in, 122–123
Pain biography of patient, 98
Pain control, balancing
    measures in, 241–243
Pain expression(s)
    amount of, 92
    appropriate, 91
    bounds of, 87
    burns and, 103–104
        management of, 104–105
    controlling
        on burn care unit, 101
        patient tactics for, 92
    mode of, 92
    patient learning when and
        how, 122–122
    patient's, 20, 40–41
        staff dealing with, 20
    social background and, 229
    staff reaction to, 92–93,
        121–122
    unacceptable, causes of, 121
Pain interactions, improving,
    279–285
Pain interference, 133
Pain legitimation, 24, 116
    crying and, 38
    patients claims of, 32
    researching, 304
Pain management; see also
    Balancing process in pain and
    Pain treatment

accountability issue, 69–70, 81
faith as part of, 285–286
force used in, 8
history of, 3–7
home, 8
interactional and
    organizational features of, 9
hospital, 8
interactional context of, 9
pain relief compared to, 20
paradox of, 273–275
patient feedback system and,
    282
research in, 12–15, 304
staff composure and, 79–80
staff tension in, 32
surgical; see Surgical pain
Pain philosophies
surgical, 66–69
varying, 280–281
Pain relief; see also Intractable
pain and Relief work
anticipation of ineffective,
    39–40
back, 118
balancing job of, 132–135
mode of, 145–149
operant-conditioning
    approach, 177
pain management compared
    to, 20
patient controlling, 152
problems in, 115–116
priorities in, 133
researching, 304
routines in, 34
rules in, 136
surgical; see Surgical pain
treatment team approach,
    174–175
Pain talk, cancer patient, 45–46,
48
Pain tasks, of surgical patient,
63
Pain thresholds, 30–31
Pain tolerance, 7
surgical, 62
Pain trajectories
changes in, rebalancing
    caused by, 249
determining factors in, 23–24
expected, 22
geriatric wards and, 182–184
unexpected, 22–23
Pain treatment; see also Pain
management
politics of, 7–9

Pain work
balancing priorities, 74–75
balancing process in, 24–25
childbirth and, 224
    complexities of, 225
consequences of, 25–26
cooperation in, 21–22
dimensions of, 20–21
on geriatric ward, 186–188
improving, 279–285
legitimate demands in, 43–44
priorities in, 24–25
staff accountability and,
    26–27, 28
in surgical pain, 61–63
Patient(s)
addicted, 124–125
attitudes of, to inflicted pain,
    88
autoeuthanasia and, 165–166
bargaining from, 90
behavioral signs of pain,
    129–130
biography of, pain trajectory
    and, 23–24
burn; see Burn patient
cancer; see Cancer patient
chronically, pain infliction
    and, 97–98
claim to pain, 50
clock-watching, 124–125, 211
control tactics used by, 89–92
controlling staff, 38–39
cooperation, 21–22
"demand schedule," 31
difficult, staff rotation in
    handling, 43
dying, 161–166
effect on other patients,
    109–110
endurance of pain, 21
experienced, inflicted pain
    and, 96
expression of feelings toward
    staff, 96–97
family of, pain and, 26
incurable, relief for, 168
judging skill of staff, 96
malingerers, 127–128
manipulators, 128–129
modes of pain relief by,
    145–149
negotiators, 128–129
nonproblematic, staff
    involvement with, 280
open awareness and, 163
pain biography of, 98

pain expression of, 20
pain relief controlled by, 152
pain users, 127–128
power of, 278
problematic, 283–285
    snowballing effect of, 284
processing, 11
psychological support of
    other patients, 106–108
response to pain, 8
setting limits for, 41
social level of, care and,
    227–228
socializing new patients, 89
staff cooperation with, 86–87
staff ratings by, 108
stereotyping of, 98, 123–124
    psychogenic, 125–127
support of fellow patients,
    111–112
surgical; see Surgical patient
terminal; see Terminal
    patient
Patient care, priorities in,
    111–112
Patient contact, tactics for
    reducing, 36–37
Patient feedback system for
    pain management, 282
Patient legitimation of pain, 116
Patient representative, in
    inflicted pain, 93
Patient reputation, 30, 79
    effect on treatment, 119
Physical rehabilitation, rationale
    for study of pain on, 307
Physician, patient's animosity
    toward, 35
Physician-nurse relationship,
    traditional, 282
Preoperative patient teaching,
    62
Priorities in pain work, 24–25
    balancing, 74–75
Processing patients, 11
Psychiatric
    cancer patient and, 47–48
    pain work and, 22
Psychiatry, 4
Public health, 4

Relief of pain; see Pain relief
Relief work
complexities in, 144–155
dimensions of, 144–155
reciprocal expectations
    concerning, 135–138

staff function in, 135
Research, in pain management,
    12–15
Rheumatoid arthritis
    covering-up pain of, 197–198
    dread in, 196–197
    eliciting help, 201–202
    hope in, 195–196
    inaction caused by,
        justifying, 199
    keeping up with normal
        activities, 198–199
    living with, 193–204
    options in, balancing,
        202–204
    pacing activities in, 199–200
    reduced activity caused by,
        adjustment to, 200–202
    renormalizing in, 200–202
    resource reduction in,
        193–195
    self-doctoring of, 196
    uncertainty in, 193–195

Sedation, snowing from,
    160–161
Sedation tactics in dying
    patients, 163–165; see also
    Drugs and Medications
Self-control of pain, 241–242
Self-hypnosis, to control pain,
    107
Sentimental order, cost of, 290
Social background of patient,
    pain trajectory and, 23–24
Social contact, as priority on
    geriatric ward, 184
Social isolation on geriatric
    ward, 189–190
Social trajectories, geriatric
    wards and, 182–184
Social work, 4
Social worker, cancer patient
    and, 48, 52–53
Social world, characteristics of,
    294
Specialists, consulting with, 10
Staff; see also Nurse
    accountability of, 276–285
        inflicted pain and, 98–99
        to pain work, 26–27, 28
        suggestions for improving,
            279–285
    attitudes of
        to pain-inflicting tasks, 88
        to surgical patient, 59–60
    communication failures of, 75

competence of, patient's
    behavior and, 105
composure of, and pain
    management, 79–80
conflicts among, 32
"in control," 33
control tactics used by, 89–92
cultural differences among,
    234
"death work," 77
incompetence or negligence
    of, patient accusations of,
    94–97
incompetent, inflicted pain
    by, 94
inexperienced
    drug doses used by, 105
    inflicted pain by, 94
interaction with patients in
    pain, 26
negligence of, patient pain
    expression and, 108
pain work in surgical pain,
    61–63
patient controlling, 38–39
patient cooperation with,
    86–87
patient rating of, 108
patient rejection of, 32
patient turning against, 37
personal experiences, effect
    on work, 122
reeducation of, 275–276
response to pain, 8
rotation of with difficult
    patients, 43
rules, patient breaking, 29
skill judged by patients, 96
stereotyping patients, 92,
    123–124
"style" of, effect on success
    with patient, 91
tension in pain management,
    32
Staff work
    legitimation of, 86
    properties of, in inflicted
        pain, 88
Status-forcing, characteristics
    of, 120–121
Stereotyping
    psychogenic, 125–127
    patient, 123–124
Suicide, 43, 165–166
Surgery
    for chronic pain, 80–81
    rationale for study of pain in,

307
Surgical pain
    drug reliance in, 65–66
    drugs used for, 62
    incisional, 62
    management, 74
        staff composure and, 79–80
    minimization, 65–66
    nonproblematic, 59–70
    pain work in, 61–63
        priorities, 74–75
    philosophy of, 66–69
    problematic, 71–81
        maximized, 80–81
    relief, 65–66
    relieving apprehension of, 61
    trajectories; see Surgical
        trajectories
    ward work and pain
        accountability in, 63–65
Surgical patient
    hospital staff attitude to,
        59–60
    pain tasks of, 63
Surgical trajectories
    controlling, 73–74
    disrupted, 76–78
    multiple, 72–73, 75
    problematic, 71
    routine, properties of, 60–61
Surgical trauma, 62

Terminal patient, and thoughts
    of death, 52
Tests, costs of, 288
Theoretical sampling used,
    306–309
Tractable pain
    ideological considerations in,
        167–171
    organizational considerations
        in, 167–171
Trajectories of pain; see Pain
    trajectories
Trajectories, surgical; see
    Surgical trajectories
Treatment, legitimating painful,
    to patient, 89–92
Trauma, surgical, 62

Vocational nurse, 53

Work and social worlds, 293–301